IMMUNOLOGY AND IMMUNE SYSTEM DISORDERS

THE FUNCTIONAL AND TRANSLATIONAL IMMUNOLOGY OF REGULATORY T CELLS (TREGS), THE ANTI-TUMOR T CELL RESPONSE, AND CANCER

IMMUNOLOGY AND IMMUNE SYSTEM DISORDERS

Additional books in this series can be found on Nova's website under the Series tab.

Additional e-books in this series can be found on Nova's website under the e-book tab.

IMMUNOLOGY AND IMMUNE SYSTEM DISORDERS

THE FUNCTIONAL AND TRANSLATIONAL IMMUNOLOGY OF REGULATORY T CELLS (TREGS), THE ANTI-TUMOR T CELL RESPONSE, AND CANCER

MICHAEL A. ALEXANDER

NOVA BIOMEDICAL

New York

Library of Congress Cataloging-in-Publication Data

ISBN: 978-1-62808-716-1

Library of Congress Control Number: 2014941041

Published by Nova Science Publishers, Inc. † New York

To Kenneth James Alexander

Contents

Foreword

Prior to the discovery and characterization of regulatory T cells (Tregs) tumor immunologist were unable to understand why anti-tumor T cells were present in the tumor mass, but ineffective at removing the tumor. Once it was understood that Tregs prevented autoimmunity, it was clear that the T cell immune response to cancer was vulnerable to regulation. Because cancer cells were previously normal functioning cells of the body, the T cell system that is responsible for immunosurveillance pauses to evaluate a situation where the cellular antigens it detects are not quite self, but part self/part non-self. These are called "neoantigens" and can be recognized by the T cell immune system. As a consequence, some of the cells are destroyed and their proteins processed by antigen presenting cells (APC). Non-self peptides associated with the tumor are presented by APC and induce a CD4 T cell response. Tregs, which arrive at this site as soon as the first CD4 T cell responds and secretes IL-2, begin their involvement in this process. All of this probably happens within the time it took to read the last few sentences. T cells have the ability to evaluate situations where cells are found that express either an irregular cell membrane or have viruses budding from them. They do what they are genetically programmed to do and that is to kill unfamiliar cells, which prepares the immune system to assimilate that cell. The assimilation part has to do with antigen processing and presentation and is the purview of the granulocyte/monocyte series of cells such as macrophages and DCs or APCs. When normal or pre-cancerous cells are killed by this process APCs also present self-antigens (peptides) that activate Tregs through their anti-self peptide T cell receptor. With that being said, the job of Tregs is to prevent the destruction of normal cells, which means preventing autoimmunity. Tregs react to the situation and respond as they do to minor inflammatory situations where they protect normal cells that are damaged until they return to their original state. Tregs protect these cells from destruction by the T cell immune system through a series of elaborate effector mechanisms. Because pre-cancerous and cancer cells express normal cellular proteins, Tregs act as if they were damaged cells and should be protected from the T cell immune system, which is determined to kill them. While this is happening the cancer continues to grow and despite the fact that the cancer cells are expressing tumor antigens recognized by the T cell immune system, Tregs continue to protect them because they are still recognized as self. They do this by eliminating responding anti-tumor T cells and in some cases, convert these responding T cells into tumor-specific Tregs. Tumor-specific Tregs attach themselves to the tumor and protect it using newly acquired effector mechanisms. This scenario occurs in almost every case of cancer because if it did not, the cancer would have been eliminated by the T cell immune system long before it became deadly.

Now along come immune-based cancer treatments (immunotherapy) that hold the promise of not only painless outpatient treatments for the disease, but also the end of chemically based treatments (chemotherapy) that have serious side effects for the patient. However, it turns out that most of the successful immune cell-based treatments (adoptive T cell therapy, dendritic vaccines, and hematopoietic stem cell transplantation) for cancer are susceptible to the influence of Tregs. In light of the information that will be described in this text, this is no surprise, but what is really important is how to regulate Treg control of the T cell immune system in a positive fashion during immunotherapy. The information to positively regulate Tregs in order to increase the effectiveness of immunotherapeutic cancer treatment is available and has to be implemented in order for these immune-based therapies to live up to their expectations. One of the many problems associated with controlling Tregs as far as cancer treatment is concerned has to do with a term called "cellular plasticity." This term refers to a cell's adaptation (execution of genetically programmed options) to different biological environments while performing specific functions. Therefore, the ability of Tregs to appear (advanced mobility) from the circulatory system (thymus-derived natural or innate Tregs) or be created (conversion from naïve/antigen-specific T cells or adaptive Tregs) at a moment's notice is a genetically programmed response and being such, it invariably is susceptible to manipulation. Despite their "cellular plasticity" and susceptibility to manipulation, Tregs play an essential role in normal functioning of the immune system. In fact, if Tregs were removed from the body, death by fatal autoimmune reactions or infection would follow shortly thereafter. In addition, there would not be any births because Tregs create maternal tolerance that allows the fetus, which is part self and part non-self to come full-term and be born.

One of the most important things Tregs do as far as the immune system is concerned is that they create homeostasis, which is the normal balance between helpful and harmful effects of the immune system as it protects the body. Homeostasis is the most salient, but almost unnoticed aspect of Treg function because Tregs silently eliminate leftover responding T cells from infections, which prevents autoimmune bystander killing of normal cells. In addition, Tregs secrete substances (lymphokines, adenosine, etc.) that reduce responding T cell division, preventing the generation of autoimmune disease-causing anti-self T cell receptors by somatic mutation. Tregs also play a positive role during anti-cancer immune-based therapy where the patient's immune system is removed by radiation and/or chemotherapy and has to recover during the treatment. In this case, despite the fact that almost all of them are removed during this procedure (lymphodepletion), the few Tregs that survive manage to control the re-population process enough to inhibit auto-reactive T cells that would induce autoimmune disease in the patient. Given this information about homeostatic control of the T cell immune response, complete removal of Tregs to allow an anti-tumor T cell response to be effective is out of the question. Tumor immunologists now realize that the creation of immunity to cancer using immunotherapy that leads to the destruction of the tumor and a remaining T cell memory to prevent a recurrence cannot occur without involvement and control of Tregs. The function of cells involved in this process is controlled by cell membrane receptor activation of intracellular translational pathways. These pathways interact with the nucleus that in turn produces transcriptional proteins, which control cellular behavior such as secretion of lymphokines, cell proliferation, or differentiation. The purpose of this text is to expose the transcriptional pathways associated with the behavior of not only Tregs, but also anti-tumor T cells, and the tumor itself. Understanding the basic biochemical pathways that govern the T cell immune response to cancer can lead to the development of new immune cell-based cancer therapies that live up to the promise of a treatment that can achieve a lifelong remission of cancer.

There are two reasons why this topic that focuses the inhibition of the anti-tumor T cell response by Tregs is so important. Those are what is happening now and what will happen in the future as far as the development and treatment of cancer is concerned. As this is being read, right now in someone's (you, me, or anyone) body a small group of cancerous cells are surrounded by T cells. Instead of trying to eliminate the cancer cells, these T cells are paralyzing and killing other T cells that have come to attack the cancer. This continues as the cancer grows and is eventually discovered by that person or their physician. More than likely, the cancer cells have escaped from their primary location and are colonizing (metastasizing) in other parts of the body. After testing comes diagnosis and sometime in the future cancer treatment is imminent. If this cancer treatment involves immunotherapeutic treatments such as bone marrow transplantation, adoptive cell (T cells or dendritic cells) therapy, chemotherapy, or a combination of both, the function of Tregs could determine if the treatment is successful (life) or unsuccessful (death). In some cases such as bone marrow transplantation, the Tregs may not even belong to the patient. In this case, donor Tregs can be used to prevent the donor's T cells from attacking the recipient's tissues while killing the tumor. The attack of normal recipient tissues by the donor's T cells is an almost always-fatal disease and side effect of this type of cancer treatment called, graft vs. host disease or GVHD. However, during other forms of immunotherapy for cancer Tregs attack the immune cells used as therapy thus inhibiting the effectiveness of the treatment. As far as cancer is concerned, what maybe happening in our bodies now and what to do about it in the future is the essence of this discussion about the immunological function and translational pathways of Tregs, anti-tumor T cells, and tumor cells. This topic is not only important for us as individuals, but also for a global society where everyone is a potential cancer victim.

This book is a natural extension of the first book called, *Immune-based Cancer Treatment. The T lymphocyte Response* for several reasons. First of all, it directly addresses one of the main problems associated with the immunotherapeutic treatment of cancer mentioned in the first book, which is caused by the regulatory T cell system or Tregs. Secondly, the first book describes the origin and function of the immune cells (T cells, NK cells, monocytes, macrophages, and dendritic cells) involved in the anti-tumor T cell response in detail. It demonstrated that all of these cells contain subpopulations, which contribute to not only how the cellular immune system functions, but also how these subpopulations are integral components of the immune system as it responds to cancer. The other similarity this book has to the first is the fact that there are no diagrams or illustrations. This is a purposeful attempt by the author to have the reader visualize in their mind the activities of cells during this very important immune response. Diagrams and illustrations do serve a purpose in that they show the reader what the author wants them to see. In this case, the imagination is used to create a world best thought of as an assemblage of cells and biochemical reactions occurring for one purpose and one purpose only and that is to eradicate a collection of cancerous cells determined to cause death. In order to really understand this struggle between the immune cells of the body and cancer, the mind has to visualize the cells and conditions they find themselves in during an anti-tumor T cell response, recreate that response based on the given information, and then use the imagination to see interactions between the cells. Mind-visualization is used by scientists to bridge gaps in information that may allow them to create alternative theories and develop new ideas based on what may happen. This book is intended to do that very same thing in the minds of not only established scientists, but also students of tumor immunology and cancer physicians. The last real chapter in the book called, *Treg Immunobiology as it Relates to the Anti-tumor T cell Response During Immune cell-based Cancer Treatment* contains information concerning the role Tregs play in the execution of immunotherapeutic treatments for various types of cancer. It suggests several ways to manipulate the translational pathways in Tregs to initiate an anti-tumor T cell immune response to cancer. The idea behind the suggestion is to temporarily turn an anti-inflammatory cell (Treg) into an inflammation-inducing cell (TH17) in order to jump-start the anti-tumor T cell immune response. Despite the fact that the T cell immune system is not a car with a drained battery when it comes to cancer (or is it?), the idea seemed like a good one at the time. The hope is that this book may inspire non-traditional thinking about a problematic topic (T cell immune response to cancer) that needs non-traditional ideas to solve.

Acknowledgments

This book unlike the first one on immunity to cancer called, *Immune-based Cancer Treatment. The T lymphocyte Response* was written entirely on the campus of Widener University. Therefore, I would like to start with the university and initially thank the student body. I was one of those students while completing a Master's Degree in Liberal Arts, which fulfilled its purpose as a way to improve my writing skills and appreciation of the world around me. More about that program later, but now I would like to thank all of the countless Widener students who were generally very nice to this older student. The staff and security that worked in the main building (University Center) were beyond nice and I would like to thank my friends Cecelia Miranda, Yvonne Williams, and Laura Edwards for their great conversations, but especially Todd Rhodes for his unwavering friendship. In addition, I would like to thank the cafeteria staff including Chuck and especially Daryl who let me eat as much ice cream as possible even after my meal plan ended. Of course my favorite shuttle drivers like Mr. Dangerfield and particularly Olaf who helped me understand why I was here. Two of my friends are campus security officers Frank, and special thanks to Rick Fountain who helped me put everything into perspective as well as a source of support and inspiration during my day-to-day existence.

The MLS program was an enriching experience because most of the teaching faculty was composed of undergraduate department heads. Therefore, as grad students we were privy to their years of experience. I'd like to thank my fellow grad students for their support of my efforts to become a better writer. However, certain faculty members such as Drs. Barbara Ryan (thesis advisor), Harry Augensen, Loyd Bastin, Rachel Batch, and especially Dr. David Ward receive a special thank you because of their kindness and willingness to discuss not only academic matters, but also life in general. However, my greatest expression of gratitude goes to Dr. Stephanie Schechner who is the Assistant Dean of the College of Arts & Sciences, Associate Professor of French, and the Director of the Masters of Arts Liberal Studies (MLS) Program. As an MLS graduate student Dr. Schechner was not only my Graduate Advisor, but also my mentor and friend. She was one of the first people I met when I came to Widener University and during the last four years someone who has taught me so much about so many things that its very difficult to describe. Not only was Dr. Schechner my Graduate Advisor and mentor, but also one of my Professors because I was fortunate enough to be a student in her graduate-level course about French Cinema. In addition, she taught me a great deal about organization and scheduling during our numerous Capstone Project meetings. Like I had mentioned previously, it is difficult to really explain how she helped me, but I do know that everything I do as a writer and academic from this point forward will be affected by the positive influence Dr. Schechner had on my career. And while still thinking about being on Widener University's campus, I would like to also that the Associate Director of Graduate Financial Aid, Diane Pelli for her guidance throughout my career as a graduate student. Finally, I would like to thank my friend, high school classmate, and landlord James Lowe for providing me shelter in his house just off campus and providing me with good memories of my stay. Thanks Jim.

Next, I would like to thank the people who are and will always be a part of my life. My friend, PhD Graduate Advisor at Penn, and mentor Dr. DuPont Guerry is by far the person most responsible for my scientific career and personality because of all the years we spent together in the lab exploring the mysteries of the immune response to human melanoma. I have DuPont to thank for my way of thinking about research and this book is a product of that thinking process. Thanks DuPont. I'd really like to thank my immediate family. They would be my sister Laurie Small, brother Kenneth, who is no longer with us, and our Mother Patricia K. Alexander. From the bottom of my heart I would like to thank them for experiencing with me the last 7 years of my career transition from a working cancer research scientist to a new author of books about cancer. I know that for them as well as me, it was not always pleasant, but I hope one day soon things will be much better. I thank you for your patience and help because without you I wouldn't have a life worth living.

Introduction

The human T cell immune system is the one of the most sophisticated biological systems in nature. T cells have the ability to literally go almost anywhere they please. If T cells are summoned to an emergency situation, which could be anything from the formation of cancer or viral infection to a benign inflammatory event, they have the ability to direct the entire cellular immune system to that site. If this is not the case, T cells along with NK cells simply make contact with virtually every living normal cell in the body. Its been estimated that normal cells come in contact with these two immune cells repeatedly over a 24hr period. This is called "immunosurveillance," which was a term first used in 1957 to describe how immune cells protected the body from cancer. Simply put, this system of immunosurveillance can detect all immunological cellular "disturbances," which tend to be minor cell surface changes in normal cells. These changes can be caused by the results of inflammation, viral infection, or pre-cancerous changes at the cell surface. The cell surface changes caused by inflammatory processes such as injuries, toxin-related inflammation, and a wide range of other temporary causes of inflammation are an important example that often leads to what is known as "tolerance." However, the T and NK cell systems are programmed (innate immunity) to destroy all cells that display irregular cell surfaces.

There are two main threats to the body and those are viral infections and cancer. The cellular immune system is genetically programmed to deal with these threats because both of them have plagued humanity for centuries. As mentioned above, these diseases also start with the appearance of cells that have irregular cell surfaces. In the case of viruses, it has to do with viral copies at the beginning stages (budding) of escape from an infected cell. The cell surface of a cancer cell changes because the DNA in the nucleus, which makes cell surface proteins, begins to mutate. This can be caused by genetic or environmentally induced DNA damage, which cannot be repaired. Consequently, the nucleus produces irregular proteins that populate the surface of the pre-cancerous cell. These proteins are called "neoantigens" because they are part normal and part abnormal in construction. Because of this tendency for these two diseases to cause cell surface changes, and the fact that they have to be killed immediately NK and T cells, these two immune cells tend to automatically attack all cells that display these types of cell surface changes. Obviously, this is not a good situation when temporary inflammation caused by bruising or insect bites induces similar cell surface changes where the cells affected will eventually return to normal. However, the T cell immune system is also programmed to deal with this situation by protecting those cells undergoing temporary inflammation from destruction. This is accomplished by making use of a specialized subpopulation of the T cell immune system called the regulatory T cell system. This system is comprised of not only T cells (Tregs), but also other cells of the immune system (macrophages, dendritic cells, and B cells) that communicate with Tregs to prevent the killing of these slightly altered normal cells by the T and NK cell systems. The regulatory T cell system has the ability to induce a state of "tolerance" that prevents the killing and gives the cells in question time to return to normal. If this regulatory system fails it can result in what is called "autoimmunity." This is where inflammation-induced cell surface proteins and in some cases, normal proteins are recognized as foreign. This situation can lead to a full-fledged autoimmune response induced against normal cells that may represent an entire tissue system. Examples would be arthritis, pancreatitis, and neurological disorders such as MS. Although the cause of autoimmune destruction in these examples is not quite as simplistic, the end result is the destruction of otherwise normal cells and tissues.

Herein lies the problem as far as cancer is concerned. Often times, not only does the cell surface of a cancerous cell become irregular, but also inflammation occurs at the tumor site from tissue crowding as the cancer begins its unregulated growth cycle. Because the cell surface changes occur first with the appearance of neoantigens, a T cell immune response has already begun to form. This response entails the processing of immunogenic cancer proteins into peptides by macrophages and dendritic cells (DCs) from cancer cells killed by the initial T and NK cell attack. Cancer-peptide specific cytotoxic T lymphocytes (CTL) are generated by this interaction and begin to kill all the remaining cancer cells. Unfortunately, while all of this is happening an inflammatory response at the site, which involves the secretion of inflammatory cytokines by macrophages and T cells is increasing and after a certain point, the regulatory T cell system is alerted and begins to take action. Pre-programmed (innate) Tregs appear first and begin to orchestrate the inhibition of the anti-tumor T cell response by secreting a number of lymphokines directed at antigen presenting cells such as the macrophages and DCs. These Treg lymphokines instruct those cells to not only purposely inhibit T cell activation, but also to begin mediating the conversion of tumor antigen-specific CTL into tumor antigen-specific Tregs. Once this conversion has taken place these converted Tregs stay physically attached to the tumor and can protect it from immune attack using several methods, which include killing newly formed attacking tumor-specific CTL. Now, a barrier that is almost impossible to breach has formed around the tumor. As soon as any of these attacking T cells approach the tumor site, they are inhibited from dividing, killed, or instantly converted into T cells that defend the tumor. This is an accelerating response because naive T cells are often converted into tumor-specific CTL off-site in draining lymph nodes and then head straight for the tumor site where they are immediately taken-over by this process. Eventually, the lymph node itself gets taken over by this expanding action of the regulatory T cell system and begins to generate even more tumor-specific Tregs within the lymph node itself. The end result of all of this activity is that the tumor now has the ability to grow without any interference from the anti-tumor T cell immune system. This type of situation occurs quite often during the development of cancer and in many cancers such as glioblastoma (brain tumor) and melanoma (skin cancer) it is a characteristic part of their development. Any successful effort to interrupt this process and allow the anti-tumor T cell immune response to occur unabated would save thousands of lives.

Every cell mentioned in this scenario was instructed to behave through normal innate instructions that involve the use of biochemical signal transduction pathways within the cell. These pathways are a part of the basic function of normal cells in the body, which includes cells of the immune system. As far as the T cell immune system is concerned, that function is to protect the body from not only diseases such as viral infections and cancer, but also from itself in the form of autoimmune diseases. All of the instructions these cells received were first initiated by the activation of cell surface receptors such as the T cell receptor complex and receptors for lymphokines. The result of this receptor activation is to induce a cascade of biochemical signals within the cell. These intracellular signals induce specific functional changes within each cell involved in this process. The signals travel through known biochemical pathways, which cause the activation or deactivation of particular cell functions like secretion of lymphokines and terminal differentiation. The coordination of these pathways toward a desired effect is called "translational regulation" and is the basis of most normal cellular activity. Translational regulation of intracellular molecules in immune cells is referred to as "translational immunology." This investigation will concern itself with the translational immunology of T cell regulation. Translational regulatory pathways associated with relevant cellular functions of Tregs, supporting immune cells, anti-tumor T cells, and the tumor cell itself will be described. It will lay out in the most simplistic terms the molecules, intracellular pathways, and the resulting cellular functions that lead to this immunological "stand-off" described above between the two (anti-tumor and regulatory) T cell systems.

The chapters will begin with the descriptions of the cellular interactions involved with a particular type of T cell regulation and their result. Then there will be a description of the signal transduction pathways associated with those interactions. In this way it should be possible to use translational immunology to not only describe the T cell "stand-off" between T cells attacking the cancer and Tregs, but also create a model. This model will consist of the activation or deactivation intracellular pathways that parallel the cellular system itself. An analysis such as this should reveal cellular functions that can be manipulated in order to bypass some of the constraints put on the anti-tumor T cell system by the regulatory T cell system. It is entirely possible that this could be done in such a way as to not induce autoimmune disease, which would occur if the entire regulatory T cell system were inhibited. Translational immunology represents a field that in the future will not only transform our understanding of cellular immunology, as we know it, but will also lead to novel anti-cancer therapies. These therapies will be used in conjunction with the newly developed immune cell-based cancer treatments of today. Understanding the regulatory T cell system as it pertains to the anti-tumor T cell response through translational immunology will allow T cell tumor immunologists to address the problems associated with the inhibition of the anti-cancer T cell response by Tregs. This should lead to the successful treatment of cancer by the use of these new immune cell-based cancer therapies that include the manipulation of intracellular transduction pathways of the T cell regulatory system.

Chapter 1

The Immunobiology and Translational Immunology of Regulatory T Cells

Origin and Importance of Regulatory T Cells

Natural (innate) and induced (adaptive) T regulatory cells (Tregs) are an essential component of the T cell immune system. This part of the T cell immune system protects the body from itself or in other words, from immune responses that are either no longer necessary (anti-viral cytotoxic T cell responses) or inappropriate (autoimmune T cell responses). The most important aspect of the regulatory T cell system is that it maintains immune tolerance by reducing or eliminating immune responses that may lead to autoimmunity. More often than not, the cell that has to be controlled in these situations is the antigen-specific CD4 or CD8 T cell. However, other immune cells such as macrophages, dendritic cells (DC), and NK cells are also the targets of the T cell regulatory system. Tregs themselves are naturally produced in the thymus (innate) and become a stable subpopulation of T cells. In addition, Tregs can be induced (adaptive) from either naive T cells from the peripheral circulation or antigen-specific T cells at the site of an active immune response (Sakaguchi 2008). Regulatory T cells (CD4+, CD25+) are further defined by their expression of the Foxhead box P3 transcriptional repressor or FOXP3 gene. Stable expression of this gene by T cells typifies the regulatory phenotype of these cells (Walker 2003). Aside from the FOXP3 gene expression being a marker for Tregs, it also plays an important role in the function of the Treg system. Defects in the either the FOXP3 promoter or coding region causes a fatal form of autoimmunity called immunodysregulation polyendocrinopathy enteropathy X-linked (IPEX) syndrome in humans (Bennett 2001) and a similar disorder in *scurfy* mice (Bunkow 2001). The severity of this disease is a testament to not only the necessary expression of the FOXP3 gene, but also to the degree or intensity of its expression on both innate and adaptive Tregs.

Dual Functional Capabilities

Tregs have been shown to markedly inhibit anti-viral responses such as HIV where Treg expansion is associated with the rapid progression of HIV in untreated individuals (Cao

2009). In addition, it was found that the expression of FOXP3 had been induced by the immune response to the infection because its expression was rapidly lost after in vitro culture, but could be re-expressed by T cell receptor (TCR) stimulation (Suchard et al. 2010). This suggests that these Tregs were not innate Tregs produced in the thymus, but adaptive Tregs formed from the anti-HIV-specific T cell population. Formation of adaptive antigen-specific Tregs can be beneficial. For instance, the gastrointestinal track harbors a plethora of bacteria that permanently reside at this location and it is the job of the T cell regulatory system to maintain tolerance. Inflammatory bowel disease (IBD) is the result of uncontrolled inflammation in response to intestinal bacteria. However, a common bacteria resident of the gut called *Bacteroides fragalis* has the ability to recruit Tregs by the production of polysaccharide A (PSA). PSA induces CD4 T cells to express FOXP3, which produce the IL-10; a powerful immunosuppressant that can reduce inflammation. Moreover, its been demonstrated that PSA alone can not only prevent, but can also cure inflammatory bowel disease in mice (Round et al. 2010). This type of tolerance induced by Tregs is what the regulatory T cell system was designed to do. However, recent findings about the function of Tregs have come to some surprising results with regard to their ability to actively participate in the very immune responses that they are supposed to be controlling.

It was found that activated T cells and hyporesponsive T cells transiently express the FOXP3 gene when cultured with TGF-β (Ziegler et al. 2007). This and other recent findings such as B cell lymphoma expression of the FOXP3 gene (Felcht 2012), led to the hypothesis that expression of the FOXP3 gene did not directly indicate the Treg phenotype (Roncarolo 2008). Despite evidence suggesting that FOXP3 gene expression under some conditions does not lead to the Treg phenotype, there is the possibly of a "flux" state in which such T cells possess the phenotypic characteristics of both antigen specific T cells and Tregs. This may explain situations where removal of T cells, based on the Treg phenotype (by anti-CTLA antibodies) during an anti-tumor T cell immune response, results in an increase instead of a decrease in tumor growth. This type of Treg removal is often associated with a reduction of tumor growth, but in this case transitioning anti-tumor T cells were also removed (Curiel 2007). Recent evidence points toward a multifunctional role of the Treg phenotype. This concept is referred to as "plasticity" (Hori 2010a) and describes the ability of this class of T cell to not only maintain states of tolerance, but also to actively participate in a positive way towards eliminating an immunological threat. In support of this concept it was found the Tregs could attract T, NK, and dendritic cells to the site of a herpes simplex viral infection by secreting lymphokines as well as the chemo attractant CCL5 during the initial stages of the infection. Removal of the Tregs resulted in a fatal infection of the virus in a mouse model (Lund 2008). Evidence that supports this protective effect of Tregs during a human viral outbreak was evident when Treg levels were elevated in patients with an acute infection of West Nile virus prior to recovery while patients whom were symptomatic for the virus, but not with a full-blown infection, had normal numbers of Tregs. A mouse model of West Nile infection confirmed these observations because not only were Treg numbers elevated during an acute infection, but also removal of Tregs resulted in a lethal rate of infection significantly higher than control mice (Lanteri 2009). From this evidence its apparent that the role of Tregs in both the control of the T cell immune response and their ability to actively participate in the immune response, puts these cells in a position just as important, if not more important, than the primary T cell immune response to infection itself (Rowe 2011). As far as their role in controlling T cell immune responses, pregnancy provides the best evidence to demonstrate the complexity and importance of the T cell regulatory system.

T Cell Regulation and Pregnancy

As far as the importance of Tregs is concerned, they play their most vital role in pregnancy and without their ability to induce tolerance there would be no births. In some sense, pregnancy can be viewed as the primordial reason why Tregs exist at all because pregnancy dictates that there has to be systemic tolerance (Schumacher 2014). Many years ago it was discovered that animals became tolerant to foreign antigens that would otherwise evoke a strong immune response if they were exposed to these antigens during fetal development. This fetal exposure type of tolerance was found to be specific because the animals were able to react normally to other antigens they were not exposed to in this way. This type of tolerance was thought to be a "specific failure of the host's immunological response." It was also observed that fertility of tolerant animals was unaffected by this failure to respond (Billingham 1953). This was the ground-breaking observation that until recently was not totally understood until the discovery of the regulatory T cell system and it's ability to induce states of absolute tolerance. Pregnancy presents several major problems for the immune system of the mother. There are three powerful antigens that the immune system is exposed to during pregnancy. Those are fetal antigens, MHC alloantigens, and male H-Y antigens. Each one of these antigens can induce a massive, if not fatal cellular immune response during non-pregnancy periods. During pregnancy these antigens are not only present locally (in and around the uterus), but also distributed system-wide throughout the circulatory system. One of the elements that initiate system-wide tolerance is the secretion of progesterone during pregnancy. Progesterone has multiple effects like down regulating MHC expression on not only target embryonic cells, which makes them harder to see by the immune system (Miech 2011), but also reduces MHC expression on dendritic cells (DC) that would be responsible for initiating an innate immune response to fetal tissue (Xu 2011). It was also found that progesterone promoted the conversion of fetal T cells into Tregs and suppressed the ability of these T cells to become Th17 T cells, which have the ability to break tolerance (Lee 2011). The down regulation of MHC class II and the costimulatory molecules CD80 and CD86 on DC by progesterone, which de-differentiates these cells to an immature version is of particular importance as far as Tregs are concerned. Immature DC have not only the ability to convert naïve T cells into Tregs, but also can facilitate their expansion during a response to alloantigens (Yamazaki 2006), which does occur during pregnancy. Therefore, the secretion of progesterone basically initiates a system-wide and organ-specific recruitment of Tregs. After this recruitment, Tregs conduct a myriad of tolerance-inducing actions that are vital to the survival of not only the mother, but also the developing fetus.

One of these actions is the induction of immune tolerance to the male H-Y antigen. As mentioned previously, this antigen can evoke a strong immune response in non-pregnant females where male skin grafts are routinely rejected (Lin 2010). The immune response to these antigens is swift because within 2 days of pregnancy tolerance-inducing Tregs specific for H-Y antigens can be detected in regional lymph nodes. H-Y antigens can also be detected in the circulation where they induce Tregs that maintain systemic tolerance (Zenclussen

2010). This tolerance to H-Y is specific to this particular antigen. However, these Tregs like many other antigen-specific Tregs are multi-talented. They posses a function called "the bystander effect," where they are able to suppress immune responses to other antigens. Removal of Tregs during pregnancy results in the loss of male offspring (Kahn 2010). In addition, to support the importance of Treg induced tolerance during pregnancy a recent study of a mouse model of spontaneous abortion revealed that the adoptive transfer of in vitro grown Tregs protected fetuses from fetal resorption (Yin 2012). Studies such as these clearly point to the importance of the regulatory T cell system in maintaining a tolerogenic state that is favorable for pregnancy to go full-term and, as mentioned in the beginning of this section, without Tregs in conjunction with the endocrine system, there would be no births.

T Cell Regulation and the Anti-Tumor T Cell Response

The next aspect of the regulatory T cell system will be that of the relationship between it and the anti-tumor T cell response. As mentioned in the introduction, Tregs pose a major threat to the enactment of a long-lasting anti-tumor T cell response. This threat to the normal functioning of the anti-tumor T cell response not only jeopardizes the natural process of tumor removal by T cells, but also can hinder or completely block efforts to treat patients with potentially effective immune-based cancer therapies. A detailed discussion of Tregs and immune-based therapies will be presented in Chapter 4, but now it is important to understand the concept of "conversion" when examining the relationship between Tregs and the anti-tumor T cell response. Often during a discussion of Tregs and conversion another word, "reprogramming" appears and often the two are used interchangeably. However, the fact is that these two words, when referring to Tregs, have different meanings. This will become clear as a detailed picture of Treg immunobiology emerges from this investigation. For the purposes of this discussion the term "conversion" means events such as naïve T cells expressing the FOXP3 gene during an immune response or induction of FOXP3 expression on antigen specific T cells in the same setting. Both of these events result in the creation of the Treg phenotype. The term "reprogramming" will refer to the phenotypical antigen specific Treg being changed back to an effector T cell by the down regulation of FOXP3. This change can result in the recreation of the anti-tumor effector function or the expression of new functional capabilities. As you will see later, the latter case where new functional capabilities are obtained has to with the creation of TH17 T cells. These T cells, that were at one time Tregs, are now proinflammatory effectors that produce IL-17 and TNF-α, which are both inflammation-inducing cytokines. By defining these two words this way is should make it easier to understand the complex relationship that Tregs have with the anti-tumor T cell response in the context of their ability to maintain immunological "homeostasis" through their ability to induce self-tolerance in the setting of a growing tumor.

As previously mentioned, Tregs play an essential role in the induction of self-tolerance by suppressing autoimmune responses and creating homeostatic conditions that allow the cellular systems to return to a normal state. A stable population of Tregs is created in the thymus as a distinct and functional lineage of T cells (Sakaguchi 2001). Many of these responses are tissue-specific (Shevach 2000) yet some are activated by the development of tumors (Drake 2006) and consequently can be detrimental to the anti-tumor T cell response unless they are removed from the tumor site (Shimizu 1999). However despite this, T regulatory cells can be converted from naïve or antigen-specific T cells in the context of a growing tumor and this "conversion" is indicative of an important anti-self tolerance mechanism that prevents the development of tumor-induced autoimmune responses. These autoimmune responses result in the destruction of normal cells that express the same or similar antigens as the tumor (Adler 2009). Even though this is not the only immunosuppressive T cell mechanism controlling the anti-tumor T cell response (Haribhai 2004), it probably represents one of the main reasons why many anti-tumor T cell responses are ineffective (El Andaloussi 2006). The activities of Tregs during an anti-tumor T cell response may be crucial to the success or failure of such a response while the tumor is growing because the tumor itself is actively inducing an environment that is tolerogenic to newly created anti-tumor T cells (Anderson 2007).

Both "innate" and "adaptive" Tregs (Bluestone 2003) play a role in the anti-tumor T cell response, but the adaptive Treg in this situation (Curiel 2007) may be a pivotal element because of the T cell-to-Treg conversion phenomenon. This conversion phenomenon takes place within the environment that the tumor has created. Sometimes it is an inflammatory setting or it can be an antagonistic situation where the tumor is shedding partial immunogenic peptides causing the T cell receptor (TCR) to negatively alter T cell function (Haribhai 2004). This situation could potentially lead to non-cancer related autoimmune responses. Tregs are not only involved with these two situations, but also when there is an unabated anti-tumor T cell response, which could potentially lead to a cancer antigen-induced autoimmune response. Conversion of naïve or antigen-specific T cells to Tregs can occur in response to viruses (Walker 2005) or tumor cells (Dumitriu 2009). In addition, natural (innate) or tumor antigen specific Tregs can be reprogrammed to become TH-17 secreting antigen-specific autoimmune effector T cells that can break tolerance by attacking normal tissues. The reprogramming process is mediated by dendritic cells (DCs), which are exposed to inflammatory conditions produced by the tumor (Bonnefoy 2011). DCs not only mediate this reprogramming process, but also are essential to the expansion and maintenance of Tregs (Yamazaki 2003). In addition to this, DC's can come under the control of T regulatory cells themselves because Tregs can cause DCs to alter their function in such a way as to benefit the continued growth of the tumor (Liang 2008). This involvement of DCs, along with the role of other immune cells in the "conversion" and "reprogramming" of Tregs, will be covered in detail in the later sections dealing with cancer induced autoimmunity and the clinical aspects related to the T cell regulatory system.

This general overview of Tregs has examined their origin, functional capabilities, and their formidable roles in pregnancy and the T cell response to cancer. From this very basic portrait of Tregs it is apparent that these specialized T cells undergo drastic changes above and beyond the differentiation stages of the average normal T cell. These changes, which many times are reversible, are quite intricate in comparison to other immune cells such as macrophages, B cells and NK cells. Another observation derived from this description of Tregs is that other cells (just mentioned) in various stages of differentiation also participate in the control of the immune responses by the T regulatory system. Despite the fact that these cell types are totally different as far as their phenotype is concerned, they play a powerful role by enabling Tregs to induce life-saving tolerogenic conditions. Most of the times Tregs dictate the behavior of these cells by causing them to in some cases, differentiate into another version of that cell or in other cases, dedifferentiate into an immature version. The idea that T cell regulation is that sole responsibility of the Treg is a misnomer. Due to the multi-cellular function of T cell regulation it should be viewed as a coordinated system with the Treg at the center.

The coordinated activities of not only the various kinds of Tregs, but also the other immune cells involved are under the control of signals each cell receives in any given situation. For instance, in the case where DC can induce antigen specific T cells to be converted into Tregs, the DCs are influenced by the tumor to essentially dedifferentiate. Normally, if DC's are aiding a positive immune response to the tumor they produce the lymphokines TGF-alpha and IL-12, which induce the development of TH-1 CD4 T cells that produce gamma interferon (INF-Γ) and activate CD8 CTL. However, some tumors can induce the same types of DC to produce TGF-beta and IL-6, which are two lymphokines that are associated with the creation of the Treg phenotype in both naïve and in this case, tumor antigen specific T cells (Dumitriu 2009). Once the TGF-beta and IL-6 receptors of these two T cells become engaged with their ligands a series of intercellular signals occur within the cells that up-regulate expression of the FOXP3 gene that consequently produces the active Treg phenotype. However, these very same Tregs can be reprogrammed into TH17 autoimmune effectors in the presence of IL-1, IL-6, and in the absence of TGF-β (Ghoreschi 2010). These intercellular pathways that are involved in this process are a part of a relatively new field of immunology called "translational Immunology," which concerns itself with the understanding and possible manipulation of these pathways in immune cells. The next section describes translational immunology from a T cell perspective and will give examples of pathways involved with the general function of the T cell regulatory system.

T Cell Regulation and Translational Immunology

Translational immunology is an emerging field and represents the combination of several scientific specialties. First, just what is translational immunology? Translational biology, as applied to immunology, is the study of intercellular biochemical pathways within cells that allow cells to function in a specific manner. Many of these pathways within the cell intersect and are influenced by external stimuli such as when a cell's receptor, say the T cell receptor or TCR, comes in contact with its ligand (peptide antigen/MHC complex). This interaction induces a series of biochemical changes within the T cell to signal it to divide, secrete lymphokines, or differentiate into another type of T cell, and many other changes too numerous to mention at this time (Birmingham 2002). Because this is an emerging field of study many basic T cell immunologist have been waiting for this science of intercellular pathways actually be applied to cellular immunology. For many biologists this is a difficult topic because it is chemically based. Cellular immunologists in the past have tended to focus on the structural components (antibodies, receptors and ligands) associated with immune cell function. However, as biochemical techniques that involved chemical alterations of these protein messengers such as phosphorylation, which could in part explain the biochemical function of immune cells, it became evident that understanding these intercellular activation pathways would lead to a more detailed understanding of immune cell function.

Translational biology has been going on for decades, but in the past few years some of the discoveries concerning immune cells have been astounding. As you read through some of the next few chapters of this book you will gain an appreciation for the biochemical processes that enable the cells of our immune system to function in a specific manner. At times, the biochemistry of these processes seems somewhat complicated, but when it is understood, there develops a deeper appreciation for the complexity and shear elegance of the cellular immune system. The T cell immune system, including all of the supporting immune cells, depend heavily on the biochemical changes that occur within each cell, especially during a T cell response to a tumor. These biochemical pathways not only direct immune cells to do what they do in a specialized manner, but also can increase a cell's sensitivity to any particular immunologic environment. As far as immunology is concerned, this field is ripe with opportunities to alter immune cell behavior to the point where, if a cell is functioning in an inappropriate manner, it may be possible to interrupt the cellular pathways that induce this unwanted behavior and correct it. It may seem far-fetched, but in the future there probably will be an entirely new generation of chemical (biochemical) compounds whose job it is to alter intercellular pathways to produce any number of beneficial cellular behaviors. This is the new frontier in immunology. One just has to examine the immunological research that is being done now to realize that understanding translational immunology may give us the means control the immune system in unimaginable ways. By using this tool, it may be possible to not only change the way the T cell immune system sees cancer, but also possibly change the way cancerous cells present themselves to that system.

This topic of translational immunology is quite complex because it involves biochemical changes that occur inside a cell and that happen almost immediately after the cell has encountered a specific stimulus such as receptor occupancy by another cell or lymphokine. Another level of complexity associated with studies such as this is the fact that these cellular pathways intersect with one another. It's similar to a "cascade effect," where if one protein is modified it sets off a series of other chemical modifications within the cell that result in a specific event occurring at a specific time. There will be numerous examples of this type activity throughout each section that deals with specific functions and settings Tregs find themselves in. These events, which ultimately control the behavior of an immune cell, are very important to understand given their role in determining how immune cells function. Initially, it would be good to just examine what biochemical intercellular changes a T cell goes through when it encounters an antigen. Next, will be an examination of the intercellular changes that occur in Tregs that are related to the specific topics (origin and importance, dual functional capabilities, pregnancy, and cancer) mentioned above, followed by a brief summary and conclusion.

Intercellular Signaling As a Result of T Cell Receptor Engagement

The T cell receptor (TCR) really is not just one protein, but a series of proteins (molecules) spanning the cell membrane of the T cell. As evidenced by their ability differentiate into at least 8 distinct subtypes, T cells are diverse and quite complex in their behavior. Each of these subtypes has a specific function (helper, CTL, regulatory, memory, etc.) that is dictated by the microenvironment present during cellular differentiation. This differentiation or functional change can not only be dictated by signals the cell receives at an extracellular membrane (outside) level, but also from within the cell, where bioactive proteins can be ingested (endocytosed) or injected into the T cells during a synaptic interface with another cell. Most of this complexity in T cell behavior is reflected in the multitude of surface receptors (locks) and ligands (keys) the T cell expresses not only on the outside of the cell membrane, but inside as well. Many of the proteins that appear on the surface of the cell have what is called an intercellular domain. The protein domains of these surface molecules extend a short distance within the cytoplasm of the cell. The reality is that these proteins, like the TCR have two faces. One of these faces is on outside of the cell membrane and the other one on the inside. However, these two parts of this same protein are quite different because they have different functions. The outside portion, as mentioned above, can function as a receptor or ligand. Its job is to interact with other cells and in the case of the TCR, a multitude of foreign antigens such as viral, MHC, fetal (pregnancy), and cancer related peptides. These peptides, which are the result of protein processing by antigen presenting cells (APC), are coupled to the TCR while attached to a self-MHC (HLA class II with CD4 T cells and HLA class I with CD8 T cells) molecules expressed by the APC. The intercellular portions of these membrane proteins (CD4 and CD8) have an entirely different function. Their job is to communicate with other proteins within the cell, which eventually, through a series of chemical interactions and sometimes through multiple pathways, directly interact with the nucleus (DNA) of the cell. After this interaction with the DNA, RNA synthesis produces specific proteins that the T cell uses as a part of its response to this outside stimuli.

As previously mentioned, the TCR is actually a complex of proteins that come together during the interaction of the cell with peptide antigens. This complex is composed of TCR-alpha, TCR-beta, and three varieties of the CD3 proteins (epsilon, delta, and gamma). These proteins not only span the cell membrane, but also protrude onto the cell surface as mentioned above. The CD3 proteins are needed to assemble the TCR alpha and beta chains on the cell surface. Two CD3-zeta proteins are associated with the ends of both the TCR-alpha and beta proteins on the inside of the cell membrane and protrude into the cytoplasm. Depending on which type of T cell (helper CD4 or cytotoxic CD8), a CD4 or CD8 protein is necessary for the contact between the APC and the T cell. If this is a CD4 T cell then there is an affinity for MHC class II (HLA-DR, DP, DQ, or DM) proteins because the CD4 protein (ligand) attaches itself to the MHC class II protein (receptor). Alternatively, a CD8 T cell has an affinity for MHC class I proteins (HLA-A, B, C) for the same reasons (Lefranc 2001). The TCR alpha and beta proteins are configured in such a way as to conform to the peptide-MHC protein complex on the surface of the APC. The TCR is now prepared to attach to the presented peptide with significant affinity to actually bind the two cells (T cell and APC) together in a semi-permanent manner. Contact is now made between the TCR-complex and the MHC-peptide complex. Included in this event is the binding of CD28 on the T cell with its ligands CD80 and CD86 expressed on the APC. Once this contact is made the T cell actually begins to spin so that all of its available receptors (TCR and CD28) are engaged to the available ligands (MHC-antigen and CD80/86) attached APC. Once the receptors are localized on the T cell surface the intercellular domains begin to interact with cytoplasmic protein messengers. These protein messengers that are described below begin to orchestrate the chemical interactions that lead to that T cells fate as either a helper, cytotoxic effector T cell.

The four CD3 subunits have what is called a conserved sequence motif (similar amino acid repeats) called immune-receptor-tyrosine-based-activation motifs or ITAMs and these serve as protein tyrosine kinase substrates. These tyrosine substrates are associated with receptors hematopoietic cells such as B cells, NK cells, macrophages, and platelets. All of the above mentioned cells have 2-3 similar sequence motifs within the ITAMs associated with their cellular receptors, but the TCR has 10 and each one is different. The increased number of ITAMs associated with the TCR is significant and thought to be associated with the individual specificity of each type of receptor. In addition, the shear number of these substrates suggests an increase in signal strength once they are activated by tyrosine kinases. The activated form of ITAMs are substrates that have been phosphorylated (PO4 added) by tyrosine kinases from the Syk family (Zap-70) and the Src family (Lck). Phosphorylated ITAMs can serve as binding sites for SH2 domains of other protein kinases that basically move off and begin to phosphorylate other proteins in a cascading manner (Underhill 2007). These descriptions very tightly focus on the TCR-CD3 complex, but there are several other steps that simultaneously involve the engagement of either the intercellular domains of the CD4 protein or the CD8 protein. These engagements result in a similar cascading effect, which involve other phosphorylation events with other kinases. These should be examined as well, but they will not be detailed here. This is to minimize the confusion due to the array of events all occurring at the same time. However, as these events occur, the reactions move closer and closer to the DNA of the T cell. As these events close in on the DNA there are at least four intercellular molecules that are important in this regard. The first is p38 MAP kinase and then NFAT, which can be activated by p38. NF-kB and NFAT are two transcription factors that can enter the nucleus and bind to the DNA. Then there is AP1, which can be activated within the nucleus and bind to DNA via the Erk and JNK2 kinase pathway. These three (NF-kB, NFAT and AP-1) can directly signal the activation or inhibition of gene expression within the nucleus itself and as will be seen later, play a major role in the functional plasticity of Tregs. The results of this gene activation or deactivation comprise the response T cells go through when they are activated (Marks 2009). The changes in gene expression in activated T cells determine the behavior of the stimulated cell. As mentioned before, they can be instructed to kill a target, divide, secrete specific lymphokines, and be instructed to perform a myriad of other functions. All of these activities determine the type and strength of the T cell response to the peptide antigens of the immunological threats mentioned above and all are induced by intercellular signals relayed down pre-determined pathways within the cytoplasm of the responding T cell.

Translational Events Associated with Thymic Development (Origin) of Innate Tregs

The development of "innate" Tregs in the thymus is understandably different from the development of normal naïve T cells. One of the standard models of their development shows how these cells begin in the thymus as single positive (CD4+CD8- or CD4-CD8+) T cells that respond to self-antigens expressed on thymic epithelial cells. Instead of being deleted as autoreactive T cells, they are selected to become innate Tregs. The reaction to self antigens expressed by the thymic epithelial cell is identical to the TCR/antigen/MHC, and

CD28/CD80, CD86 interaction described above except in this case the peptide antigen is not foreign, but of self origin (Josefowicz 2009). The selection of T cells that are to become Tregs is mostly based on the strength of the signal transmitted (as above) by the TCR. T cells responding strongly to self are eliminated, whereas moderate responses and minimal responses lead to the positive selection of Tregs and normal T cells respectively (Caton 2004). This occurs through the engagement of the TCR and the subsequent translational events, which will be mentioned below, result in the creation of the innate Treg.

As mentioned above, NF-kB is an important transcription factor because of its access to the nucleus. The NF-kB pathway comprises a family of transcription factors or components such as PKC-Theta, Bcl-10, CARMA1, Malt-1, IkB kinase 2, and c-Rel. The NF-kB pathway plays a role in not only general CD28-CD80/86 TCR engagement, but also the development of innate Tregs in the thymus. CARMA1, Bcl10, and Malt1 (CBM complex) constitute adaptor components that allow the TCR to associate with NF-kB. Once the TCR is engaged with the self-peptide MHC complex PKC-Theta is activated, which leads to the construction of the CBM complex and this results in the activation of NF-kB. It was found that the assembly of the adaptor molecule was necessary for the development of innate Tregs in the thymus, but not adaptive Tregs that originate from the peripheral circulation. Transgenic mice that lacked CARMA1 were devoid of innate Tregs while having a normal functioning conventional T cell population. The creation of adaptive Tregs was not negatively affected because they are created from the conventional T cell pool (Barns et al. 2009). Therefore, it was determined that the assembly of the CBM complex after TCR engagement and subsequent NF-kB activation was an activity specifically associated with the creation of innate Treg precursors, which occurred at an early stage of their development (Molinero 2009).

The involvement of the NF-kB pathway implicitly involves the interaction of the NF-kB complex with the DNA of the T cell and in this case the FOXP3 locus. It has been shown that FOXP3 expression in innate T cells from the thymus is associated with the demethylation of a conserved coding sequence within the FOXP3 genetic loci. This sequence element, which is characteristic of developing innate Tregs, is referred to as the Treg-specific demethylation region or TSDR (Huehn et al. 2009). Another member of the NF-kB family, cRel has been shown to play a pivotal role in the initiation process associated with the "remodeling" of the FOXP3 locus. Transgenic mice, which were c-Rel negative, were almost devoid of innate Tregs. It was determined that during the development of innate Tregs that it was c-Rel, but not NF-kB that bound directly to the FOXP3 gene and initiated further modification of the gene thereby creating innate Tregs (Hori 2010b). The resulting innate Tregs were thought to be a source of "stable" T regulatory cells created for the purpose of responding to situations (inflammatory responses) that required them to induce tolerance in a systematic fashion. However, that was found not to be the case when newly formed Tregs were transferred to mice that were devoid of lymphocytes. After transfer a subpopulation lose the ability to express the FOXP3 gene and are able to function as normal helper CD4 T cells. It was also found that some of these Tregs that had lost FOXP3 expression regained it under conditions that were identical to their creation, namely TCR/CD28 engagement. This method of re-activation of the Treg phenotype in these cells is distinct from the creation of adaptive Tregs in that it was TNF-beta independent. In addition, the re-activated innate Tregs possessed the characteristic demethylation pattern of innate, but not adaptive Tregs (Komatsu et al. 2009).

Despite the fact that NF-kB does not directly interact with DNA during this process, the NF-kB pathway is crucial if not completely necessary for the production of innate Tregs. The NF-kB pathway, as mentioned above, is activated by the two signals produced during T cell activation (TCR and CD28 signals). However, the proinflammatory cytokine TNF-alpha specifically activates the NF-kB pathway in Tregs (Nagar et al. 2010). Therefore, the NF-kB pathway itself is a developmental innate Treg regulator. It has been shown that more innate T cells are produced in the thymus during inflammatory conditions where there are significant amounts of proinflammatory cytokines in the circulation (Long et al. 2009). From the data presented here and above it is clear that creation of innate Tregs in the thymus is specific and separate from the creation of the Treg phenotype from normal or antigen specific T cells in the periphery. Adaptive T cells can be created without activation by TCR/CD28 engagement or the need for cell division (Walker et al. 2005), which are two essential steps in innate Treg development. As will be seen in progressive sections of this part of the book, the function of these two types of Tregs are essentially, but not exactly the same, which may be related to their developmental origins.

Translational Control of Functional Duality in Tregs

As mentioned previously Tregs have the ability to not only induce "states" of tolerance, but also to actively participate in immune responses to pathogens and in many cases, autoimmune responses. The dual functional capability of these cells is accompanied by phenotypic changes within the cells through the aforementioned functions of "conversion" and "reprogramming." These phenotypic changes are associated with the "plasticity" of the Tregs that is a characteristic of these cells. This plasticity allows them to control immune responses that would otherwise lead to death via a series of unregulated autoimmune responses where vital organs and tissue systems are destroyed. As mentioned earlier, phenotypic changes that are associated with the conversion process (naïve/antigen specific T cell to Treg and Treg to helper T cell) are simply the expression of FOXP3 (naïve/antigen specific T cell to Treg) or the loss of expression (Treg and Treg to helper T cell). This loss of FOXP3 expression and subsequent creation of helper T cell phenotype has only been found in a subpopulation of innate Tregs (mentioned above) that loose FOXP3 expression and can function as traditional helper T cells (Komatsu et al. 2009). Here, as per the definition of "conversion," which was provided earlier, the change is not of function with regards to phenotype of the converted T cell. Reprogramming, which does involve conversion of one cell to another is accompanied by the expression of a different function not associated with the "classic" phenotype of a CD4 helper T cell or CD8 effector cell. An example of this would be the reprogramming of CD4+, CD25+, and FOXP3+ Tregs into TH17CD4 helper T cells, which now have the ability to secrete the proinflammatory cytokine IL-17, a function not associated with either CD4 Tregs or normal CD4 T cells (Hirahara 2010). Both conversion and reprogramming of T cells associated with T cell regulatory phenotypes and functions make use of different intercellular translational pathways to achieve the various phenotypes and functions that result from these two transforming events.

Conversion

Some of the translational events surrounding the conversion of naïve T cells to adaptive Tregs are very similar to those associated with the creation of innate Tregs in the thymus. They are dissimilar in that once a naïve or antigen specific T cell has been converted into a Treg; it is entirely possible that the same cells can revert back to their original phenotypes by the loss of FOXP3 expression. This is unlike the majority of innate Tregs in that once these cells are created as Tregs they remain that way over the lifetime of the cell. It is not quite clear why this is, but more than likely it has to do with the modifications made on FOXP3 gene during the development of Tregs in the thymus. It was mentioned earlier that during innate T cell ontogeny the NF-kB family member c-Rel was the initiator of the remodeling of the FOXP3 gene, which was associated with a specific pattern of demethylation of the Treg-specific demethylation region or TSDR (Hori 2010a). In addition it was found that innate Tregs displayed demethylation patterns within the TSDR that were almost complete. Where as adaptive or "converted" Tregs showed only partial demethylation (Janson 2008). The reason adaptive Tregs are only partially demethylated is related to how these Tregs are created or converted from naive T cells.

T cell growth factor beta (TGF-β) has been found to specifically mediate the conversion of naïve T cells into adaptive Tregs (Chen et al. 2003). TGF-β is able to induce several intercellular pathways that not only regulate cell growth during conversion, but also directly interact with sites on the FOXP3 gene causing its expression in normal T cells, which now have the functional capabilities of Tregs. The first of these pathways is the mitogen-activated protein kinases (MAPKs), which play an essential role in signal transduction in response to growth factors, cytokines, and lymphokines. There are at least 11 members of the MAPK superfamily and these kinases can control proliferation, differentiation, and cell migration, which makes them essential for immune cells to function normally (Adler 2008). Of the members of the MAPK superfamily, p38, which induces cell cycle arrest, plays a major role in the induction of adaptive Tregs. It is selectively activated (phosphorylated) in response to TGF-β, which in turn coincides with the activation of another pathway involving the SMAD transcription factors. Once TGF-β binds to type II and then type I TGF-β receptors on the T cell a series of events occurs (Huber 2008).

Immediately, the SMAD2 and SMAD3 proteins are phosphorylated, which allows them to join with SMAD4 to form a heterodimer. This SMAD complex directly interacts with the FOXP3 gene; inducing its expression and subsequent formation of the adaptive Treg (Gorlelik 2002). Another of these proteins (SMAD7) is an inhibitor of this process and once activated by TGF-β, the FOXP3 gene down regulates its expression (Fantini 2004). This is possibly the reason why the MAPK/p38 pathway is activated in order to arrest the cell cycle. This would allow for the down-regulation of the SMAD7 inhibitor. These are just two events where transcriptional factors activate the FOXP3 gene within a region of the gene that contains the FOXP3 promoter and two enhancer regions. The transcription factors that bind in this region are the TCR activation induced factors NFAT, AP1, Sp1, and STAT5 (FOXP3 promoter region), NFAT (TCR activation) and the TGF-β-induced SMAD complex (Enhancer 1). Proximal to the FOXP3 gene itself is Enhancer 2 where STAT5 and CREB-ATF bind (Boehmer 2008). CREB-ATF is a transcriptional activator that binds to a TGF-β-induced demethylated site in this enhancer region and actually drives the expression of the

FOXP3 gene (Kim 2007). The translational immunology related to the conversion of either normal or antigen specific T cells into Tregs seems complex, but it is the result of several simple interactions such as the engagement of the TCR/CD28 complex and TGF-β interaction with its receptor on the T cell surface. Unlike the "conversion process" the "reprogramming process" requires additional translational events to occur in order to change the functionality of the reprogrammed cell.

Reprogramming

As mentioned above reprogramming involves an alteration of the functional capability of the cell after it has been changed from either a normal functioning T cell or Treg to a T cell that takes on a different function it did not have prior to this change. A classic example is the change of a Treg into a TH17 CD4 T cell (Koenen 2008). This conversion of Tregs into TH17 T cells is dependent on the presence of lymphokines IL-6, TGF-β, and IL1β. IL1β is not necessary for the conversion of naive CD4 T cells into TH17 T cells, but is essential for the conversion of Tregs into TH17 helper T cells (Ghoreschi 2010). TH17 CD4 T cells are quite different from CD4 helper T cells in that these cells are proinflammatory in that they instead of producing IL-2 and INF-γ like TH1 CD4 T cells; they produce the cytokine TH17, which does play a role in protection against pathogens such as bacteria and fungi (O'Quinn et al. 2008). However, TH17 CD4 T cells have been implicated in the induction of Rheumatoid arthritis (Adamopoulos et al. 2010) and a series of other inflammatory diseases (Park et al. 2005). In addition, TH-17 CD4 T cells have the ability to be effector T cells (CTL) with the ability to damage cells in organ tissue systems. The functional capability of these cells will be discussed in the next section that deals with autoimmunity, T cell regulation, and the anti-tumor T cell response. The important functional aspects of Treg to TH17 T cell reprogramming related to the translational pathways involved in their development will now be examined.

As far as the genetic characteristics as they relate to the function of the TH-17 T cell is concerned, the expression of the retinoic acid-related orphan receptor (RORgammat) is essential (Ivanov II et al. 2006). The RORgammat transcription factor protein is encoded by the RORC gene and is a member of the NR1 subfamily of nuclear receptors (Benoit 2006). RORgammat controls expression of a chemokine receptor (CCR6) that allows the TH17 T cells to migrate to inflammatory sites (Singh 2008). Both Tregs and TH17 T cells express the CCR6 receptor regardless of whether the TH17 T cells were differentiated from naïve CD4 helper T cells or converted from Tregs. CCR6 receptor's only known ligand is the chemokine CCL20 (macrophage inflammatory protein or MIF). TH17 T cells secrete CCL20 at inflammatory sites to attract Tregs and other inflammatory cells (Yamazaki et al. 2008). As mentioned previously, this inflammatory reaction occurs as the tumor begins to "crowd-out" the space occupied by normal cells, but the result of this response is dependent on the this very important reprogramming of Tregs into TH17 T cells. One inflammatory characteristic of a significant Treg to Th17 T cell reprogramming event is the destruction of normal cells that share antigen-specificity with the tumor. Since many of the Tregs at a tumor site were converted from tumor specific T cells (CD4 helper T cells and CD8+ CTL) that posses an anti-tumor T cell receptor, these newly created TH17 T cells can have an affinity for not only the tumor itself, but also the normal cells the tumor was derived from because of the recognition of neoantigens. TH17 T cells that have been converted from tumor specific CTL by IL-6 or IL21 plus TGF-β have been shown to have a reduced ability to kill the tumor, but at the same time secrete IL-17 and the above-mentioned chemo-attractant CCL20 (Huber 2009). Th17 T cells that are the result of the reprogramming of Tregs and secrete IL-17 still express the FOXP3 gene and are capable of reverting back to Tregs, but more importantly these cells can both participate in pathogen defense and inhibit autoimmune responses (Voo 2009).

This type of complex "plasticity" involved with Tregs and TH17 T cells is just being understood. This unique cellular function is a critical factor in the outcome of not only autoimmune disorders such as intestinal colitis, but also anti-tumor T cell immunity. In the tumor microenvironment, where on one hand Tregs can inhibit tumor specific T cell activity and on the other, IL-17 secreting TH17 T cells can contribute to the anti-tumor response by killing the tumor themselves, how this modulation of T cell types plays out can determine if the host lives or dies (Muranski 2008). At the center of this activity is the transcription factor STAT3, which is involved with T cell activation in general, but here specifically with Tregs and TH17 T cells. This transcription factor is pivotal when it comes to this balance between Tregs and TH17 T cells mentioned above. STAT3 binds to most of the genes involved in the Treg/TH17 reprogramming and de-reprogramming by regulating T cell survival genes such as *Bcl2, Fos, and Jun* (Durant 2010). In addition, STAT3 is directly involved in the conversion of Tregs into TH17 T cells by virtue of its ability to bind to both IL-17 and IL-17f promoters. During the process of TH17 conversion DNA elements such as histone H3 (within these promoters) is demethylated allowing STAT3 to bind. STAT3 binding to the IL-17 promoter initiates transcriptional activity of the IL-17 genes (Wells 2012). The expression of the IL-17 genes is a TH-17 T cell lineage commitment activity, which must occur as these cells differentiate from Tregs into TH-17 T cells. This is an example where transcriptional regulation of gene function during the reprogramming phase directly results in a change in cellular function, namely the secretion if IL-17 by T cells that used to be Tregs. This type of differentiation (phenotype and functional change) is the hallmark of this unique cellular activity possessed by T cells of the T cell regulatory system. Reprogramming is a specialized function utilized by the T cell immune system to quickly adapt to changes within the microcellular environment without the need for the creation of a new T cell linage via cell division and T cell differentiation. The steps that occur during the reprogramming process require no cell division and as a matter of fact, cell division is inhibited during this period. In the previous section when discussing the transcriptional regulation of the conversion process, activation of the MAPK/p38 pathway is responsible for halting cell division (Huber 2008), which is supported by the mobilization of the cell survival genes mentioned above. The function of reprogramming of naïve T cells or Tregs into TH17 T cells involves a complex array of translational intercellular processes. This function that has many of the attributes of the conversion function such as the mobilization of the MAPK/p38 pathway by TGF-β depends entirely on the expression of RORgammat. It is an essential function of the T cell immune system that seeks to achieve a balance between Tregs and TH17 inflammatory T cells. Both functions of conversion and reprogramming will be revisited in the proceeding sections of this book because of their importance in autoimmunity, Treg effector functions, and the inhibition of the anti-tumor T cell response.

Translational Events Associated with Tregs and Pregnancy

As mentioned in the *T cell regulation and pregnancy* subsection above, pregnancy presents a multitude of problems for the T cell immune system without the aid of the T cell regulatory system. In a sense, pregnancy represents the ultimate challenge for Tregs because of the complex nature of the T cell responses that must be regulated for the fetus to come to full-term. Also as previously mentioned, there are three major T cell responses, which are against MHC antigens (alloantigens), H-Y (male antigens), and fetal antigens (primordial half self, half non-self). All three of these antigens are powerful T cell immunogens and if seen in any context other than pregnancy would elicit a very strong and almost anaphylactic-type of T cell response. Therefore, many transcriptional regulatory events associated with Tregs and pregnancies occur as Tregs control the T cell responses to these powerful T cell immunogens. Many of the transcriptional events that are associated with conversion of naive or antigen specific T cells to Tregs and the reprogramming of Tregs into TH17 T cells occur during this process. As far as pregnancy is concerned, the most important aspect of the induction of tolerance to these antigens is the balance between the Tregs and TH17 T cells. In this situation, translational events that control the ratio of Tregs to TH17 T cells are critical to the outcome of the pregnancy.

The primary role of Tregs in pregnancy is to control the T cell response to the antigens mentioned above by creating and environment of tolerance. Fetal alloantigens have been the focus of studies that arrived at these conclusions by demonstrating that not only the number, but also the strength of the inhibitory capacity of Tregs increased during early pregnancy. By mid-gestation this increased inhibitory capacity of these active Tregs begins to fall to preterm levels prior to delivery. Once labor begins all high-affinity IL-2 receptor (IL-2R) positive Tregs disappear, leaving only low affinity IL-2R Tregs (Zhao 2007). Not only would a decrease in Treg numbers during this initial process be detrimental to the pregnancy, but also an increased ratio of proinflammatory TH17 T cells would jeopardize the survival of the fetus.

Recently, several pregnancy-related abnormalities such as recurrent pregnancy loss (RPL) and preeclampsia have been attributed to an increased ratio of TH17 T cell to Treg cell, where the TH17 T cell dominates. Normally, TH17 do exist in a minority because of their anti-microbial importance (Ishigame 2009). However, from a translational immunologic point of view, the balance between these two types of T cells begins with their signature gene expression, which for Tregs is FOXP3 gene and for TH17 the RORgammat gene. Both genes are induced in the presence of TGF-β and IL-2. However, it was determined that the FOXP3 protein has an affinity for that of the RORgammat gene. The interaction between these two proteins inhibits the development of the TH17 T cell phenotype leading to stable expression of the Treg phenotype (Zhou 2008). In addition, it was also determined that the FOXP3 gene itself could interact with the RORgammat gene through DNA-DNA interactions that can prevent RORgammat from transactivating the IL-17A promoter. This also inhibits the development of the TH17 T cell phenotype. However the opposite occurs when proinflammatory cytokines such as IL1B (humans), IL-6, IL-21, and IL-23 are present. When these conditions are present FOXP3 expression is diminished and the inhibition of the TH17 T cell phenotype is blocked. This results in the conversion of Tregs directly into proinflammatory TH17 T cells (Ichiyama 2008). Since Tregs and TH17 T cells share a similar lineage and to a certain extent have opposing activities, external factors that influence the signal transduction pathways of either type of cell can skew the ratio between the two.

As mentioned above, several disorders that result in problem pregnancies have been reported to involve an increased ratio of TH17 T cells to Tregs. In RPL both TH17 T cells and TH17 cytokine levels in the peripheral blood and deciduas (uterine lining during pregnancy) of women with RPL compared to non-RPL women were significantly elevated. Levels of Tregs in these same locations were not only low, but also the inhibitory effect of the Tregs that were found at these sites was less powerful when compared to the control group of women. These differences were highly significant and are now indicators in the diagnosis of RPL (Lee 2012). Almost the exact immunopathology was found in preeclampsia, which is a condition that often leads to preterm abortion (Toldi 2011). One possible cause of such situations may be progesterone. In the *T Cell Regulation and Pregnancy* subsection it was mentioned that progesterone creates conditions favorable to the creation of Tregs by creating Treg producing immature DC. Also mentioned was the fact that TH17 T cells can be created in the presence of IL6 (IL-1β in humans) in conjunction with STAT3 binding to the IL-17A promoters (Wells 2012). It was found that progesterone not only actively induced the STAT5 response (increase in phosphorylation) to IL-2, which is favorable to FOXP3 expression, but also decreases the phosphorylation of STAT3 in the presence of IL-6, thereby inhibiting the formation of TH17 T cells (Lee 2011). In this case, where the formation of the fetus brings along with it an initial inflammatory response as fetal antigens are exposed to the mother's immune system, progesterone forces the mother's T cell immune system to create tolerizing Tregs and inhibit proinflammatory TH17 T cells.

Therefore, situations that affect the level or ability of progesterone to perform this function are a threat to a successful pregnancy and may be related to the pathology of both RPL and preeclampsia. It has been shown that over 80% of women with RPL and preeclampsia develop an immune response (skin sensitivity) to progesterone. This suggests that there is interference with the function and possibly the amount of available progesterone to induce tolerance (Itsekson 2007). In fact, progesterone has been used to treat RPL despite there being a need to study the treatment in detail (Walch 2008). Another mechanism related to the inability of progesterone to function properly may be the existence of deleterious polymorphisms of the progesterone receptor. These polymorphic changes in the receptor block the ability of the hormone to properly bind and enter the cells of not only the immune system, but also other tissues (Mei-Tsz 2011). Immunologic regulation of pregnancy is complex and involves not only Tregs, but also a host of other immune cells and the cytokines they produce such as NK and B cells, as well as antigen presenting cells such as dendritic cells and macrophages (Chen 2012). However, at the center of all of this is the Treg cell because of its unique ability to induce senescence in responding T cells and thereby creating a state of immune tolerance.

Translational Events Associated with Tregs, Dendritic Cells the Anti-tumor T Cell Response

"*Treg Effector Mechanisms*" is the title of the third chapter of this volume the signal transduction pathways associated specifically with Tregs, as they control inflammation and the anti-tumor cell T cell response, will be discussed in detail at that time. Therefore, this subsection will discuss translational events associated with Tregs through another important immune cell type. The dendritic cell or DC has already been mentioned in passing during this first introductory chapter about Treg immunobiology. DCs play a major role in the induction of tolerance in not only the control of autoimmune responses, but also in the unwanted immune tolerance induced during the anti-tumor T cell response. The DC is probably the second most important cell aside from the Treg in preventing autoimmune responses. In order to understand how important these cells are one must understand their origin, function, and their multipurpose role as the preverbal "guardians" of the cellular immune system. As you will see, the DCs are one cell type, but in fact these cells can function in many different tissue/organ systems and in some cases, take on the appearance of the cells that inhabit the specific organ system the DC happens to find itself in. These cells make use of a specialized function called "oligopotent end stage differentiation," which allows these cells to take-up residence anywhere in the body. After the basic information about DCs and the relationship between DCs and T cells (Tregs) is presented an introduction to the translational pathways responsible for the DC's role in Treg-mediated inhibition of the anti-tumor T cell response will be described.

Origin, Types, and Basic Functions of DCs

Dendritic cells come from the myeloid lineage of the bone marrow. The myeloid lineage gives rise to the monocyte and the macrophage. This lineage of immune cells is probably one of the most diverse groups of cells in our bodies. Briefly, the initial cell to emerge from the bone marrow is the monocyte. This is basically a circulating undifferentiated cell that has an immediate function in the blood, which is to congregate at sites of tissue damage or inflammation. But if called upon, the monocyte can enter the tissues and turn into a multitude of different cells that have multiple duties to perform. Once the monocyte leaves the circulation and stops on a blood vessel wall or in any tissue it differentiates into a macrophage. This differentiation brings with it several physical and functional changes. One of the physical changes is that the macrophage begins to resemble an amoeba where there is a distinct change in the nucleus (DNA) to cytoplasm ratio. When the macrophage was a monocyte it resembled a typical circulating lymphocyte that is made-up of 90% nucleus and 10% cytoplasm. Once the change to macrophage occurs these cell proportions change to 30% nucleus and 70% cytoplasm.

This is because the macrophage has an increased ability process and present antigen to T cells during an immune response. This process requires much more cytoplasm because this metabolic system of breaking-down engulfed proteins into smaller peptide units and then associating them with cellular class II and I histocompatability antigens on the cell surface is a complex multi-step process (see below).

Macrophages that enter specific tissues on a permanent basis terminally differentiate into DCs and take on the appearance of the resident cells. For instance, when they take up residence in the brain they are called microglial cells. Under the microscope, one of these cells would look like a neuron to an untrained eye. In the liver, they become Kupffer cells and in the skin they become Langerhans cells. In every organ system they all turn into one type of cell (DC) regardless of what they look like. That simple change a monocyte goes through once it stops and turns into a macrophage represents a profound change as far as the T cell immune system is concerned. The macrophage is a somewhat more specialized cell in that it has the ability to eat (phagocytosis) debris. That debris includes bacteria, dead cells, dead viral-infected cells, and other pathogenic and non-pathogenic material. In other words, everything it comes across. As mentioned earlier, once this material that is usually protein in nature is ingested (encapsulated inside membrane vesicles), it's acidified into protein subunits called peptides. These peptides are associated with above-mentioned MHC-class II and class I self-proteins and expressed on the cell surface for T cells (CD4 and CD8 respectively) with the appropriate receptor to respond to. This activity is called antigen presentation (Alexander 2011).

Dendritic cells are basically created from either the monocyte or the macrophage when they interact with two lymphokines, which are secreted by T cells. These lymphokines are IL-4 and granulocyte-monocyte colony stimulating factor, or GMCF. There are two phenotypic classes of DCs: the tissue DC, which is the subject of this discussion, and the plasmacytoid DC (pDC). The pDC mainly circulates in the bloodstream but can inhabit the liver. The standard DC can also be found in the blood and in almost every tissue-organ system in the body. Both these cells have antigen-presentation capabilities, but the pDC has a heightened ability to create Tregs in situations when autoimmune/inflammatory conditions are present (Lombardi et al. 2009). This will be examined in detail during the discussion how DCs induce Tregs.

DCs also tend to create homeostatic conditions within the immune system (Merad and Manz 2009). Aside from their function in anti-tumor T cell responses, they are involved in a myriad of other immune responses. Many of these functions (including antigen presentation) have to do with refining the T cell response to pathogenic organisms, viruses, and inflammatory responses.

Because DCs can induce Tregs, they can control autoimmune reactions that could lead to diabetes, arthritis, and lupus. For instance, if a person takes steroids, the steroids tend to alter cells slightly, such as islet cells in the pancreas. The cell membrane of these cells becomes irregular in response to the steroid. The immune system notices this and initiates an inflammatory response. This response requires that macrophages, mast cells, and a host of other cells appear at the site to protect the body from a widespread autoimmune anomaly that could threaten life. These cells don't know why this is happening and that it is just a local phenomenon, but the inflammation call still comes out in the form of chemo attractant cytokines secreted by cells in that area. Once the islet cells change to the point where the immune system thinks they are not self an autoimmune response can occur. This type of autoimmune T cell attck can lead to damage or the destruction of the islet cells that support insulin-producing beta cells and therefore lead to the development of type 1 diabetes. Autoimmunity will be discussed in detail during the next chapter. Now however, the relationship between DCs and Tregs as far as the anti-tumor T cell response is concerned, must be understood in detail. This will occur before the description of DC-related translational induction pathways during the inhibition of the anti-tumor T cell response by Tregs in order to get a clear picture of the role DCs play in this important T cell response.

Interactions between T Cells and DC During the Anti-tumor T Cell Response

The first area to examine when it comes to discussing the functional interactions and relationships between T cells, Tregs, and DCs should be how DCs affect T cells and Treg development. T cells that respond to cancer cells secrete a large array of lymphokines such as INFγ and IL12 (for Th1 development) as well as IL-4 and IL-10 (for Th2 T cell development) and many others including GM-CSF during the activation phase of the response (Hung 1998). As these lymphokines find their receptor on the surface of the appropriate cell they are internalized and this event begins a cascade of intercellular transcriptional activity within those cells that results in a specific action that cell must perform. Once monocytes stop moving and begin to differentiate into macrophages, then are stimulated with IL-4 and GM-CSF lymphokines, they are immediately signaled to differentiate into DC. This differentiation actually is in two stages. The first stage, which is the development of the immature DC, occurs with a minimum signal from these lymphokines. Immature DCs frequently induce T cells to become Tregs by the secretion of TGF-β and IL-10. However, if this lymphokine signal is constant then mature DCs develop that have increased expression of MHC-class I and II antigens as well as CD80 (B7.1) and CD86 (B7.2) receptors. What mature DCs can do and immature cannot is enter a tissue where there is an ongoing immune response, sample or absorb (phagocytosis) the proteins and then find their way to the nearest lymph node. Once they reach this important immunological organ the DC begin to not only present the immunogenic peptides from the tumor site to T cells, but also begin to instruct T cells.

IL-12, IL10, and gamma interferon (INF-γ) are three very important lymphokines. These proteins, two (IL-12 and IL-10) of which are secreted by both DC and T cells are pivotal during the anti-cancer T cell response. T cells are responsible for most of the secreted INF-γ, but under special circumstances DC can also secrete this lymphokine. IL-12 activates type-1 helper T cells and leads to a productive anti-cancer T cell response, which includes induction CD8 killer T cells. IL-10 however, induces suppressive responses and has been shown to directly induce Tregs with another lymphokine called transforming growth factor beta or TGF-β, which also is secreted by immature DC. INF-γ secreted by CD8 T cells during a T cell immune response has the ability to increase expression of MHC class II proteins on DC. This is important because it increases the DC's ability to present tumor peptides to responding T cells. Once CD4 T cells begin to respond to these peptides presented by the DC, they secrete more INF-γ and IL-12, which can accelerate the response (Cohen 1990). However, there is a caveat to this situation. Tregs can be cancer-peptide specific as well (Wang 2005). As a matter of fact, some of these Tregs were at one time anti-cancer responding T cells (Liu, 2009) and they turned into Tregs because DCs converted them. Tregs secrete IL-10 (Jonuleit 2000) and once DCs stimulate them under these conditions they begin to secrete massive amounts of this lymphokine. This in turn causes DC to secrete TGF-β and more Tregs are created (Marguti 2009). In a situation where there is a brisk anti-tumor T cell response with DCs entering the cancerous mass, and there are large numbers of Tregs present, a productive anti-cancer response is not possible. This is another very important aspect of the relationship between DC and T cells that is crucial to understand and control during T cell-based immunotherapeutic treatment of cancer with DC vaccines.

As previously mentioned, the plasmacytoid dendritic cell (pDC) cell tends to immediately induce Tregs. The pDC does this in a specialized manner by the secretion of an enzyme called indoleamine 2, 3-dioxygenase (IDO), which interferes with the ability of T cells to metabolize tryptophan. Tryptophan metabolism is essential for T cell function because without it, all T cell based activity ceases. IDO is a powerful immunosuppressant all by itself, but most importantly it can convert normal naïve T cells into classic T regulatory cells capable of secreting the immunosuppressive lymphokine IL-10 (Baban 2009). As discussed before, IL-10 in combination with TGF-β can convert even more T cells into Tregs. Unfortunately, tissue DCs can also secrete IDO when the B7 on the DC surface is cross-linked by a Treg expressed protein called cytotoxic T cell lymphocyte antigen-4 or CTLA-4. Once the B7 protein on the surface of DCs is cross-linked this way IDO is released by DCs, which again has the same effect. That effect being the conversion of normal T cells into T regulatory cells. However, fortunately this IDO pathway is well known because when it breaks down tryptophan there are certain metabolites produced, which are thought to actually induce the conversion of T cells to Tregs (Munn 2004). This pathway has a pharmacologic inhibitor, which will be discussed in the section on how to improve the ability of therapeutic DCs to induce a positive anti-cancer T cell response.

The next area to concentrate on is the ability of T cells to control DC. This is accomplished by cell-to-cell contact using the series of ligands (keys) and receptors (locks) mentioned above. One of these situations is with a receptor called CD40 expressed by the DC. Its ligand CD154 (high) is expressed by activated T cells like activated effector CD8 and CD4 helper T cells as well as platelets. Ignoring platelets and focusing on T cells, contact between CD154 on T cells and CD40 on DCs result in maturation of the DCs. This enables DCs to secrete the type-1 CD4 helper lymphokine IL-12 and present antigen at a much more efficient rate. It has been also shown the Tregs begin to express the CD154 ligand after activation. However, the expression of this ligand is at minimal levels on Treg cells (Ma 2009). Perhaps the strategy here is for the Treg to only minimally mature the DC allowing them to continue to induce Tregs, as immature DCs are able to. Despite that, the main purpose of this interaction is to amplify the anti-cancer T cell immune response. Another thing that occurs as a result of this interaction between activated T cells and DCs is that if any DCs that are induced into the immature (Treg-inducing) state they may not stay at that stage for and extended period of time. However, as mentioned above, once they are exposed to CD154 (high) T cells they quickly get pushed into the mature DC phenotype. Again, this is where they can begin to induce the type of T cell response that invariably will lead to the destruction of the cancer. This is called "licensing", where basically activated CD8 killer T cells and helper T cells give DCs a license to do what they are supposed to do, which is to continually induce a productive immune response against the cancer (Haning 2008). This is why it is very important that the DCs arrive at a cancer site where there are a dominating number of anti-cancer T cells. In this way they actually join the battle. However, as mentioned before, if DCs arrive at a cancer site dominated with Tregs the results are quite different.

To a certain extent DC are at the mercy of not only antigen-activated T cells, but also Tregs through their elaboration of lymphokines that affect the direction of the DC's differentiation pathway. However, several of the ways T cells, and particularly Tregs control DC function are not by lymphokines, but are dependent on cell-to-cell contact.

It is important to understand how Tregs control DC function in a way that is detrimental to the anti-cancer T cell response. Tregs express a gene called lymphocyte activation gene-3 (LAG-3 or CD223) that is a protein that is in the same family as the identifying CD4 protein found on normal helper T cells, which participates in MHC-class II binding during antigen specific CD4 activation by APC. This protein, once expressed is a ligand. Its receptor is the MHC class II protein expressed by not only DC, but also by tumor cells and activated T cells as well. The expression of MHC-class II by tumor cells and its interaction with LAG protein of T cells is important because in the next section concerning autoimmunity, this interaction can increase tumorgenicity. However, it is important to understand this lymphocyte LAG/MHC-class II interaction because it causes a lot of problems when DCs are used during anti-cancer immunotherapeutic treatments, which will be discussed at length in the future. Once DCs mature there is an increase of certain cell surface proteins that enable the DC to communicate with T cells in a positive manner. These are the receptors CD80 (B7.1) and 86 (B7.2). There expression is an essential part of the maturation process that the DC must go through in order to sustain a productive anti-cancer T cell response. Many times, Tregs usually encounter DCs arriving at a cancer site in an immature state because the lymphokine concentration that drew them there was not strong enough to fully mature them. For reasons to be explained later that have to do with increased mobility of Tregs, the Tregs are drawn to these DC like magnets. The LAG-3 ligand immediately connects with the MHC class II of the DC and something happens.

This interaction between LAG-3 and MHC class II induces the association of the cytoplasmic (inside of the cell) domain of MHC class II protein with some other intercytoplasmic molecules called ITAM, which was previously discussed associated with T cell activation and will be discussed in detail later. Once this interaction occurs there is a negative signal sent to the DC and that signal tells the DC to lower it's expression of CD80 and 86 to a level that make it virtually impossible to communicate with T cells in a positive fashion (Liang, 2008). As mentioned before, there are "innate" Tregs that are created in the thymus and there are the "adaptive" Tregs that are created from existing cancer-specific T cells (Bluestone 2003). It turns out that both of these types of Tregs can perform this type of DC inhibition, but the Tregs created from the anti-cancer T cell pool can do it even more efficiently. Published reports reveal that it takes ten-fold less cancer-specific Tregs to inhibit DC maturation that it does compared to innate Tregs. Another unfortunate thing that Tregs do to DC is that once they have basically de-differentiated (mature to immature) the DCs, Tregs have the ability to reprogram the DCs to go to the nearest draining lymph node (Liu 2009b). This is a problem because what is going on is that inside that lymph node is that antigen-presenting DCs are activating T cells to respond and kill the tumor. Once fully matured in the lymph node the tumor-specific T cells are instructed by chemokines to go into the cancer mass and destroy the tumor. Therefore, because of this Treg-induced DC de-differentiation that occurred at the tumor site, this process is interrupted. Consequently, the draining lymph nodes begin to fill-up with Treg altered DC ready to turn those productively produced anti--cancer T cells into more Tregs (Bayry 2007). These newly transformed anti-tumor Tregs essentially use the same chemokine trail to go back into the cancer mass and stop any true anti-cancer T cells from doing their job. In addition, this is a bidirectional event because engagement of the LAG-3 ligand negatively affects early T cell activation events (Macon-

Lemaitre 2005). This is just one example of several cell-to-cell contact methods Tregs use to control the behavior of DC. Both of the activities (CD40 DC licensing and Treg/LAG de-differentiation of DCs) and resultant functions mentioned above and a few others are the result of the activation of intercellular signal transduction pathways in both cell types. This next section is important because for the first time translational pathways will be described that occur in two cell types at the same time.

Translational Events that Affect DC after Their Interaction with Tregs

This is one of the many translational events that occur in DCs that results in the DC's ability to convert either naive CD4 T cells or tumor antigen specific T cells into Tregs by direct cell-to-cell contact with activated Tregs. This would be a scenario where DCs would arrive at the site of a newly formed cancer and would encounter not only activated innate Tregs, but also activated Tregs that were converted from the anti-tumor T cell responders. As mentioned before in the TCR example, engagement of receptors that cells poses initiate the activation of intercellular pathways that can either activate or deactivate cellular functions. One of these events that occur in DCs that was previously discussed, which involved a ligand on an activated T cell (or Treg) called lymphocyte activation gene-3 protein or LAG-3 and its receptor (MHC class II protein) on the DC is an important translational event. Because LAG-3 is part of the CD4 family of ligands it has an affinity for MHC class II proteins. What happens is when the LAG-3 comes into contact with the MHC class II protein on the DC cell surface intercellular changes begin to occur on the inside of the cell membrane (Liang 2008). Several complexes are attracted to the intercellular portion of the MHC class II protein. These are lipid rafts (Cho 2010) and Fc receptor domains, which contain the protein kinase substrates that were previously mentioned and called, immune-receptor-tyrosine-based-activation motifs or ITAMs. Unlike the positive situation with the T cell receptor phosphorylation of ITAMs, this situation induces a negative signal because ERK and SHP-1 are recruited. This is due to the fact that the protein tyrosine kinase *syk* (same as Zap-70 with the TCR) is not involved with ERK phosphorylation in this situation as it is with other ITAM-mediated activation signaling cascades in B-cells and T cells. The recruitment and phosphorylation of ERK is particularly inhibitory because it has been shown reduce the ability of DC to activate Th-1 CD4 T cells by secretion of IL-12.

This is called an ITAM inhibitory pathway and the end result for the DC is that it inhibits DC activation and suppresses maturation of these cells (Liang 2008). Both of these inhibitory actions (suppression of maturation and inhibition of IL-12 secretion) prevent DCs from inducing a productive anti-tumor T cell response and in fact may be conducive to the creation of even more Tregs. It was found that this activity, due to the cross-linking of MHC class II by LAG-3, could be inhibited by methyl-B-cyclodextrin a lipid metabolism inhibitor (Cifuentes 2008), which interferes with a proteins association with lipid rafts that SHP-1 is attached to. Furthermore, ERK had to be phosphorylated as an upstream event in order for SHP-1 to associate with the lipid rafts because once ERK was inhibited with a compound called PD98059 the association did not occur (Liang 2008). These and other pathway inhibitors, which are important as far as manipulation of these pathways, will be discussed in detail in the last chapter. However, in support of the fact that this particular type of pathway inhibits the ability of DC to activate CD4 T cells and induce Tregs, it was found the activation of ERK induces the increased secretion of IL-2 and IL-10 (Slack 2007), which are both involved in the induction of Tregs. As far as the inability of DCs to active CD4 T cells, once this ITAM inhibitory pathway is activated it was found that MHC class II expression in these cells was decreased by degradation of recycled MHC class II molecules. Therefore, these degraded molecules were not replaced on the cell surface and unavailable to be used by potential antigen-specific CD4 T cells as a stimulus (Graham 2010). In this example where LAG-3 expressing Tregs have the ability to alter DC maturation, the result is not only to reduce the ability of CD4 T cells to be activated by the reduction of both the secretion of IL-12 and the degradation of MHC class II molecules, but also to increase the conversion of more Tregs by the secretion of two lymphokines (IL-2 and IL-10) used in their creation.

Translational Events that Affect Both (Bi-directional) Tregs and DC

One recent investigation revealed a quite complex series of intercellular events that occur in all T cells as they migrate through the tissues and make contact with other cells of the immune system (Hogg 2011). It has to do with the T cell's ability to move from one place to another through tissues and organs of the immune system, such as lymphatic vessels and lymph nodes. Much of this movement involves a cell surface protein expressed on T cells called leukocyte function-associated antigen-1 or LFA-1. It is a ligand found on activated T cells and has its receptor (ICAM-1) expressed by cells of the myeloid series such as DC. The motility aspect of the this issue is related to how rapidly Tregs move toward activated DC when compared to the speed of naïve antigen-specific T cells that need to reach the DCs in order to start a productive anti-tumor T cell response. The activation of LFA-1 on Tregs by DC can increase their motility. This increases their ability to reach DC first. The interaction between this ligand and its receptor on Tregs can not only block naïve T cell access to DC by simply causing Tregs to get in the way, but can also prevent full maturation of DCs from occurring by down-modulating the B7.1 (CD80) and the B7.2 (CD86) proteins. DC's express these proteins at maturity and are needed by the same naïve T cells to initiate anti-tumor cell T cell proliferation. Because this activity cements these two cells together, dealing with this phenomenon it the setting of immunotherapy is very important. LFA-1 expression does play a major role in T cell motility and the de-differentiation of the DC (Onishi 2008). Controlling this activity and understanding these pathways, generated inside the T cell via LFA-1 and inside the DC via ICAM-1, can be very an important tool used to control the fate of naïve tumor antigen-specific T cells.

This is an important concept to understand because not only does LFA-1 contact with ICAM-1 affect the DC, but affects the T cell expressing LFA-1. This is called a bi-directional pathway affecting both cells, but in different ways and using different intercellular mediators. This activity within the T cell is generates what is called an "inside-out" signal. As mentioned before LFA-1 is highly expressed on activated T cells (Tregs), but it is in a low-affinity state in resting T cells (naïve). One of the many events that change LFA-1 into a high-affinity state is the engagement of CD4 with MHC II or CD8 with MHC I, both receptors of these T cell ligands. In other words, T cell activation must have occurred in order for this high-affinity state of LFA-1 to take place. This aspect of intercellular activation pathways was left out of the section in this chapter about TCR signaling. That is until now, because controlling T cell motility is an essential function as far as cell-to-cell contact is concerned and must be considered a major factor in future anti-cancer immunotherapeutic design. This is a normal process because the LFA-1/ICAM-1 interaction basically stabilizes the interaction between the T cell and DC. Once this process begins and LFA-1 is converted to the high-affinity state by CD4/CD8 engagement and then forms an immunological synapse (IS) between the T cell and the DC. Within the T cell Lck is activated and phosphorylates Zap-70, which in turn does the same thing to an adapter called SLP-76. SLP-76 then associates with not only the ADAP/SKAP55/RIAM complex, but also the GTPase RAP1 is activated. This entire complex locates itself at the IS just after T cell activation. This leads to an increase cytoskeleton activity where the actin cytoskeleton is remodeled, which leads to increased cell motility. The cytoskeleton of the T cell controls its ability to move (motility). The motility of T cells rapidly increases as a result of this intercellular pathway activation (Horn 2009).

Importance of the DC, Treg, and T Cell Translational Events in This Chapter and Beyond

The information that has been presented so far concerns the signal transduction pathways involved with the activities of DC and Tregs during the anti-tumor T cell response. These pathways are vital to the basic understanding of how the T cell immune system fails to attack and remove cancerous cells. It is apparent that the interactions, which result in the specific induction of these pathways, originate from lymphokine/receptor and cell-to-cell contact signals received and sent by both the DC and Treg. The resultant cellular behavior caused by the activation of these pathways in both cells can redirect the T cell response to the tumor and make it quite ineffective. The conversion of anti-tumor T cells into Tregs and the inhibition of the anti-tumor T cell response by mediators such as IDO are only several of the inhibitory effects brought about by the induction of intercellular translational pathways in these two cells. Others specifically associated with Tregs will be covered in detail later. These include the direct attack (killing) of anti-tumor T cells through cell lysis or injection with adenosine and are a direct result of the activation of induction pathways that are specifically designed for those purposes. The involvement of TH17 autoimmune T cells in the inhibition of the anti-tumor T cell response is many times a consequence of the interactions between DCs and Tregs. Some, but not all of the induction pathways responsible for the rise of the TH17 T cell population in relation to the Treg population have been mentioned.

These pathways are related and the consequent failure of a positive T cell response is often caused by the activation of induction pathways in DCs and Tregs by the presence of the tumor. There are several ways the tumor can do this such as secrete immunosuppressive lymphokines, shed cell-free immunogenic proteins, and express altered normal proteins (neoantigens). However, the most important factor involved in the induction of this anti-tumor T cell inhibition is the perception by the T cell immune system that the initial response to the formation of a new tumor is an autoimmune response that must be stopped. The next chapter looks at this issue of autoimmunity from the viewpoint of both the general T cell immune system and the specialized regulatory T cell system in relation to not only the formation of a tumor, but also as it relates to established tumors that may have left (metastasized) the original site.

This first section of this text was intended to impart the necessity, complexity, and sheer eloquence of the regulatory T cell system. As previously mentioned, this system frequently calls upon other cell types such a macrophages, DCs, NK cells, and occasionally B cells to regulate the responses of the T cell immune system. If left unchecked these responses can lead to serious tissue damage and complete deregulation of immunity, which is characteristic of the autoimmune disease such as the IPEX syndrome caused by genetic defects in the promoter or coding regions of the FOXP3 gene. Also mentioned earlier was the fact that the regulatory T cell system is needed to create tolerogenic conditions in order to maintain immunological homeostasis. This system is not only complex on a cellular level, but also complex as far as translational immunology is concerned. In general, intercellular pathways in non-immune cells (normal tissues and tumor cells) are complex because these pathways can intersect in a cascading fashion resulting in a particular cell function. The regulatory T cell system brings another level of complexity to translational pathways by virtue of the fact that many of the resulting cell functions that are caused by the activation of these pathways are reversible. Two familiar examples of that would be the ability of Tregs to revert back to antigen-specific T cells by loss of FOXP3 expression and DCs being de-differentiated by signals from other T cells. Despite its complex nature, the regulatory T cell system, when working properly, is rapid and efficient at what it does.

Understanding and controlling the regulatory T cell system will lead to new treatments for not only cancer, but also a host of other diseases related to autoimmune responses. The chapters that follow will examine Treg translational immunology, autoimmunity, Treg effector mechanisms, the translational immunology of the direct control of the anti-tumor T cell response by Tregs, and most importantly how intercellular pathways could be modified to aid immune-based cancer treatment. Many of the same issues related to the relationships between the various cell types in the regulatory T cell system that were mentioned in this chapter will be revisited in a different context as they relate to the specific areas mentioned above. There may also seem to be some redundancy in the activation of certain induction pathways as the book progresses. This is due to the fact that there is redundancy in translational pathways such that the activation of the same pathway can have a different outcome depending upon which cell is involved or what stimulus induces it. This will become apparent as additional cells in the regulatory T cell system such as macrophages, DCs, and tumor cells are introduced in the proceeding chapters. From an examination of these areas it should be possible to get a clear understanding of why and how the anti-tumor T cell response under the control of Tregs becomes ineffective not only in the presence of a growing tumor, but also during the immunotherapeutic treatment of established tumors.

Chapter 2

Autoimmunity, Tregs, and the Anti-Tumor T Cell Immune System

Simply put, autoimmunity is the recognition by the immune system of self, which includes cells and tissue systems, but every thing else is recognized as non-self. Despite this fact there is a basic definition of autoimmunity; it contains two powerful words and they are "immune" and "self." As far as the T cell immune system is concerned, T cells that recognize self are eliminated in the thymus as a result of their reactivity to self-peptides presented either by epithelial cells or antigen presenting cells (APC) derived from the bone marrow such as macrophages and DC (Sprent 1988). However, this is an oversimplification of a complex process that occurs in the thymus where some T cells, which are weakly reactive to self, become positively selected for a specific purpose. In certain situations, the immune system must also recognize self in the context of non-self (Lo 2012). For instance, when T cells respond to antigenic peptides presented by APC they must do it in the context of self-MHC antigens. This recognition of self (autoantigen) by the T cell is the result of the selection process mentioned above. An exception to this rule is the positive selection of FOXP3 expressing T cells, which are selected based on a strong response to self (Caton 2004). As mentioned in the previous chapter, Treg selection in the thymus involves the presence of TGF-β and IL-2 and the cross-linking of CD28 on the T cell by CD80/86 (B7) on the APC. In contrast, Tregs that develop in the periphery do so as the TCR recognizes autoantigens in the presence TGF-β and very little IL-2 (Josefowicz 2009). In addition, it was determined that despite the fact that both thymic epithelial cells and bone marrow derived APC can present self antigens during this process, APC are more efficient at it. The reason is that unlike epithelial cells, APCs in this situation express high levels of both B-7 and a Treg chemo attractant called CCL22 (Roman 2010).

Why the development of Tregs both in the thymus and the periphery is important to autoimmunity has to do with the TCR specificity of the cell. The specificity of the Treg TCR is focused on self-peptides; the exception being those adaptive antigen-specific Tregs that were converted from responding T cells to Tregs. All of the innate Tregs and a major proportion of adaptive Tregs fit this self-specificity profile. The adaptive Tregs that have been converted from naive or conventional T cells are in fact, derived from the population of T cells that were positively selected in the thymus for their weak reactivity to self-peptides. Another important aspect of both innate and adaptive Tregs that is pertinent to autoimmunity is the fact that both of these types of Tregs cannot secrete IL-2, but express the high affinity form (Alpha) of the IL-2 receptor (IL-2RA). This IL-2 receptor, unlike the traditional IL-2 receptor, can be activated by minute amounts of IL-2, which would otherwise be ignored by naïve T cells that encounter immunogenic peptide and MHC on the surface of APC (Cheng 2011).

These two characteristics of Tregs (recognition of self and high affinity IL-2 receptors) allow Tregs to interfere with autoimmune responses. Inflammatory damage to cells can induce a T cell response to peptides that have been processed from APC that represent cellular proteins that have been disfigured by the death of cells during inflammation. As T cells respond to those altered proteins two things happen. The first thing is that these T cells release large amounts of IL-2 and chemo attractants as they become activated. The second thing that happens is that as normal cells are destroyed, self-peptides are released into the bloodstream. Innate Tregs possessing TCRs specific for normal peptides of that cell type are attracted to the site by those same chemo attractant chemokines, become activated by the IL-2 released by autoantigen responding T cells, and then attach themselves to the damaged cells via the TCR. Once this occurs, Tregs can protect the cells from being killed and effectively shutdown or control the autoimmune response. This process is a basic example of how innate Tregs prevent autoimmune T cell responses that occur on a regular basis, but it is the failure of this process that can lead to autoimmune disease.

This examination of autoimmunity, as it relates to a growing tumor, the T cell response to it, and the involvement of the regulatory T cell system will initially focus on the very early stages of a growing tumor and how precancerous cells are dealt with by the T cell immune system. Later effects of cancer-induced autoimmunity that involve both Tregs and TH17 T cells, which play a role in its prevention or promotion, respectively will also be examined. This dual function, which actually can be derived from normal tumor antigen specific T cells that have been converted into Tregs and then reprogrammed into a TH17 T cells, depends heavily on the use of the TCR during these phase-shifts from normal CD4 T cell to Treg, and then to TH17 autoimmune effector T cell. Many of the autoimmune problems associated with the development cancer are due to the changes that the cellular immune system goes through as it deals with the shifting nature of the cancer cell itself.

When a cancer is formed, the normal cells that it develops in are reduced to their simplest form. In a sense these cells become primordial. The extent and continual nature of the DNA damage that becomes a part of the malignant phenotype of cancer sends the cells back to a more primitive state similar to their embryonic origins. For all intents and purposes, the cells are no longer lung cells, liver cells, or skin cells, but are a form of cancer stem cell, which is sent back in time to an embryonic condition where only the semblance of the original cell remains. Once back there, these newly formed cancer cells have a new mission. That mission is to grow unabated until all the resources of the host are depleted. Differentiation of a cell is its ability to change into another type of cell (Schjeide 1970). However, this is a type of de-differentiation is actually going forward. It just appears to be differentiation in the forward sense because the cell mass is changing in response to its environment. One of the main forces in the cancer stem cell environment is the T cell immune system, which can unfortunately force the cancer to be even more virulent. For the first time, these new cancer cells have what their normal counterparts did not and that is the ability to differentiate at an incredible rate, but this differentiation is sometimes fueled by the immune system. Other than NK cells and B-cells, the T lymphocyte is the main enforcer of the cellular immune system because of its ability to attack any foreign invader, which includes cancer cells and leave an immunologic "memory" in the form of memory T cells. T cells recognize and kill most of the cancerous cells, but what is left over cannot be seen by the T cell immune system.

The tumor mass has several different options when it comes to evading the immune system. The first two are obvious, but the third is not. Stopping the production of recognizable cancer proteins is probably the first one. The second is to stop production of the self-proteins (MHC-classI and II) needed by T cells to target cancer-specific proteins expressed by the cancer. The third option, which is due to the increased metabolic rate of the tumor, would be to increase the production of altered immunogenic self-peptides that are associated with MHC molecules on the tumor cell surface. When this happens, Tregs are attracted and begin to protect the cancer from the T cell immune system. Every single one of these options can be forced upon the cancer by selective pressure put on it by the immune system. This is the process called "immunoediting" where both the innate and adaptive T cells of the immune system eradicate all of the susceptible tumor cells and those that remain continue to grow (Kim 2007). The continual differentiation of these cells is what allows the cancer stem cell to thrive in the face of imminent attack by the T cell immune system (Schatton 2009). This is a dynamic process where the T cell immune system is coping with these and many other changes the cancer stem cells are forcing on the system in order to take over the person's body and cause death. However, all of this begins with those first initial stages that a cell goes through as it becomes pre-cancerous and is first noticed by the immune surveillance system and recognized as possibly foreign.

Therefore, this chapter will focus on examples of cancer-induced autoimmunity from its early stages to the later ones, which will take into account the interplay between the T cell response and the regulatory T cell system. In order to fully understand the underlying relationship between cancer and the immune system a description of the stem cell nature of cancer as it relates to autoimmunity, Tregs, and the anti-tumor T cell response will be included in the cancer-induced autoimmunity section. In addition to focusing on cancer-induced autoimmunity, the next section in this chapter will discuss defects in the regulation of the T cell immune system by Tregs and their conversion into TH17 T cells, which are associated with the inflammatory process of autoimmunity. As a part of that discussion, the participation of T cells and Tregs in autoimmune diseases and chronic inflammation that is associated with the development of cancer will be examined. Finally, autoimmune diseases associated with the failure of Tregs that predispose those patients to developing cancer-related autoimmune diseases such as vitiligo, will be highlighted in order to understand the relationship between Tregs and cancer. As per the first chapter, the cellular interactions will be described and in a separate section the transduction pathways in Tregs, anti-tumor T cells, and tumor cells relating to that cellular behavior will be examined in detail. This dual approach to examining autoimmunity, Tregs, and the anti-tumor T cell response should demonstrate the problems associated with the tenuous balance between non-self and self that the T cell immune system has to deal with while being confronted a developing tumor. In addition, the question of what happens when Tregs fail to control autoimmune responses that are a consequence of the interaction between the tumor and the anti-tumor T cell response will be examined as it relates to inflammation and autoimmunity.

Immune Cellular Interactions

Cancer-Induced Autoimmunity

There is one classic example of a cancer-induced autoimmune disorder, which was mentioned earlier and that is the condition called vitiligo. Vitiligo itself is a well-known skin disorder that affects 0.5% of the world's population with men and women being equally affected. The cause of generalized vitiligo has been thought to be associated with genetic, autoimmune, and neurological factors and there are various treatments for it such as ultraviolet light therapy as well as steroid treatments. Two immediate problems associated with the disorder are sunburn of affected areas and because it is disfiguring in appearance, psychological problems are often associated with it appearing on areas such as the face (Njoo 2001). However, melanoma-associated vitiligo was definitively ascribed to be an autoimmune by-product of the T cell response to melanoma in humans. This is supported by the observation that when melanoma patients were treated with melanoma-associated peptide, specific CD8 T cell clones induced depigmented areas around melanoma lesions where there were none before treatment (Yee 2000). In fact, one of the diagnostic features of primary melanoma is what is called a "halo" of depigmentation surrounding not only primary melanomas, but also the precancerous lesions; acquired/congenital nevi, dysplastic nevi, Spitz nevi, as well as halo nevi (Kolm 2006). Often these halos are associated with early melanoma lesions that are receding and are thought to be the evidence of a brisk cellular immune response despite the fact that they are rare (Rubegni 2009). Since melanoma-associated vitiligo is a result of the immune response to melanoma, an examination of that response is warranted in order to understand the autoimmune properties of the anti-tumor T cell response that causes this skin disorder and other cancer-induced autoimmune reactions. Moreover, this examination will involve the examination of the ability of a growing tumor to control the T cell response and describe the autoimmune consequences as they relate to the T cell immune response to cancer and the role Tregs play in this response.

Melanoma

Melanoma is a type of cancer that develops from the melanocyte, which is a pigment-producing cell that produces and packages melanin in response to ultraviolet light exposure. Melanocytes develop from what is called the neural crest, which are ectodermally derived cells that appear along the outer surface of the neural tube in the early stages of embryonic development. In addition to giving rise to melanocytes these cells give rise to spinal, cranial, enteric, sympathetic ganglia, Schwann cells, and cells of the adrenal medulla. These are all cells of the nervous system, which makes the melanocyte an immune privileged cell. Immune privilege is a phenomenon where certain tissue systems such as the central nervous system (CNS) and reproductive organs that are sensitive to inflammation, restrict the movement and abilities of immune cells to enter and function normally (Mrass 2006). This situation complicates the immune response to melanoma because T cells have difficulties entering neural tissues, which a growing melanoma might appear to be. Once melanomas develop they may metastasize to other parts of the body and are the most malignant of all the skin cancers.

Melanomas tend to occur in predominantly in white women and men usually, but not always, over the age of 40 who are light in complexion and have a lot of moles. However, people of color do get melanoma usually on the palms of the hands and soles of the feet. There is a greater incidence of melanoma in people who have what is called dysplastic nevi, which are complex (irregular shape) moles thought to be the beginning stages of melanoma. There are four major types of melanoma. They are superficial spreading melanoma, nodular melanoma, acral lentiginous melanoma, and lentigo maligna melanoma. Intra ocular melanoma is a rare type of melanoma affecting the eye (Turkington 1998).

To aid in the determination of the prognosis of melanoma a staging technique was developed by Dr. Wallace Clark, Jr. of the University of Pennsylvania. It is called Clark's classification system (Clark 1986). It classifies melanomas by how deeply they penetrate the layers of the skin and is very accurate in the prediction of the lethality of any melanoma lesion that appears in the skin. This development was an invaluable tool because histological sections of melanomas not only revealed the invasion depth of the cancer, but also showed the presence of a lymphocytic infiltrate (Clark 1984). There was an extreme correlation between the presence of this lymphocyte infiltrate and survival of this type of skin cancer (Kornstein 1983). Scientists were able to determine not only the type of lymphocyte (T cell) infiltrating the cancer mass, but also the method the T cells used to attack the cancer cells. It turns out that the T cells were responding to formally melanocyte-specific proteins that were altered during the change from normal cell (melanocyte) to cancer cell (melanoma) and now recognized as foreign and called melanoma-associated antigens (MAA). Some of these MAA are closely related to normal melanocyte antigens and are thought to induce melanoma-related autoimmune responses during treatment (Palmer 2008). These antigens are numerous and can be markers used to identify different pathological stages of melanoma (Graf 1989).

The T Cell Response to Melanoma

As mentioned previously, CD4 T cells must see foreign proteins in association with a self-protein called HLA-DR. As melanocytes make the transition from normal to dysplastic and then to cancerous, they start to express the HLA-DR proteins (Guerry 1984). This in combination with the MAAs induces a CD4 T cell immune response that includes the formation of CD8 killer cells (Guerry 1987). Both of these T cells (CD4 and CD8) could be visualized in sections of the tumor mass. The killer T cells could be detected because they secreted INF-Γ when they attacked the melanoma cells. This response, seen in the skin was reproduced in the laboratory using melanoma cells cultured in the lab and purified T cells from the patients the cultured melanoma cells came from (Guerry 1987). Other studies in this laboratory demonstrated that primary melanoma cells, but not metastatic melanoma cells were able to not only present melanoma-specific proteins, but also proteins such as tetanus toxoid. This was a significant finding because it showed that early malignant cancer cells were able to alert the immune system of their presence by acting like normal antigen presenting cells. These and other in vitro studies were the framework and model for not only melanoma and its treatment, but also many other types of cancer (Alexander 1989).

Antigen Presentation by Melanoma Cells

The ability of melanoma cells to induce a CD4 T cell response that also generates a cytotoxic CD8 T cell response against the tumor is possible and does occur in early primary melanoma. This is supported by the fact that an immune response, which includes both CD4 and CD8 T cell responses, has been detected against primary, but not metastatic melanoma cells in vivo and in vitro (Guerry 1984). In mouse models advanced melanoma cell lines, which previously did not express MHC-classI (HLA-A, B, C) or class II (HLA-D) proteins, were able to present melanoma tumor antigens only after both MHC proteins were genetically inserted into the cell lines. This led to the immunologic removal of the tumor from mice that had received the genetically altered melanoma cells (Chen 1994). As far as presentation of tumor antigens in human melanoma cells is concerned, the process of antigen presentation itself had to be re-evaluated in order to understand why late-stage melanoma cells do not present immunogenic melanoma-associated antigens to either CD4 or CD8 T cells. Antigen presentation by "professional" antigen presenting cells such as macrophages and DC occurs in two stages. One stage of the process occurs within the cell where intercellular proteins or extracellular proteins (class I and class II pathways) find themselves inside intercellular membranes called vesicles. While inside, these vesicles the proteins are processed into smaller peptides and then associated with the appropriate MHC-class I or MHC-class II molecule. There is also something called a "chaperone" protein, which would be the MHC-class II invariant chain for class II processing and a similar protein called a "transporter" protein called TAP for class I processing. These proteins attach themselves to the peptide to be presented and then through another process transfer the peptide to the MHC-class I or II molecule that is destined to be expressed on the surface of the cell where it is detected by either CD4 (class II) or CD8 (class I) responding T cells (Alexander 2011). Since melanoma cells are not lymphocyte lineage cells this process is slightly different, more complex, and sensitive to disruption.

Alternate Antigen Presentation Pathways Used by Melanoma Cells

For some time it has been known that MHC-class I antigen presentation in human melanoma through the TAP transporter system during antigen processing is defective in early melanoma and can led to the progression of metastatic disease (Cresswell 2001). In addition, the down regulation of the TAP transport system occurs specifically in primary melanoma lesions that lack signs of spontaneous regression as if the tumor is exploiting this phenomenon to escape destruction by CD8 cytotoxic T cells (Dissemond 2003). This particular activity by melanoma cells that results in immune escape is related to the nature of the tumor cell itself. This is caused by the stem cell nature of melanoma, which will be discussed in more detail later as it relates to the T cell immune response. Despite this characteristic of melanoma, it was shown that inserting the genes of TAP into TAP deficient melanoma cell lines made these cells susceptible to CD8 cytotoxic T cells, which were previously unrecognizable by human melanoma peptide specific CTL (Tao 2008). This type of replacement of a defective or down regulated gene product in order to induce specific immunity to melanoma is a tool used to understand why melanoma cells are not recognized by T cells that would otherwise kill them.

As far as MHC-class II antigen presentation by melanoma cells is concerned, the evidence related to it, and the successful eradication of melanoma, seems to only pertain to early melanomas. After this early period, MHC-class II expression by melanoma cells seems to be an indicator for a poor prognosis for outcome of the disease. There are several reasons for this and most of them are related to the negative effects that occur as the MHC molecule, which is a receptor, makes contact with either the TCR or the LAG-3 ligand. This is similar to the situation, which was discussed earlier where the LAG-3 (CD4 family member) of the T cell made contact with the MHC-class II molecule of the DC. This interaction resulted in the down regulation of key cell surface proteins (CD80/86) needed by the immune system (CD4 T cells) to respond to tumor antigens presented by DC. In this case, once the MHC-class II proteins of the melanoma cell are exposed to the LAG-3 ligand they develop a resistance to FAS-mediated and drug induced cell death through the activation of the MAPK/Erk and P13K/Akt pathways (Hemon 2011). Of course this is a bidirectional event because as previously mentioned, engagement of the LAG-3 ligand negatively affects early T cell activation events (Macon-Lemaitre 2005). Another aspect of this LAG-3 and melanoma situation is that a separate subpopulation of Tregs that express high levels of LAG-3 are detected in tumor masses and in the circulation of melanoma patients (Camisaschi 2010). This subset of Tregs constitutively secretes IL-10 and TGF-β that are two previously mentioned lymphokines, which modulate DC function and convert T cells to the Treg phenotype. It is evident that the expression of MHC-class II by melanoma presents problems for the T cell immune system that may overshadow the potential positive effect its expression may have on the induction of a CD4 T cell response to the tumor.

Negative Effects of Alternate Antigen Processing and Presentation of Antigens by MHC-Class II Proteins Expressed on the Cell Surface

As mentioned above melanoma cells have the ability to process and present tumor-associated and autoimmune self-antigens in association with MHC-class II molecules on the surface of the cell. In early melanomas, the consequences of the interaction between antigen specific CD4 T cells and these MHC-class II antigen complexes can be the induction of a productive T cell immune response, which includes the induction of melanoma specific cytotoxic CD8 T cells. One of the major questions is why does this CD4 T cell response fail in response to late stage melanomas that are still producing these MHC-class II antigen complexes on their cell surfaces? This is a complex question, but some of this failure has to do with the development of alternate MHC-class II antigen peptide processing pathways that are developed by melanoma cells as the continue down the tumorgenesis pathway to late-stage disease. The causes can be selective pressures brought about by the T cell immune system itself (immunoediting) or related to the stem cell nature of melanoma, which will be discussed in this section. These alternate peptide-MHC-class II processing pathways can alter the nature of the T cell response to the tumor by not only altering the antigenic peptide selection the responding T cells must see, but also unleashing inhibitory activities associated with the tumor by engagement of the MHC-class II molecule.

Antigen processing of peptide MHC-class II complexes in APC involves distinct stages that involve the association of the peptide, which is chaperoned by the invariant chain, to the peptide-binding grove of the MHC-class II protein. Once this occurs, the complex arrives on the cell surface and is associated with cholesterol-dependent lipid microdomains or lipid rafts (Khandelwal 2010). These are the same lipid rafts mentioned during the description of the TCR assembly process and the ITAM inhibitory pathway in DCs and as mentioned in both of those instances, these rafts are sites where translational pathways interact (Cifuentes 2008). In addition to that fact, lipid rafts control the clustering of the MHC-class II peptide complexes on the cell surface and therefore control the strength of translational signals that are produced just below the cell membrane. Once these signals are initiated the cell responds accordingly such as in the case with DC where CD80/86 is down regulated, which diminishes the CD4 T cell response to DC presented peptides. Late-stage melanoma cells also display MHC-class IIpeptide complexes on their surfaces associated with lipid rafts, but once contact is made with the T cell receptor a higher level of aggregation of these complexes occurs when compared to normal APC. This immediately has several immune suppressing implications regarding what was already discussed. The first is with LAG-3 activation in T cells where it was mention that LAG activation negatively affects early T cell activation events (Macon-Lemaitre 2005), but also it was determined that LAG engagement by MHC-class II can induce down regulated T cell proliferation to the point where the level of T cell activity is below normal homeostatic conditions (Workman 2005). The second immune suppressing implication would be the interaction of LAG-3 expressing Tregs (Camisaschi 2010) with the MHC-class II peptide complex mentioned earlier, which for all intents and purposes functions as a receptor on the surface of the tumor cell.

It has already been established that signaling through the MHC-class II complex on the cell surface of DCs causes them to revert to a more immature state that can induce the creation of adaptive Tregs. In addition, similar signaling through this complex on monocytes can induce T cell anergy with classic T cell anergy-related up-regulation of cell cycle inhibitors P27Kip1 and P21Cip1 (Kriegel 2008). However, when the MHC-class IIof melanoma cells is cross-linked with antibodies that mimic the TCR the MHC-class II proteins begin to aggregate as the lipid rafts coalesce in clusters that are much larger than those found in APC during similar antibody ligation. In addition, it was determined that the c-Jun NH2-terminal kinase or JNK (a member of the MAP kinase family) was phosphorylated (activated) during this process (Barbieri 2011). This is a significant observation because JNK activation contributes to the growth rate and increased tumorgenesis of melanoma by up-regulating phosphoinositide-dependent kinase 1 (PDK1), which induces Akt and protein kinase C (PKC) activation (phosphorylation) that leads to tumor growth (Lopez-Bergami 2010). Both the increased clustering of MHC-class II proteins and the induction of the JNK pathway are two negative aspects of the interactions of the TCR with the melanoma-associated expression of MHC-class II. The increased clustering of these proteins is particularly damaging to the T cell response if the melanoma cell does not express the second signal (CD80/86 or B7) for CD4 T cell activation. T cell activation to peptide antigens presented by MHC-class II must also include the interaction of the CD28 ligand on the T cell with its receptor (CD80/86 or B7) on the APC. If the T cell receptor is activated without the second signal (CD28/B7) the T cell becomes anergic and cannot secrete IL-2 or proliferate (Mondino 1994). This also occurs with melanoma because many melanomas do not always express the second signal necessary for T cell activation to occur. This is called clonal anergy where the absence of this second signal renders the responding T cells tolerant to further activation (Becker 1993). Therefore, MHC-class II expression in late-stage melanoma can contribute to the progression of the disease rather than its destruction as it does in early-stage melanomas. Much of this has to do with the increasing genetic instability of the melanoma cells as they change in response to their environment. This genetic instability is related to the stem cell-like nature of many solid tumors.

The Relationship between the Stem Cell Nature of Cancer, Autoimmunity, Tregs, and the Anti-Tumor T Cell response

As the T cell immune system approaches a site where precancerous cells are forming what it sees it a group of cells that are distinctly different from the surrounding normal cells of any given tissue system. Those differences, which were mentioned earlier, include the presentation of distorted self-peptides by MHC molecules on the precancerous cell surface. These peptides are derived from mutated proteins produced as a consequence of tumorgenesis. This is a process that is the result of a series of unrepaired or disrepaired DNA breaks that occur in the nucleus for a number of reasons. One of these reasons has to do with the general genetic instability of the human genome, which is defined as the accumulation of DNA breaks due to mild or severe defects in genes responsible for DNA repair (Hsu 1983). Another form of genetic instability that has relevance to tumorgenesis is called chromosomal instability, where this type of genetic instability increases the rate of gross chromosomal genetic rearrangements during each cell division (Michor 2005). This type of damage to the chromosome over a period of time is what invariably leads to the combination of DNA errors (mutations), which are typical of a tumorgenic even that leads to cancer. Chromosomal damage of this type is the result of what is called DNA double-strand breaks, which actually occur quite often, but are normally repaired quickly (Mills 2003). As mentioned above, if problems arise with the repair mechanisms the process of tumorgenesis may begin. Another way that tumorgenesis occurs is by DNA damage brought about by environmental factors, some of which are natural and some manmade. This is called "carcinogenesis" and is a model of how tumorgenesis begins in normal cells and often is the starting-point of the cancer stem cell.

Carcinogenic Induction of Tumorgenesis and the Development of Cancer Stem Cells

There are two types of carcinogens and those are natural carcinogens and manmade carcinogens. Two natural carcinogens are ultraviolet light and radon gas. Two manmade carcinogens are benzene and dioxin. All of these can induce cancer (tumorgenic) by similar mechanisms, which act on sensitive cells of the body. Skin damaging ultraviolet light radiation comes in two forms. UVA (315-400nm) and UVB (280-315nm) are separate wavelength forms that have both been shown to cause skin cancer, which the most prominent form is melanoma. (Brem 2010). There are other forms of skin cancer such as basal cell carcinoma that are also caused by these forms of ultraviolet light (Burke 2009), but melanoma is the most deadly and prone to occur during extended exposure to UV radiation. The melanocyte is the target cell of UV radiation, which causes DNA damage (oxidative) to the cells. Melanocytes have been shown to have a deficiency in repairing this type of DNA damage (Wang 2010). The genes responsible for the repair are called nucleotide DNA excision repair genes or NER. Evidence suggests that once mutations occur in these genes the process of tumorgenesis in melanocytes begin. In addition, it was found that some of these mutations were congenital, which means that they can be passed down to prodigy (Rass 2008). This would support the fact that melanoma is often a familial form of cancer.

The next natural carcinogenic agent is radon gas. The element radon (radon-222) is a radioactive gas formed by the decay of trace quantities of uranium. It seeps through the pores in subterranean rocks and ends up accumulating in dwellings that have poor ventilation. It is most prevalent in geographic areas where radium (precursor of radon) can be detected in the soil (Teichman 1988). Exposure to radon gas not only in the home, but also uranium and hard rock mines can cause lung cancer by creating what is called oxidative free radicals in epithelial cells in the lungs (Steck 1999). However, radon gas can also cause leukemia, lymphoma (Rericha 2006) and a rare form of leukemia called monocytic leukemia (Eatough 1993). Free radical formation inside of cells induces the same type of oxidative damage to DNA as mentioned above and the induction of cancer is governed by the same inability to repair the DNA by the NER genes.

Dioxin is a manmade chemical, which is a part of a family of compounds that are by-products of the manufacturing process of such products as plastics. There are 200 of these family members and they are classified as dioxins and furans. These compounds are not only toxic and carcinogenic, but are also resistant to decay and dispersal in the environment (Frontier 2000). The main compound is called 2,3,7,8-tetrachlorodibenzo-*p*-dioxin (TCDD) and works its way through the environment by attaching to a cellular receptor called AH (Tuomisto 2005), which is distributed throughout the bodies of most species on the planet. However, the way dioxin moves into our bodies is not only through the food chain, but also through the lower-level atmosphere. Factories that produce products such as plastics, rubber, and a few others are or have been responsible for dioxin dispersal through the air. It gets deposited in the fat of not only mammals, but also fish that are part of the food supply (Leino 2008). As far as dioxin-induced cancer is concerned, breast cancer was one of the cancers that were focused on the most. Laboratory studies demonstrated that when this xenobiotic (biologically foreign substance) chemical, dioxin bound to the AH receptor of cells it induced the activation of genes that were able to differentiate that cell into a cancer cell. A human breast cancer cell, which was grown in the laboratory was very sensitive to dioxin receptor binding, and they theorized that the cell been created by exposure to dioxin (Rivera 2006). In addition, it was found the female mice fed high fat diets with dioxin during the height of their estrogen cycle developed breast cancer at a significantly higher rate than those that did not, but were also on a high fat diet (Merrill 2010). The evidence concerning human cancers was evident when epidemiologists examined the prevalence of not only breast cancer, but also prostate cancer within areas located near factories that routinely discarded dioxin into the environment through the air. There was a significant increase in the diagnosis of both cancers when compared to individuals who lived in remote sites.

Benzene, which is another manmade compound, starts out as a clear liquid that has a sweet odor. It has a high evaporation rate and quickly becomes airborne. This is a completely different type of chemical when compared to dioxin for several reasons. First of all, it is in active use by industries that produce such things as plastics, synthetic fibers like nylon, some types of rubber, detergents, dyes, and a long list of other products used on a daily basis. The second thing is that unlike dioxin, which can be dispersed through the air and the food chain, benzene is mostly an airborne pollutant. Finally, benzene does not accumulate in the body like dioxin does. The dangerous aspect of benzene with regards to health and its ability to cause cancer is that it is found almost everywhere. It's found in even remote regions because it has the ability to attach itself to water in the form of rain or snow. Then it can become airborne when the water evaporates. The major sources of exposure to benzene are automobile exhaust, industrial emissions, tobacco smoke, paint, furniture wax, and evaporation of gasoline from cars and service stations. Breathing high levels of benzene can cause immediate death, while slightly lower levels can cause drowsiness, elevated heart rate, headaches, and unconsciousness. As far as cancer is concerned, all of the leukemia's originated from chromosomal damage induced not by native benzene, but it's metabolites. There are several pathways of metabolism in humans, but both of these pathways begin with the enzymatic breakdown of benzene into benzene oxide. After this there are a series of complex steps that produce at least 10 different metabolites of benzene. One of these metabolites (1-4 benzoquinone) interferes with a replication and maintenance gene called Topoisomerase II and this is where benzene begins to damage chromosomal activity (Rappaport 2009). These benzene metabolites such as benzene oxide have been shown to cause DNA lesions, which are distorted segments DNA that have to be repaired by enzymes like the topoisomerases. Bone marrow progenitor cells are the cells that leukemia develops from. They tend to repair their DNA more because these cells often respond to lymphokines that change them into several different types of white blood cells. This process often starts and then stops. In order for these bone marrow cells to revert to their original primordial state, the DNA must be returned to its original configuration by repair enzymes. (Hartwig 2010). These are continuous adjustments bone marrow cells have to make to their environment to supply the body with a variety of white blood cell types. When benzene attacks these cells it interferes with not only the genes for the repair enzymes, but also increases the number of "DNA mistakes" that have to be repaired. As a result mutant DNA remains and once expressed, leukemia is formed.

These examples of carcinogenic induction of tumorgenesis were given in order to understand not only the causes and mechanisms associated with cancer formation, but also to highlight the diversity of cell types sensitive to cancer-inducing carcinogens. It is important to understand that the T cell immune response to each of the types of cancers mentioned here are different in the sense that these T cell responses encounter situations where carcinogens cause these cancers over a long period of time. In some instances, many decades pass by during exposure to these carcinogens as the cells slowly make the transit from normal to precancerous and finally to full-blow cancer. During this period and particularly the normal to precancerous period, autoimmune responses occur because Tregs begin to lose specificity for the self-antigens of the precancerous cells as they become more and more unrecognizable through the mutation processes associated with tumorgenesis. Once this occurs, normal cells from which the tumor is forming and that share tumor associated antigens, such as with gp100 (melanocyte and melanoma shared antigen), autoimmunity begins (Chang 2011). However, during the total time period between normal cell and actual cancer the T cell immune system has made numerous adjustments to the changes the cell has gone through, but these adjustments made by the T cell immune system pale in comparison to the ones that accompany the cancer stem cell phase of a tumor's existence.

Cancer Stem Cells

Cancer stem cells, which have also been called "tumor initiating" cells were first theorized to exist around the time that there was definitive proof that hematopoietic stem cells were indeed a reality and that an undefined embryonic-like primordial cell (stem cell) gave rise to the multiple cell types of the hematopoietic system. The initial properties ascribed to these cancer stem cells (CSC) were that the cells had self-sustaining properties and gave rise to populations of tumor cells that became distinctly different (differentiated) from the CSC through genetic mutations. CSC are a minority population, which have the ability to drive the tumorgenesis process. As part of the definition of CSC, these cells not only had to have the ability to self-renew (repeated passage in xenogenic host while retaining genetic identifiers), but also in this setting, had to give rise to non-stem cell tumor populations that were a mirror image of the original patient tumor populations (Reya 2001). As time went on there was much confusion and speculation about where CSC originated. The reason for this is because it was difficult to determine if these cells originated from transforming mutations in multi-potential stem cells, tissue-specific stem cells, progenitor cells, mature cells, or malignant cancer cells. There was even debate about whether CSC caused cancer similar to how carcinogens induce tumorgenesis or that these cells were ultimately the result of carcinogenesis. More study had to be done on the genetic basis of self-renewal and tumor cell differentiation in order to answer those questions (Wu 2008).

One of the major characteristics of CSC was the fact that they were resistant to chemotherapy. Melanoma was chosen as a chemo-resistant tumor system where there was the identification of an ATP-dependent efflux transporter P-glycoprotein called ABCB1. This glycoprotein is a member of an ATP-binding cassette (ABC) superfamily that function as energy-dependent efflux pumps for transport of small compounds between cells (van Helvoort 1996). It was also determined that these P-glycoprotein are involved in multi-drug resistance of malignant cells (Ueda 1986). In melanoma it was determined that the P-glycoprotein ABCB5 identifies CD133+ progenitor cells associated with human epidermal melanocytes and it is expressed in a subpopulation of malignant melanoma cells (Goldstein 1989). It was determined that the ABCB5 glycoprotein plays a major role in the ability of melanoma cells to be resistant to doxorubicin (a cationic chemotherapeutic agent) by specifically removing it from ABCB5+ melanoma cells. Even though ABCB5+ cells are approximately 10 percent of the tumor population, this cell type is present in a majority of highly malignant human tumors. In addition, ABCB5+ cells have been associated with not only the phenotype of metastatic melanoma, but also the physiologic phenotype of cancer stem cells (Frank 2005). The resistance to chemotherapeutic agents is just one of the ways these cancer stem cells survive. Another way is to directly alter the T cell immune response.

The cancer stem cells described above are a model for other cancer stem cell systems associated with other types of malignancies such as myeloid leukemia (Bonnet 1997). These cells directly interface with the T cell immune system in ways that are not only detrimental to the anti-tumor T cell response, but also the entire immune system, which is degraded by a series of interactions between T cells and CSC. Some of the immunomodulation effects on the anti-tumor T cell response such as tumor-expressed MHC-class II signals that induce T cell anergy have been mentioned. There are some of these mechanisms that have been exclusively associated with CSC such as the induction of TGF-β and IL-10 production in T cells that come in contact with the CSC in a B7-specific manner (Schatton 2010). As mentioned earlier, production of these lymphokines by responding T cells creates Tregs and immunosupressive DC and since these are soluble these effects go beyond the tumor site. In fact, in another tumor system (squamous cell carcinoma) CSC, which were CD44 positive not only produced the inhibitory cytokines TGF-β and IL-10, but also proinflammatory cytokines such as IL-1a, IL-6, and GMCF. In addition, CD44+ CSC in these particular types of cancers (laryngeal squamous cell carcinomas) display reduced HLA class I and II expression, which is due to previously mentioned down-regulation of TAP (Chikamatsu 2011), that makes them "invisible" to class I and II antigen specific cytotoxic T cells (Ogino 2006).

Alteration of the T Cell Immune System by Cancer Stem Cells That Lead to Autoimmunity

From this information, and the information provided above about the way tumor cells interact with the T cell immune system, it is apparent that the tumor, and in this case CSCs, basically reek havoc with the system. All of these activities directed at the T cell immune system have wide-ranging effects on the ability of the T cells in the system to maintain immunological homeostasis within the body. One of the many examples of this phenomenon is the effect of excessive lymphokine release as cancer patients respond to their tumors. This is called a "lymphokine storm." In colorectal carcinoma, patients present with a marked increase in the disregulation of T cells, which is brought about by increased amounts of IL-4 secreted by T cells during the anti-tumor response. IL-4 induces a type-2 T cell response (antibody formation) and actively inhibits type-1 T cell responses (cytotoxic T cell). This can lead to not only autoantibody responses, but also susceptibility to infections (Pellegrini 1996). A very similar situation occurs in patients with hematological cancers such as myeloma and chronic lymphocytic leukemia. In these cases there is a skewing of the CD4+ repertoire toward type-2 T cells and reduction of type-1 CD4 activity (Christopoulos 2011). This again can induce autoimmunity via the production of autoantibodies to tissues related the original cancer. The induction of an autoimmune response in this way may seem problematic, but in the case of patients who have melanoma and have developed vitiligo, it in many cases proved to be a positive prognostic indicator related to the immune-induced regression of the tumor.

As these autoantibodies attach themselves to normal cells a natural part of the immune response occurs. This is called "phagocytosis" and is primarily a macrophage function, but monocytes and DCs can also do this. Antibodies attach to cells via the F(ab) portion of the molecule (the Y end) and what's left protruding is the Fc portion (stem of the Y) of the molecule. Macrophages, and both DC and monocytes (APCs), express an Fc receptor, which can attach to the protruding Fc portion of the attached antibody. Once this occurs a series of events occurs within the APCs that lead to not only the death of the antibody-coated cell, but also its internalization. This process of phagocytosis leads to the processing and presentation of antigen and in these cases, self-antigens. In this situation, where a patient with cancer produces autoantibodies, there are several separate, but similar things that occur within the T cell immune system. These events directly impact not only the anti-tumor T cell response, but also the health of the patient as far as autoimmune disease is concerned. As mentioned earlier, the TCR of Tregs is largely specific for self-peptides. This increased phagocytic activity of APC caused by this skewing of a cancer patient's T cell response to antibody production can systematically activate Tregs, which are a minority population of the total T cell pool. Once this occurs, this small population of T cells are either non-responsive through hyper activation or spread too thin to respond to type-1 CD4 T cells that begin to successfully attack normal tissues like the melanocyte. Part of this CD4 activation to melanocyte/melanoma antigens is the generation of antigen-specific CD8 CTL. These cells in turn attack melanocytes and are thought to cause both melanoma-related and generalized vitiligo (Garbelli 2005).

Recent studies have supported the theory that Treg activity associated with vitiligo is defective and in relation to how cancer cells alter the T cell immune system, several of these defects will be mentioned now. A more complete discussion of Treg defects and autoimmunity will be discussed later in this chapter and in a subsequent chapter concerning Treg effector mechanisms. However, the defect in Treg activity described below is not associated with the general effector function of Tregs from either melanoma-related or generalized vitiligo patients. In one study, the inability of functional Tregs to move (home) into vitiligo skin was reported and was related to the absence of Tregs in these areas of the skin where melanocyte damage was occurring. It was found the Tregs from these patients expressed the necessary chemokine receptors (CCR4, CCR5, CCR8, and CLA) needed to enter the skin and were found to be able to migrate towards CCR4 via the homing chemokine CCL22. Despite this, there was very little expression of the chemokine (CCL22) in vitiligo skin. Therefore, it was concluded that the absence of Tregs in the lesions allowed for the destruction of melanocytes by CD8 CTL, which target melanocyte/melanoma antigens such as MART-1 and gp100 (Klarquist 2010). Despite this finding associated with the inability of Tregs to home to the vitiligo lesions, another more substantial study revealed that there was indeed a functional defect in Tregs among generalized vitiligo patients. This study demonstrated that Tregs failed to maintain peripheral tolerance during to the rapid expansion of self-reactive CD8 CTL. In addition, it was determined that both CD8 CTL and Tregs were present in vitiligo skin. Furthermore, it was found that these CD8 T cells were hyperactive because they produced more INF-γ and TNF-α compared to non-vitiligo CD8 T cells when stimulated in vitro. When the same comparison was done concerning the ability of Tregs to inhibit CD8 INF-γ production, the Tregs from the vitiligo patients were unable to suppress INF-γ production (Lili 2012). This is similar to the concept mentioned above as far as Tregs becoming non-responsive due to hyper activation during an antibody response to autoantigens, but in this case it is cased by this global expansion of melanocyte specific CD8 CTL.

The Importance of Autoimmunity during the Anti-Tumor T Cell Response and Its Relationship to Treg Dysfunction and the Predisposition of Autoimmune and Cancer Patients to Contract Other Autoimmune Diseases

Many melanoma patients who have been treated for their disease have developed vitiligo. Clinically, the development of this autoimmunity related to autoantibody production (Maire 2013) and vitiligo (Uchi 2006) has been associated with a positive prognosis for late-stage melanoma patients undergoing treatment. Many studies have suggested that this positive prognostic indicator was due to the fact that the T cell response to melanoma included antigens that were also present on normal melanocytes. It was thought that since the tumor also expressed these normal melanocyte-specific antigens such as Mart-1 and gp100, the T cell response was more inclusive in scope (Yee 2000). This means that the inclusion of normal melanocyte antigens would lead to the destruction of the tumor. In a certain sense this is true, but the mechanism of this response has just been recently elucidated. One of the basic concepts involving the T cell response is the generation of population of T cells that retain the genetic memory of the initial encounter with antigen. There are two types of memory T cell populations that are generated during a T cell immune response. The first is the central memory T cell (Tcm), which is predominantly a CD4 T cell that is CD45R0+ and expresses CCR7 and CD62L. These cell surface proteins allow the Tcm to migrate through endothelial veins and into secondary lymphoid organs. Tcm cells have a higher response to antigen; produce large amounts of IL-2, INF-γ, and IL-4 upon stimulation when compared to naive T cells. Tcm also upregulate CD40L, which allows them to instantly interact with DC and B cells during an immune recall response. The other type of memory T cell is called an effector memory T cell (Tem) and represents both CD4 and CD8 phenotypes. These memory T cells lose expression of CCR7, but have other chemokine receptors that allow them to home to inflamed tissues. The Tem contain large amounts of perforins, which is a cytotoxic agent used by CD8 CTL to destroy targeted cells. The most important thing about this population of memory T cells is that it can produce Th-1 and Th-2 CD4 T cells as well as, CD8 CTL (Sallusto 2004). This is an important aspect of the anti-tumor T cell response because after the initial attack of the tumor, these two types of memory T cells are created. These memory T cells are thought to play a role in tumor-associated autoimmunity as well as the eradication of the tumor itself.

As far as melanoma-associated vitiligo is concerned this is the case. Recently, it was determined that in cases where there was vitiligo associated with the T cell immune response to melanoma there was also the appearance of circulating Tem cells. On the other hand in the reverse situation where there was no induction of vitiligo during the anti-melanoma T cell response, there were only circulating Tcm and very few Tem. Apparently, the autoimmune response to normal melanocytes by anti-melanoma T cells was in large part due to the maintenance of the Tem cells over time. Since these Tem cells are maintained through this autoimmune reactivity, they become a source of anti-melanoma effector T cells over a very long period of time (Byrne 2011). As mentioned above, the Tem cells are a source of CD8 CTL specific for melanocyte/melanoma-shared antigens. This type of effector CTL has a high affinity TCR and the original CD8 T cells that became part of the Tem pool may have escaped clonal deletion in the thymus. Characterization of CD8 CTL from non-melanoma vitiligo patients reveals that such CTL are Th-1 CD8 effectors that kill melanocytes via the granzyme/perforin pathway (Oyarbide-Valencia 2006). It was also determined that these memory T cells did not suffer from T cell "exhaustion." This is a common characteristic of anti-viral and anti-tumor T cells that are usually derived from the Tcm T cell pool. This type of exhaustion, which is called "hierarchical exhaustion" is brought about by chronic exposure of antigen-specific T cells to antigen and can lead to deletion or T cell anergy. T cell anergy is brought about by the some of the mechanisms previously mentioned such as the lack of the second signal by the tumor, which is thought to occur early in the T cell response. However, exhaustion usually occurs during an anti-tumor T cell response as the tumor begins to metastasize and immunogenic tumor antigens begin to appear at various locations throughout the body (Kim 2010). Therefore, since these anti-melanoma Tem cells do not suffer from exhaustion they are very effective at removing the tumor and this is why autoimmune responses such as melanoma-related vitiligo are positive indicators associated with T cell-induced removal of the tumor.

This concept concerning the apparent benefit to the anti-tumor T cell response to melanoma by the appearance of an autoimmune response to melanocyte begs the question: why is this occurring at all given the presence of Tregs, which are supposed to prevent the destruction of melanocytes in the first place? This question and its answer points right back to the dysfunction of Tregs, which was addressed previously. Those issues regarding Treg dysfunction (inability of Tregs to migrate to vitiligo skin and skewing the T cell response to a Th-2 antibody pattern) are probably the result of a larger array of genetically based autoimmune defects that originate from multiple locations within the human genome (Zenewicz 2010). In addition, definitive studies in mice point toward the absence of Treg influence during the development of generalized vitiligo (Chatterjee 2013). The basic evidence for this comes from studies that were done to determine if patients with vitiligo and their siblings suffered from other autoimmune diseases such as systemic lupus erythematosus (SLE), inflammatory bowel disease (IBD), or hypothyroidism. In a study looking at over 2000 siblings of generalized vitiligo patients it was determined that they were 20 times more likely to suffer from the above autoimmune disorders that the general population (Alkhateeb 2003).

This is a very complex issue and many of the instances related to autoimmune disease can be traced back to the dysfunction of Tregs or the resistance to their influence by autoimmune effector T cells. For instance, Tregs isolated from type 1 diabetes patients showed a reduced ability to express the FOXP3 gene in the presence of IL-2. This response to IL-2, which is contrary to Treg function, was found not associated with the IL-2 receptor, but its ability to deliver a positive signal that supports FOX-P3 expression (Long 2010). The translational pathways involved in this Treg defect will be discussed in detail later in this chapter, but suffice it to say, this is just one aspect of a complex series of events that lead to the development of a myriad of autoimmune diseases associated with Treg dysfunction. These dysfunctions of Tregs can not only originate from the Treg itself, but can also be manifested in T cell resistance (mentioned above and in a future chapter concerning Treg effector mechanisms), cytokine insensitivity, or just inadequate numbers of Tregs (Buckner 2010) as in the case with the global expansion of anti-melanocyte CD8 effector T cells in vitiligo. Since multiple defects in Treg function exist, new methods must be developed to not only detect them, but also in some cases like the inhibition of the T cell response to a developing cancer, induce them. Understanding these alterations in Treg immunobiology and applying them to both autoimmune disorders and the T cell response to cancer will allow cellular immunologist to manipulate the cellular immune system in a basic and positive way.

Autoimmune Responses, Inflammation, and the Induction of Cancer

This topic is very important as far as relating autoimmunity, the T cell response, and Tregs to cancer itself. Earlier it was mentioned that children of patients who had generalized vitiligo were 20 times more predisposed to having a separate autoimmune disease such as SLE, IBD, or hyperthyroidism. This is thought to be genetic evidence of a generalized autoimmune defect within the human genome. And as vague as that sounds, the defect is probably based in the T cell immune system with its complex array of activities such as the recruitment of inflammatory cells such as mast cells, tumor-associated macrophages (during an anti-tumor T cell response), dendritic cells, NK cells, neutrophils, and eosinophils. These cells appear not only during inflammatory events associated with relatively normal inflammatory responses to bacteria and viruses, but also during the growth of a tumor. These cells mentioned above arrive at an inflammatory site and secrete a number of cytotoxic proinflammatory mediators such as reactive oxygen (ROS) and nitrogen species (RNS), which are involved in oxidative DNA damage mentioned in the environmental carcinogenesis section. Serine and cysteine proteases, as well as the cell membrane perforating agent matrix metalloproteinase are also released into this inflammatory environment. These proinflammatory mediators can cause significant damage to normal tissues and that is why homeostasis must be maintained by the immune system (Tregs), but then there is this struggle between Tregs and responding T cells. Responding T cells and Tregs also contribute to this inflammation by secreting proinflammatory cytokines such as IL-1, IL-6, and IL-8. Continual inflammation (chronic inflammation) of normal cells has detrimental effects that not only could lead to autoimmune diseases such as diabetes, but also to the development of cancer (Vendramini-Costa 2012).

A rudimentary example would be how infectious agents such as human papillomavirus (cervical cancer) (Bosch 2002) and *Helicobacter pylori* (stomach cancer) (Graham 2000) that induce inflammatory conditions can lead to the development of cancer. Here the process, which is called innate inflammation that leads to tumorgenesis is similar to the process of carcinogenesis in that it involves not only transcriptional changes within the target cells or tissues (to be described in detail later), but also similar DNA repair damage that leads the affected cells down the cancer pathway (Trinchieri 2011). This again is another very complex issue that if examined closely, can shed light on this relationship between autoimmune inflammation and the development of cancer. It was discussed earlier how chemical carcinogens induced tumorgenisis in normal cells and how the inability of DNA to repair itself led to cancerous genomic mistakes. This phenomenon also occurs in a natural setting related to autoimmune gastritis. In this model, chronic inflammation of the gastric tract is associated with the development of gastric polyps and gastric carcinomas. An autoimmune CD4 T cell that was specific for a peptide expressed by cells in the stomach (ATPase proton pump) induced the induction of tumorgenesis and the formation of pre-cancerous cells by secreting proinflammatory agents in response to the peptide. As a consequence of the secretion of these agents, which are discussed below, normal cells of the gastric tract become inflamed. This is the initial step in tumorgenesis. This type of CD4 T cell that caused cell changes associated with the progression of human gastric cancers, such as hyperplasia and dysplasia of gastric epithelial cells is a model that can be applied to autoimmune responses in general (Nguyen 2013). This is how an autoimmune response targeted at a specific cell associated peptide can lead to cancer. From a simplistic point of view it may seem that many instances of autoimmunity are opportunities for the formation of cancer. This would not be an illogical assumption given the important role that Tregs have to control such T cell responses.

One of the more complex aspects of how inflammation may lead to cancer is the role that lymphokine IL-17 plays in the continuance of the inflammatory response. As noted earlier, TH17 T cells can be created from both innate and adaptive Tregs under conditions that favor the secretion of IL-6 and TGF-β. This conversion process does have a functional purpose and that is to aid the host in defense of fungal and bacterial infections. However, when this response is examined from an inflammatory autoimmune disease point of view, it is clear that the elaboration of IL-17 by converted TH17 T cells plays a major role in the severity of the autoimmune response. In fact, because of the synergy between other inflammatory cytokines such as tumor necrosis factor alpha (TNF-α), IL-17 has been shown to play an essential role in the pathogenesis of several autoimmune diseases such as rheumatoid arthritis (RA) and multiple sclerosis (MS) (Zhu 2012). Critical translational signal pathways, which were mentioned earlier, and will also be discussed in this section, control not only the conversion of Tregs to TH17 T cells, but also the secretion of IL-17. The formation of TH17 T cells from resident Tregs has a special significance because of the formation of granulomas. By definition a granuloma is a structure formed by the immune system that has the purpose of isolating material such as infectious organisms like bacteria and fungi and inert material like silica from the rest of the body. Typically, this process starts with macrophages, which are full of the substance through phagocytosis. Their membranes fuse together and form a typical granuloma mass. However, Tregs have been shown to infiltrate granulomas and play a critical role in impeding their growth. However, when Tregs appear in sarcoidosis lesions, which are granulomas of the lung and other organs, they seem to be unable to arrest their growth (Taflin 2009). The possibility of TH17 conversion from resident Tregs may play a role in this type of Treg dysfunction because granulomas of this type tend to induce chronic inflammation, which in turn can initiate the conversion process of Tregs to TH17 T cells. It has been found that cutaneous granulomatus disorders, which include sarcoidosis, granuloma anulare, psoriasis, and other cutaneous granulomas are detected months or years before the development of cancer in these tissues (Alexandrescu 2011).

Chronic inflammation can not only cause cancer, but it can also be a contributing factor in how cancer cells continue to mature and eventually spread (metastasize) throughout the body. As mentioned previously, both Tregs and DC secrete the lymphokine IL-6 in the tumor mass during the anti-tumor T cell response. It was shown earlier how this lymphokine could cause Tregs to be reprogrammed into TH17 effector CD4 T cells. It was found that this lymphokine affects cells other that lymphocytes. Apparently, IL-6 is able to activate or increase the expression of DNA methyltransferase-1 (DNMT1). This enzyme has the ability to methylate stretches of DNA called CpG islands, which represent fully functional genes and their promoters. Once these islands are hypermethylated by DNMT1 the gene products (proteins) can no longer be expressed. In effect, this activity silences gene expression and some of these proteins control cellular growth. In colorectal cancer it was found that this type of gene silencing mediated by IL-6, silenced genes associated with adhesion, which in effect allows the tumor cells to migrate throughout the body (Foran 2010). How tumor cells have the ability to travel to distant sites in the body is another by-product of chronic inflammation. Since inflammation is part of the healing process of the body, part of its role and the roles of the cells involved is to remodel damaged tissues to a functional state. Part of this remodeling process involves the induction of new blood vessels and is the process as angiogenesis. This is a useful process because often, damaged tissues cannot be repaired if there is no blood supply to oxygenate the tissue. Oxygen facilitates the regeneration and remodeling of the damaged tissue. However, this process is subverted during the growth of many solid tumors. Normally, when cells are deprived of a blood supply through injury, a process called hypoxia occurs and the cells secrete chemokines that alert resident macrophages. Once the macrophages appear they begin to secrete pro-angiogenic factors and chemokines, which begin the angiogenesis process. In the inflammatory environment of a tumor mass, these macrophages are the previously mentioned tumor-associated macrophages (TAM) and their development is dependent on the presence of angiopoetin and vascular endothelial growth factor or VEGF. The secretion of VEGF's, chemokines CXCL1 and CXCL8, as well as hypoxia inducible factor 1 alpha (HIF1a) by TAMs is regulated by transcription factors NF-kB, STAT3, and AP-1 (Grivennikov 2010). Involvement of these transcription factors in the angiogenesis process is an important aspect of the tumor inflammatory microenvironment. Many of these transcription factors such as NF-kB and STAT3 are also involved in the conversion of Tregs into TH17 T cells via the activities of these TAMs and DCs that are actively involved in the anti-tumor T cell response.

Given this background on the inflammatory autoimmune response it is clear that there is a strong link between autoimmune disease and cancer. Recently there was a meta-analysis of literature published between 2001 and 2011 on the risk for cancer development in patients with autoimmune and chronic inflammatory diseases (Franks 2012). The authors reported a statistically significant association between 23 separate autoimmune and chronic inflammatory diseases and cancer development in those patients. The authors also point out that many of these autoimmune disorders that lead to cancer have various pathologies such a celiac disease that involves direct participation of the T cell immune system or Crohn's disease, which is due to the formation of macrophage granulomas as discussed above. Another aspect of these diseases is that they have systemic effects such as in rheumatoid arthritis (RA), which can affect multiple tissue systems (Turesson 2007). Despite the apparent causal effect of theses diseases as far as can cancer is concerned, some like multiple sclerosis (MS) do tend to lead to cancers of the central nervous system (CNS), but also prevent other cancers from forming based on the type of immune response they engender such as increased immune surveillance in this case (Bahmanyar 2009). The authors of this meta-analysis also pointed out that just like with vitiligo and melanoma, many patients who developed primary cancers also developed autoimmune disorders related to the T cell response to the primary malignancy. This was an important study from a clinical point of view because many of these cancer patients will be treated with immune-based immunotherapies. These types of therapies, which are often inhibited by Tregs that immediately take control of antigen presenting DCs, may have a profound effect on the patient's T cell immune system. Often immunotherapies that use DCs as antigen presenting cells redirect Treg activity, which in effect, leaves the patient vulnerable to autoimmune attack by self-specific T cells that are generated during the anti-tumor T cell response.

This association with autoimmunity and cancer is a complex one when looked at from a cellular (T cells, Tregs, and tumor cells) point of view. The interactions of the translational pathways that dictate these cellular behaviors are at this point, very complex, inter-related and almost beyond our ability to understand them in relation to "the big picture," which in this case is the relationship between T cells, Tregs, and tumor cells. The operative word here is "almost" because our knowledge of these translational pathways is increasing daily. It's a known fact that these pathways, which become activated within the cells mentioned above, actually work together within single cells and possibly shared between cell types. The response of these cells to their environment is controlled in some instances by the genetic predisposition of that particular cell, which as previously mentioned is referred to as an innate response. On the other hand, there is the adaptive response, which is based on genetic information like the innate response, but is also controlled by positive or negative genetic alterations such as somatic mutations. For instance, this allows a T cell to behave in a way that it was not genetically programmed for such as its reaction to self or the conversion/reprogramming processes of naïve T cells, Tregs and TH17 T cells. This too is a natural response to the T cell's environment and must be understood. Tumor cells also utilize this feature as mentioned in the cancer stem cell section of this chapter.

Underlying all of this cellular behavior is the activation of intercellular pathways that direct that cell, based on external stimuli, to behave in a particular purposeful manner. The next section of this chapter will outline some of these pathways. In some cases it will show how their intersection inadvertently induces the activation of other translational pathways that are detrimental to a positive outcome of the T cell response in this setting of autoimmunity, inflammation, and cancer. In addition, there will be a discussion of the participation of the gene products of oncogenes, which were mentioned earlier as the genetic remnants of viral infections that became part of the human genome. During a discussion in the next chapter, which has to do with Treg effector functions, an attempt will be made to identify translational pathway elements that may be transferred or shared between different immune cell types. Particular attention will be paid to not only beneficial purposes, but also purposes that lead to negative behavioral responses in the cells involved in the transference or sharing of transcription factors. However, in the next section the functional areas that will be covered will include translational events associated with T cells and precancerous chronic inflammation, T cell immune-related cancer-induced autoimmunity, Treg dysfunction, and the translational pathways involved with the formation of cancer stem cells. Just as autoimmunity, inflammation, and the induction of cancer are interrelated so too are the translational pathways that are involved in these processes and the hope is that this interrelationship will become apparent as this next discussion of translational pathways proceeds.

Translational Pathways Associated with Tregs, Anti-Tumor T Cells, and Cancer Cells in the Autoimmunity/Inflammation Process

The description and purpose of the translational pathways discussed in this section will encompass not only the activities of anti-tumor T cells and Tregs, but also those of cancer cells and other cells that participate in the autoimmunity/inflammation process. The reason for this is to get broader understanding of how the activation of the same pathways in different cells can produce completely different or the same cellular behaviors. The pathways that will be examined here may follow the same sequence in terms of what substrates get phosphorylated or modified, but the resulting cellular activity is dependent on which type of cell is being discussed such as a T cell or malignant cancer cell. There is a certain commonality between the translational pathways in these two types of cells that in some sense begs the question: is there a reason for this? The similarities in the activation of intercellular pathways between these two completely different cell types (T cells and cancer cells) will be examined closely and the possible answer to the above question will be addressed. As pointed out in the previous section, there is an intimate relationship between autoimmunity, inflammation, tumorgenesis, the responses of anti-tumor T cells, and Tregs. To a certain extent, this relationship is reflected in these apparent similarities in translational pathway usage by the cells involved in this process. This will become important in the final section where the use of inhibitors or modifiers of translational pathways to increase the effectiveness of immune-based cancer therapies will be discussed. Some of these agents will not only operate on the target cells (anti-tumor T cells or Tregs), but may also interact with normal or cancerous cells. A careful understanding of these relationships is vital to the success of altering translational pathways to improve cancer therapies.

Translational Events Associated with the Development and Progression of the Cancerous Cell

There is a plethora of information about the translational pathways associated with both the development (tumorgenesis) and the progression (metastasis) of cancer. An attempt will be made to limit this discussion to translational events within tumor cells that impact the T cell immune system. This includes the development of cancer-induced autoimmune reactions. It is quite clear from the previous section of this chapter that as cancer cells change, the anti-tumor T cell immune response changes. Sometimes these changes in the anti-tumor T cell response result in the development of T cell anergy. This type of T cell anergy involves the activation of specific translational pathways in T cells that the cancer cell has induced during contact (Abe 2013). The translational immunology of T cell anergy will be discussed later in this section, but now attention should be focused on the specific activation of translational pathways that cause this and other negative phenomenon such as cancer-induced autoimmunity, defective memory T cell development, and the inability of Tregs to control autoimmune T cell responses.

Translational Events Associated with Tumor Cell MHC-Class II Expression

MHC-class II expression by tumor cells and particularly by late-stage melanoma cells, can present the T cell immune system with several problems. These problems are not only associated with the loss T cell function after T cell interaction MHC-class II molecules with out the second signal (CD80/86), but also an acceleration of the tumorgenesis process as a result of ligation of the tumor cell MHC-class II complex by either the TCR or the T cell's LAG-3 molecule, which is an MHC-class II ligand. There are two separate translational events within the tumor that result in the progression of the tumorgenesis process. The first one has to do with the ligation MHC-class II molecules using a monoclonal antibody (L243) as a surrogate for both the TCR and LAG-3 ligation. Once ligation of MHC-class II proteins occurs, the proteins aggregate through the formation of the previously mentioned lipid rafts. While in the lipid raft configuration, the c-Jun NH2-terminal kinase or JNK (MAP kinase family) is phosphorylated (Barbieri 2011). The phosphorylation/activation of JNK induces the up-regulation of phosphoinositide-dependent kinase 1 (PDK1) expression. The up-regulation of PDK1 leads to the activation of Akt and protein kinase C (PKC). The JNK-induced phosphorylation of both Akt and PKC has been associated with increased tumor cell growth and is the basis of c-Jun's oncogenic activity (Lopez-Bergami 2010). There is evidence to support the fact this transcriptional pathway to leads to increased tumorgenesis. In addition, the observation made earlier about carcinogenic substances and how they can induce cancer is directly related to the JNK/PKC/Akt pathway. It was determined that Akt activation via the

JNK signal pathway is involved with arsenic-induced tumor formation in human bronchial epithelial cells. Here, instead of JNK activating PDK1 in response to arsenic, it phosphorylates STAT3 at a specific amino acid residue (serene 727). This phosphorylation of STAT3 leads to Akt activation and the secretion of vascular endothelial growth factor (VEGF) by the cells. This growth factor initiates the angiogenesis process, which allows in this case, newly formed cancer cells to escape from their primary site in the lungs. In this situation, the activation of Akt is an extension of the carcinogenic process initiated by arsenic (Liu 2012).

The other translational events that occur within the tumor that result in the acceleration of the tumorgenesis process are a direct result of the interaction of T cells with MHC-class II molecules on the tumor cell surface. The LAG-3 protein expressed by T cells is a member of the CD4 family and a natural ligand of MHC-class II proteins expressed by APC. This protein serves to stabilize the interaction between the T cell and APC during normal T cell responses to antigens. However, as mentioned previously, the interaction of the LAG-3 protein with MHC-class II molecules induces a bidirectional effect on both the T cell (Workman 2005) and APC (Liang 2008). When T cell expressed LAG-3 or a soluble form of the protein comes in contact with the MHC-class II molecules of the tumor cell several transcriptional events occur.

The activation of these pathways can induce resistance to not only chemotherapy-induced death, but also the natural process of cell death mediated by the Fas/Fas ligand interaction. One of the two translational pathways activated is similar to the situation where DC maturation is inhibited by the DC's interaction with LAG-3. This Treg-creating inhibition of DC maturation involves the ITAM inhibitory pathway via the activation of the MAP kinase ERK, but not the P13k/Akt pathway (Liang 2008). Using MHC-class II melanoma cells as a model, the LAG-3/MHC-class II interaction resulted in the activation of both the MAPK/ERK and P13K/Akt pathways. As discussed previously, the activation of Akt promoted tumorgenisis by the induction of VEGF secretion. This initiates the angiogenesis process that leads formation of new blood vessels, which allows the tumor cells to escape or metastasis.

In this case, the activation of both MAPK/ERK and P13K/Akt pathways results increased survival of melanoma cells by allowing them to be resistant to two types (chemotherapy and Fas ligand) of cell death (Hemon 2011). Both of these interactions (TCR or anti-class II antibodies and LAG-3) with the MHC-class II proteins of the tumor directly impact the anti-tumor T cell response. Not only does this interaction induce resistance to tumor cell death and promotion of metastasis, but also the T cells that expressed the LAG-3 receptor can no longer maintain immunological homeostasis (Workman 2005). This inability to control other T cell responses, particularly when it comes to Tregs, which have a defined LAG-3 positive population (Camisaschi 2010), is of critical importance to other T cell responses not related to the tumor.

Once LAG-3 expressing Tregs come in contact with tumor-bound MHC-class II proteins these cells that are supposed to regulate T cell-based autoimmunity are rendered useless. This is one of the reasons why autoimmunity and immune disregulation occur during the growth of a tumor.

Translational Events Associated with Lymphocyte and Tumor Secreted IL-6

The examples above demonstrate how the T cell immune system itself can contribute to the progression of tumorgenesis. This immune system-induced progression of tumorgenesis directly impacts the T cell response to the tumor. In keeping with that theme is the role that the lymphokine IL-6 plays in not only the progression of cancer, but also in chronic inflammation, which was discussed earlier as an inducer of primary tumors. As far as its role in inflammation leading to cancer is concerned, the natural role of IL-6 in T cell differentiation starts with the activation of the Jak/STAT-3 and MAPK Ras/Erk pathway. This pathway enables T cells to resist programmed (Fas/Fas ligand) cell death and controls the conversion of Tregs into TH17 T cells. Recently it was discovered that blocking IL-6 during inflammatory responses such as IBD, MS, and RA was beneficial in terms of reducing the incidence of inflammation-associated cancer (Neurath 2011). As mentioned earlier, IL-6 is responsible for activating the DNA methylation enzyme, DNA methyltransfease-1, which has the ability to silence genes that regulate tumor growth and adhesion (Foran 2010). Related to these findings is the fact that cancer stem cells (CSC) or tumor-initiating cancer cells have the ability to quickly adapt to the T cell immune response by producing altered non-immunogenic non-CSCs. It turns out that IL-6 may play a role in the creation or more specifically, the recreation of CSCs.

The gene Oct-4 codes for a transcriptional factor that is expressed in embryonic stem cells an embryonal carcinomas. It is thought to be largely responsible for the growth-burst of normal hemopoietic stem cells. It was found that in CSCs, this gene was silenced by retinoic acid (RA) treatment of these cells. This is because retinoic acid receptors form a complex with a hormone response element (HRE) within the Oct-4 promoter (Schoorlemmer 1995). As discussed earlier, T cells and DCs secrete IL-6, but tumor cells can also secrete this proinflammatory lymphokine. Breast cancer cells that have an over expression of the HER-2 (human epidermal growth factor receptor-2) gene begin to express the high levels of IL-6. Secretion of IL-6 by these tumor cells is associated with the activation of STAT-3 in what is called an "autocrine" loop where there is the perpetual release and use (IL-6R engagement) of the same IL-6 secreted by the tumor cell (Hartman 2011). This situation contributes to cancer-induced inflammation that can lead to the recruitment of natural Tregs and the conversion naïve or tumor antigen-specific T cells into Tregs and then into TH17 T cells. In addition to the inflammation induced by IL-6, it was also discovered that in this very situation, where breast carcinoma cells are producing IL-6, activation of the Oct-4 gene was occurring. This activation of the Oct-4 in non-CSC allows them to regenerate into CSC. The signal transduction pathway in this case results in the direct activation of STAT-3, but starts with a signal transducer called Janus-Activated Kinase-1 or JAK-1 (Kim 2013b). However, the most interesting aspect of how this contributes to the regeneration of CSCs lies in the fact that when JAK-1 is activated, it phosphorylates the IL-6 receptor, which then leads to the concomitant phosphorylation of STAT-3. When dimerization of phosphorylated STAT-3 occurs in the cytoplasm, these complexes head straight for the nucleus. Once there, the STAT3 dimers activate STAT-3 target genes that control cell cycle regulators such as cyclin-D1and c-MYC, as well as inhibitors of cell death (apoptosis) and survival such as BCL-xl (Ahmad 2008). Once these cell cycle regulators and inhibition of apoptosis genes are activated, these tumor cells that were not stem cell-like become self-generating CSCs like their parents.

As mentioned earlier, many of the translational events that occur in cells start from a common activity such as in the case of the formation of lipid rafts in both MHC-class II positive tumor cells and T cells in response to the ligation of the MHC-class II proteins and the TCR, respectively on the surface of these cells. However, the pathways that are generated are completely different depending upon which cell is involved in this process. In addition, there are situations where completely different transduction pathways are activated, but lead to the activation of an identical transduction pathway such as the P13K/Akt pathway. As shown above, this pathway that leads to increase tumorgenesis by both inducing angiogenesis and allowing the tumor to escape from the primary site. In addition, it can increase tumor survival via activation transduction pathways associated with survival and proliferation such as activation of the RhoA-P13K/Akt-Erk pathway, which is activated by fibronectin in embryonic stem cells. The activation of this pathway by fibronectin is also associated with the increased expression of the oncogenes c-fos, c-myc, and c-jun as well as the cell cycle regulators cyclin D1/CDK4 and cyclin E/CDK2 (Park 2011). Despite the fact that these are embryonic stem cells, it is apparent that the activation of these cell survival pathways, which include inhibitors of cells death such as BCL-xl mentioned earlier, have a commonality associated with them that can be found in not only cancer cells, but also hemopoietic stem cells and lymphocytes.

Translational Events Associated with the Anti-Tumor T Cell Response (T Cell Memory) and Treg Control of Autoimmunity

The response of anti-tumor T cells is very complex. Even though it seems rather straightforward where T cells, which have a TCR for tumor antigens attack the tumor; this response has some lingering aftereffects. On of the most important of them is the development of T cell memory populations. As mentioned earlier in *The importance of autoimmunity during the anti-tumor T cell response and its relationship to Treg dysfunction and the predisposition of autoimmune and cancer patients to contract other autoimmune diseases* section, there are two types of memory T cells that are crucial for not only preventing a recurrence of the tumor, but also inadvertently causing cancer-induced autoimmunity. Effector memory T cells (Tem) home to areas of inflammation and immediately begin to kill targets expressing antigens recognized by their TCR. These memory T cells are considered "protective," but the "reactive" memory T cells, called central memory T cells (Tcm) reside in the lymphatic system. When activated by specific antigen, they give rise to not only CD4 helper T cells (Th-1 and TH-2), but also cytotoxic CD4 effectors (Sallusto 2004). As far as the response to a growing tumor is concerned, the Tcm cells can present a problem with autoimmunity because they need low-level stimulation to exist in the body. To a certain extent, it's not usually a problem because antigens related to the tumor are readily available and expressed on the normal cells that the tumor was derived from. This expansion of memory T cells does not a priori result in cancer-induced autoimmunity because it's a simple expansion phase that has more to do with increasing numbers than it does with generating effector T cells. However in some instances, such as in cases of melanoma-induced vitiligo where normal melanocytes specifically express melanoma tumor antigens, an effector T cell response is generated. The reason for this has to do with the fact that several immunogenic melanoma-specific peptide antigens recognized by responding T cells such as gp100 are expressed in an identical form on normal melanocytes. In this case, CTL are generated and this results in the destruction of melanocytes and causes the pathology of melanoma-induced vitiligo (Byrne 2011). The creation of these two types of memory T cells is a very important aspect of not only the response to a tumor, but also T cell responses to viruses and pathogens depend heavily on generation both types (Tem and Tcm) of memory T cells.

Signal Transduction and CD4 Memory T cells

One thing that is important to understand about memory T cells is the fact that they have the ability, unlike naïve T cells; to respond rapidly to the reoccurrence of whatever antigen their TCRs are specific for. After sustained antigen stimulation, naïve CD4 T cells begin to secrete not only IL-2, but also INF-γ, which as discussed earlier, can increase the expression of MHC-class II proteins on APC and tumor cells and thereby increase the ability of these cells to present antigens (Alexander 1989 and Guerry 1987). This activity by naïve T cells is regulated by the T-bet transcription factor, which induces INF-γ production by binding to the INF-γ promoter. However, memory CD4 T cells have the ability to immediately secrete INF-γ upon contact with the target antigen. This pathway to INF-γ secretion turns out to have nothing to do with T-bet expression or it's ability to bind to the INF-γ promoter, but has to do with a member of the NF-kB family of transcription factors. NF-kB has been discussed earlier when talking about the translational pathways associated with antigen-specific TCR activation of T cells. Its been known for quite some time that NF-kB controlled T cell signaling associated with antigen specific activation (Hayden 2008), but recently it was determined that the P50 subunit of NF-kB was responsible for this rapid INF-γ secretion of the memory CD4 T cells by binding directly to the INF-γ promoter (Lai 2011).

One of the areas of interest mentioned in the beginning of this section had to do with signal transduction events associated with the development of defective T cell memory responses. As mentioned previously, expansion of naïve CD4 T cells results in the formation terminal effector cells (Teff), effector memory T cells (Tem) or central memory precursor T cells that eventually become long-lasting central memory T cells (Tcm). Naïve T cells decide on what path to follow first based on the strength and duration of TCR signals it receives, which leads to the development of Tem. Central memory T cells are created as central memory precursors enter the lymphatic system such as lymph nodes and are exposed to weak MHC-class II signals. This division of labor, which also involves exposure to lymphokines as mentioned above is similar to the fate of CD8 memory T cells (Pepper 2011). It has been known for some time now that T cell proliferation is controlled by the kinase activity of cyclin-dependent kinase (CDK) complexes, but that the activity of these CDK complexes are inhibited by cyclin-dependent inhibitors called CDKIs. One of these inhibitors called p27kip1 when activated interrupts the S and G2/M phase of the cell cycle and induces cell quiescence (Sherr 1999). However, recently it was discovered that p27kip1, which can control T cell differentiation, migration, and apoptosis could degrade the CD4 memory precursor T cell pool during an immune response. Over expression of p27kip during an immune response not only inhibits program that controls the differentiation of the CD4 precursor memory pool, but in the process of inducing apoptosis in CD4 Teff effectors, which under steady-state conditions is a normal process, the long term T cell memory or Tcm get reduced in numbers (Jatzek 2012).

This is an important finding regarding the anti-tumor T cell response because if the pool of CD4 Tcm gets reduced during the process of the T cell immune response to the tumor, a recurrence of the disease is sure to follow. Earlier it was shown that often during the growth of primary tumor inflammatory conditions are created. This inflammatory reaction included the secretion of IL-6 and in conjunction with secreted TGF-β Tregs are created. In addition, it was also shown that IL-6 is not only secreted by lymphocytes (DC and T cells), but also by a wide variety of tumor cells and in fact can induce a CSC-like state in tumor cells through the JAK-1/STAT3 signal transduction pathway (Ahmad 2008). In contrast to these findings, it was shown that IL-6 could induce senescence by inducing G1 arrest in tumor cells through the specific induction of p27kip1 (Mori 1999). In addition, IL-6 also has the ability to arrest the G1 phase of the cell cycle in T cells that are exposed to *H. Pylori*, which again is due to the up regulation of p27kip1 (Schmees 2005). It is highly likely that the pathway involved with IL-6 and cell cycle arrest involves the Janus-Activated Kinase (JAK)/STAT3 pathway induced by the phosphorylation of the IL-6 receptor.

The interesting thing about this is that there are 3 forms of JAK (JAK-1, JAK-2, and JAK-3) and all three forms in conjunction with STAT3 induce increased proliferation of the cells. Another interesting aspect is the fact that inhibition of the JAK-3/STAT3 pathway in colon carcinoma cells induces not only cell cycle arrest, but also apoptosis and the specific up regulation of p27kip1 (Lin 2005). Therefore, if the IL-6/STAT3 pathway is involved with the up regulation of p27kip1 and T cell quiescence in the example above, somewhere along this pathway STAT3 is inhibited or only allowed to activate p27kip1 alone. One possibility is the activation of protein tyrosine phosphatases such as PTPN2, which have been shown in T cells to specifically inhibit the Janus kinases JAK1, JAK2, and JAK3 because they are substrates of these protein tyrosine phosphatases (Simoncic 2002). Therefore, inhibition of these JAK substrates by PTPN2 would diminish STAT3 activation and allow p27kip1 to induce senescence in T cells. In support of the fact that diminished expression of STAT3 promotes T cell senescence, it was found that patients with autosomal dominant hyper-IgE syndrome posses a dominant negative STAT3 mutation that makes them susceptible to bacterial and fungal infections. It was determined that these patients had significantly lower numbers of CD4 and CD8 Tcm when compared to healthy control subjects (Siegel 2011).

This supports the possibility that the inhibition of JAK by PTPN2 and the subsequent reduction of STAT3 can lead to the upregulation of p27kip1 and the consequent reduction of the T cell memory pool. However, despite the fact that the exact IL-6 to p27kip1 pathway is unknown at the present time, this ability of p27kip1to degrade memory T cells is not a good situation for the anti-tumor T cell response. There is another curious caveat to this situation and it has to do with the cancer-induced autoimmune response to melanocytes, namely vitiligo. It was determined that melanoma-induced vitiligo was due to the presence and maintenance of CD8 effector memory T cells (Tem) that were circulating in the peripheral blood of melanoma patients with vitiligo and those that did not have the autoimmune disease only had circulating Tcm (Byrne 2011). This, in addition to the fact that a diagnosis of vitiligo in a melanoma patient is a positive prognostic factor (Uchi 2006), would lead one to believe that in fact, this reduction in the CD4 or CD8 memory precursor pool does happen.

There is a high probability that this happens in most cases since a minority, but not the majority of cancer patients are affected by chronic cancer-induced autoimmune reactions such as vitiligo, which would indicate the loss of the Tem population of memory T cells.

Signal Transduction and CD8 Memory T cells

The activation of naïve CD4 T cells and the development of memory T cells, their subsequent ability to rapidly respond to recall antigens, whether they be bacteria, viral, or tumor antigens is the first step in the memory T cell response. The re-activation of memory CD4 T cells leads to an effector stage and this is where CD8 T cells come in. Proliferation of CD8 T cells by antigen and INF-γ/IL-2 secreted by memory CD4 T cells results in the generation of two distinct populations of CD8 T cells. First there are the short-lived effector cells (SLECs) that become terminally differentiated and once they clear the system of the treat, undergo apoptosis and disappear. The other population is the memory precursor effector cells or MPECs. These cells give rise to a persistent and long-lived population of self-renewing memory T cells (Tem) that when called upon rapidly become cytotoxic CD8 effector cells. Understanding the transcriptional pathways that are involved in their development and activation is essential to the development of immune-based therapies. The reason for this is that the goal of these therapies is not only to re-direct the immune system to remove the treat (viral or tumor), but also leave behind active memory effector cells to guard against recurrences of the disease.

As discussed earlier, activation of the P13K/Akt pathway in tumor cells and embryonic stem cells was associated with cell survival, which allowed tumor cells to become resistant to cell death (Hemon 2011) and embryonic stem cells to proliferate in response to fibronectin (Park 2011). In addition, activation of MAP kinase family member JNK led to increased tumorgenicity by first activating Akt and PDK1, which in turn phosphorylated PKC (Lopez-Bergami 2010). In terms of the regulation and differentiation of CD8 SLECs and MPECs, the P13K/Akt pathway is at the center of a complex series of signal transduction pathways that are initiated as a consequence of the activation of this pathway. Some of this was covered earlier when discussing T cell activation, but it begins with TCR, CD28, and lymphokine receptor engagement at the T cell surface. Once P13K is activated by receptor tyrosine kinase (RTK) signals via engagement of these receptors, phoshytidylinositol-4, 5-bisphosphate (PIP2) is phosphorylated to generate phoshytidylinositol-3, 4, 5-triphosphate (PIP3). PIP3 then interacts with pleckstrin homology (PH) domains on the proteins Akt and phosphoinositide-dependent protein kinase (PDK1).

PDK1 and the mammalian target of rapamycin (mTOR) complex 2 (mTORC2) must further phosphorylate Akt in order for it to travel into the cytoplasm and eventually to the nucleus. At both of these locations Akt can interact with transcriptional pathways that influence CD8 metabolism by turning it off or on. Akt can also interact with transcriptional regulators that control cell quiescence (dormancy), which is important for MPECs long-term existence. As Akt enters the cytoplasm it is phosphorylated again and then sets off a series of events that activate mTORC1. The mTORC1 transcription factor positively or negatively regulates protein synthesis, cell metabolism and growth, all of which are essential for SLECs function or the MPECs quiescence state. As far as the dormancy state of CD8 memory T cells is concerned, this happens as Akt enters the nucleus and phosphorylates the forkhead box O or FOXO transcription factors, which inhibit them from entering the nucleus and activating target genes associated with proliferation, apoptosis, motility, and metabolism (Kim 2013a). In other words the action of Akt inhibits these processes allowing memory CD8 cells to exist in a steady state for an extended period of time.

Transcriptional Regulation of Tregs and Its Impact on Autoimmunity

As mentioned in the earlier section of this chapter that had to do with Tregs and autoimmunity, the current thinking about the source of many autoimmune disorders focus on the inability of Tregs to control autoimmune T cell responses. There are three Treg-associated conditions that can lead to autoimmunity by the dysfunction of Tregs. Those are insufficient numbers of Tregs at the site of an inflammatory response, defective Treg function, and the resistance of autoantigen-specific T cells to inhibition by Tregs (Buckner 2010). Normally, Tregs interfere with autoimmune T cells (CD4 and CD8 responder/effector T cells) through a variety of mechanisms prior to their contact with normal cells. Since resistance to Treg interference is related to Treg effector mechanisms, this topic will not be covered in this section, but in the next chapter, which is about the translational immunology of how Tregs inhibit autoimmune T cell responses. This section will describe in detail the translational pathways involved or potentially involve with the failure of Tregs to respond to autoimmune T cell responses.

Transcriptional Pathways That Lead to Diminished Numbers of Tregs

The first Treg-associated condition that can lead to autoimmunity is related to the number of Tregs at any given site where autoantigen responsive T cells mount an attack on normal tissues. This was discussed earlier when it was mentioned that a system-wide expansion of anti-melanocyte CTL occurred (Lili 2012) in patients with generalized vitiligo, thus reducing the ratio of Treg to autoimmune CTL. Another mechanism that results in fewer numbers of Tregs has to do with the high affinity IL-2 receptor (IL-2R) these cells express (Cheng 2011). Once IL-2 engages this high affinity receptor, a series of transcriptional events gets initiated that result in the activation and expression of the FOXP3 gene. It begins with the phosphorylation of tyrosine kinases Janus kinase 1 (JAK-1) and JAK-3, which is followed by the phosphorylation of tyrosine residues on the IL-2R ß-chain. This results in the phosphorylation of STAT5 and Shc, which leads to continual FOXP3 expression. This series of events is regulated by protein tyrosine phosphatases such as protein tyrosine phosphatase N2 (PTPN2) that can control the strength and duration of this IL-2/IL-R pathway (Simoncic 2002).

In human type-1 diabetes it was found that patients had a decreased responsiveness to IL-2 in both innate and adaptive Tregs. Despite the fact that the absolute numbers of Tregs in the periphery of normal controls and diabetic patients was the same, this is a situation where a limited number of functional Tregs results in the development of an autoimmune disease. The reasons for this is that the IL-2 Tregs respond to is secreted by T cells at the site of inflammation, which in this case would be the pancreas where ß-islet cells are inflamed. Because the Tregs of these patients are unable to expand in response to IL-2, which means continual expression of FOXP3, their numbers are reduced at the inflammatory site. It was found that diabetic patients displayed a decrease in the expression of phosphorylated STAT5 (pSTAT5) in response to IL-2. This reduced expression of pSTAT5 was found to be associated with increased levels of PTPN2, which is consistent with the role of protein tyrosine phosphatases to inhibit signal transducer and activator of transcription factors (STATs) phosphorylation (Simoncic 2002). Reduced expression of pSTAT5 results in the inability of the IL-2R ß-chain to respond to IL-2 secreted by T cells at the site of inflammation. This decrease in IL-2 responsiveness was also detected in CD4 cells of diabetic patients and may be associated with genetic factors (Long 2010). It was recently discovered that many of these patients have a single nucleotide polymorphism (SNP) in a gene that encodes PTPN2 and is called PTPN2rs1893217. It is called a "risk" allele because of its association with the disease. However in this case, the presence of this PTPN2 SNP causes a reduction in both PTPN2 expression and pSTAT5, but with the same result, that being non-responsiveness to IL-2 by Tregs during the inflammatory response in the pancreas. This is in contrast to what was found above where an increase in PTPN2 expression and a decrease in pSTAT5 led to the autoimmune pathology of the disease. This is an indication that the role of PTPN2 in regulating IL-2 responsiveness is complex. It also points to the possibility that multiple intercellular transduction pathways are affected by these protein tyrosine phosphatases (Long 2011).

Transcriptional Pathways That Control Treg Function

The second Treg condition that can lead to autoimmune disease is a functional defect in the ability of Tregs to control autoimmune T cell responses. As far as the functional capabilities of Tregs are concerned, most of it is controlled by the FOXO transcription factors. In general, this family of transcription factors controls a vast array of cellular processes, is distributed in wide variety tissues, and can control or is involved with multiple translational functions (Monsalve 2011). There are four members of the FOXO family of transcription factors and they are FOXO1, FOXO3, FOXO4, and FOXO6. FOXO4 is expressed throughout the cells of the body and FOXO6 expression is limited to the nervous system and like FOXO1 and FOXO3, they target genes in the nucleus that inhibit cell cycle entry and can induce apoptosis. T cells express FOXO1 and FOXO3, which play a major role in the control of T cell homeostasis, but as far as Tregs are concerned the FOXO transcription factors have control over the expression of the FOXP3 gene (Hendrick 2012).

Most of this happens in the thymus as FOXO1 and FOXO3 transcription factors in concert with cRel bind to the FOX3 promoter and induces the expression of FOXP3 in T cells selected in the thymus to become Tregs. The conversion of either naïve or antigen-specific T cells into Tregs does not require cell division and a part of the conversion process demands, through the activation of the MAPK/P38 pathway, that cell division does not occur (Huber 2008). During the proliferative phase of the T cell response to antigen, cyclin-dependent kinases (CDKs) control cell-cycle entry and cell division (Sherr 1999), but in adaptive Tregs proliferation is inhibited by activation of the MAPK/P38 pathway and the upregulation the of cyclin-dependent kinase inhibitors (CDKIs) such as P27kip1 (Adler 2008). P27kip1 also has the ability to T cell induce senescence, which is an essential cellular state associated with the long-lasting T cell memory pool. However, over expression of P27kip1 can diminish numbers of memory T cells through apoptosis (Jatzek 2012). This can occur as a direct result of the continual activation of the P13/Akt transduction pathway because of what Akt does to intercellular FOXO3 (Kim 2013a). FOXO3 not only induces the expression of FOXP3 in concert with cRel during thymic differentiation, but also plays a role in the conversion of peripheral T cells into adaptive Tregs. In order to induce a state of non-proliferation during the conversion process, FOXO3 positively controls the expression of CDKIs P15, P19, P21, as well as P27kip1 (Hendrick 2012).

Once these CDKIs are activated cell division ceases, FOXP3 expression occurs, and adaptive Tregs are created. However, Akt has the ability to phosphorylate FOXO3, which prevents it from entering the nucleus; thus preventing not only the creation of adaptive Tregs, but also diminishing the expression of FOXP3 in already established Tregs. Apparently, this Treg reducing activity of the P13K/Akt pathway is the result of hyperactivation of the pathway through the combined ligation of the TCR, CD28, and the IL-2R and can play a role in converting Tregs into autoimmune effector cells. This process results in the reverse-conversion of Tregs back to their original state (autoimmune effector cells) before TGF-β and IL-2 converted them into Tregs. However, because FOXO3 cannot enter the nucleus and induce the expression of CDKIs, which would halt cell cycle entry, Treg proliferation can be induced by Akt activation of mTORC1. In situations where just the TCR and the IL-2 receptor are engaged a lower level of P13K activation is induced by specific receptor tyrosine kinase (RTK) signals from this interaction that lead to Treg proliferation and continued maintenance of the Treg phenotype (Soond 2012). As P13K is activated by this receptor combination (TCR and IL-2R) it results in the limited phosphorylation of Akt (pAkt) by PDK1 and mTORC2. However, this amount of pAkt is enough to inhibit the tuberous sclerosis complex (TSC1/2), which is an inhibitor of mTORC1.

mTORC1 activation leads increased cell growth, protein synthesis, and cell metabolism (Laplante 2012). However, there is not enough pAkt to phosphorylate FOXO3 and prevent it from inducing and maintaining FOXP3 expression. Despite the fact that FOXO3 still has the ability to induce T cell senescence by its control of CDKIs, there is T cell proliferation because the growth signals provided by mTORC1 probably override the ability of the CDKIs activated by FOXO to inhibit cell cycle entry. In fact it has been shown that partial phosphorylation of Akt at Ser473 was a characteristic of the state of the P13K/Akt pathway in Tregs. In order for Akt to be fully active (able to phosphorylate FOXO3) it must be phosphorylated at not only Ser473, but also at Thr308. Despite the fact that this condition can be reproduced as above (TCR, CD28, and IL2-R ligation) in both Tregs and normal T cells, Tregs normally only express the partially phosphorylated version (Ser473) of Akt. Forced expression of fully phosphorylated Akt in Tregs results in the reversal of their suppressive activity (Crelin 2007). In addition, it was also determined that continual stimulation of the TCR in this situation leads to a significant decrease in FOXP3 gene expression. This is because during continual TCR stimulation there is the loss of permissive histone modifications found in the 5′ untranslated region (UTR) of the FOXP3 gene, which are characteristic markers for FOXP3 gene expression. In contrast to this situation, where there is little or intermittent TCR engagement, this leads to continual FOXP3 expression and supports the role of limited Akt phosphorylation in maintaining the Treg phenotype (Sauer 2008). The intermittent engagement of the Treg TCR is how Tregs keep in contact with the cells they are protecting and therefore is a mechanism designed to support their continued maintenance at inflammatory sites. The type of continual stimulation that involves the Tregs three most important receptors (TCR, CD28, and high-affinity IL-2R) can lead to functional failure of their ability to control autoimmune T cell responses and as mentioned above, Tregs may be transformed or converted back into the very autoimmune T cells they were attacking. Therefore, this type of situation can lead to the functional inability of Tregs to control autoimmune T cell responses because the Tregs lose their effector functions during the proliferative transition period when Tregs are being converted back into autoimmune effector cells.

Transcriptional Pathways That Control T Cell Anergy As It Relates to Autoimmunity and the Anti-tumor T Cell Response

The basic concept of T cell anergy and autoimmunity was born out of the laboratories of the influential immunologist Charles Janeway. In combination with the work of other scientist, Charles Janeway was able to theorize and prove the "second signal" requirement for T cell activation (Gayed 2011). Janeway theorized that their had to be a second signal associated with the T cell response because in many cases where T cells responded to microbial pathogens, an adjuvant-like substance such as lipopolysaccharide (LPS) had to be added to achieve antigen-specific T cell proliferation (Janeway 1989). Then there was his discovery of the role that APC-expressed CD80 (B7.1) and CD86 (B7.2) played in providing that crucial second signal in order to activate T cells through the TCR (Wong 1995). The reason why this "second signal" hypothesis is so important is that it has direct implications concerning the fate of autoreactive T cells. In order for successful T cell activation and proliferation to antigen to occur not only does the TCR have to be engaged with a peptide antigen presented in the context of MHC-classI/II on the APC, but also the CD28 receptor on the T cell must interact with its ligand CD80/86 (B7.1 and B7.2) on the APC.

However, prior to the knowledge of these CD28 ligands it was discovered that when T cells responded to antigen (Cytochrome C) presented by APC that were treated with a cell membrane cross-linker (1-ethyl-3-(3-dimethylaminopropyl)-carbodiimide) or ECDI they became anergic to further stimulation for a finite period of time (Schwartz 1987). In effect, what the cross-linker did was destroy the ability of the CD80/86 molecules of the APC to make contact with the T cell CD28 receptor. It was later determined that T cell anergy could be induced using immobilized anti-TCR antibodies (anti-CD3) without the second signal, which in this case were anti-CD28 antibodies. The use of these two antibodies together resulted in those T cells being responsive to antigenic challenge, unlike the anergy induced by using the anti-TCR antibody alone (Jenkins 1990).

This finding led to the hypothesis that this was yet another way the immune system was able to eliminate self-reactive autoimmune cells by causing them to become anergic after encountering autoantigens expressed by normal cells, which do not normally express the APC ligands CD80/86. This is a basic fundamental function of the T cell immune system that not only has implications related to autoimmunity, but also the T cell response to tumors where T cells and especially CD4 helper T cells are rendered anergic by the presence of immature DC that express diminished amounts of CD80/86. As previously mentioned, this very thing occurs as T cell or Treg expressed LAG comes in contact with MHC-class II molecules of DC and activate the ITAM inhibitory process during the anti-tumor T cell response (Liang 2008). However, the induction or creation of T cell anergy in the context of autoimmunity is very important not only from the standpoint of inducing anergy in autoreactive T cells, but also critically important for the function of Tregs that prevent unwanted autoimmune T cell responses. During this discussion of translational events that control the anti-tumor T cell response and Treg control of autoimmunity it was mentioned that in order for Tregs to function properly, cell division had to be halted, except during their expansion phase. For all intents and purposes Tregs are anergic T cells, which display many, but not all of the characteristics of anergic T cells (Li 2005). These characteristics of Treg anergy will be discussed in detail later, but now the transcriptional pathways involved with the establishment of peripheral T cell anergy will be described.

Transcriptional Pathways Associated with TCR-Only Interactions That Induce Anergy

There are three major transcriptional pathways involved with the two-signal (TCR and CD28) successful activation of T cells. Some of this was discussed during the description of T cell activation through the TCR in the previous chapter and in this chapter when discussing P13K activation leading to Akt phosphorylation. Again, all of this begins with the general signal induced in lipid rafts caused by receptor tyrosine kinase (RTK) signals due to the engagement of both the TCR and CD28. There are three transcriptional activators that enter the nucleus as a result of the RTK signals that cooperate in the successful activation of T cells to this two-signal stimulus. They are the nuclear factor of activated T cells (NFAT), activator protein one (AP1), and nuclear factor *kappa B* (NFkB). Through the RTK signals an important series of events occurs at the cell membrane. As discussed previously phospholipase C (PLC) is recruited and hydrolyses the PIP2, which forms diacylglycerol (DAG) and cytoplasmic IP3. The creation of DAG is important because it controls the activation of downstream pathways toward the activation of AP-1, NFkB, and Akt. These three nuclear transcriptional factors can rapidly enter the nucleus with NFAT to induce T cell activation. The previously mentioned P13k signals from the ligation of CD28 assist the activation of NFkB. During the one-signal stimulus (TCR-only) NFAT production is an essential step in the production of anergic T cells. However, with regards to the induction of T cell anergy the most important player in its creation is the activity of diacylglycerol kinases or DGKs. These kinases can catalyze (phosphorylate) DAG into phosphatidic acid (PA) or prevent phosphorylation, which is dependent detection of the second-signal contribution by the interaction of CD28 with the CD80/86 (B7) ligand on the APC. This activity by DGKs either terminates the control of downstream events that lead to T cell activation or promotes them. DGKs are complex enzymes that have ten isoforms. These enzymes are very important to the one-signal/two-signal fate of the T cell response because they cannot only increase the ability of DAG to induce the three (AP-1, NFkB, and Akt) nuclear transcription factors that lead to T cell activation, but can also diminish their expression by converting (phosphorylation) DAG into PA (Joshi 2013). There are two critical pathways involved with the induction of T cell anergy. The first is the induction or inhibition of AP-1 expression. DAG controls AP-1 by activating RasGRP1. This promotes activation of Ras, which leads to the activation of the Raf1-Mek1/2-Erk1/2 pathway that leads to the activation of AP-1. NFAT is activated by the hydrolization by PLC of PIP2 into IP3 and DAG. DAG goes on to activate the pathways mentioned above while IP3 induces Ca++ influx that leads to the activation of calcineurin. Calcineurin dephosphorylates NFAT, which allows it to enter the nucleus. If DAG activation of AP-1 is successful, then NFAT forms a complex with AP-1 and in conjunction NFkB induces the cascade of events that lead to T cell activation. However, if two of the DGK isoforms are activated to suppress the ability of DAG to induce AP-1 by converting it into PA, NFAT can enter the nucleus and begin to induce genes that promote T cell anergy such as those two DGK isoforms (Zhong 2008). Not only does NFAT control the expression of DGK genes, but it also induces the expression of over 100 other genes directly responsible for long-lasting T cell anergy (Baine 2009).

Transduction Pathways That Sustain the Anergic State

The induction of T cell anergy is not a fleeting condition that last for a brief moment in time, but a persistent state that can last for an extended period. It is of interest to understand the molecular pathways that contribute to this persistent state of anergy. While these T cells are incapable of responding to antigen, the entire immune system is compromised. The reason why the T cell immune system is compromised has to do with the nature of the TCR. This is the most important cellular receptor possessed by the body because without it, there simply would be no immunity. Life as we know it cannot exist without the ability of the body to defend itself. As immunologists know, this receptor possessed by T cells is controlled by the expression of series genes. These TCR genes are complex and have both inherited and adaptive qualities that allow T cells to respond to antigens that are both coded for within the gene pool and many that are not. The recognition of antigenic peptides that are not coded for in the genetic make-up of the TCR are recognized through an adaptive process that involves somatic (real-time) mutations of the TCR genes. These mutations are a result of rapid multiplication of the T cell as it becomes activated by an immunological threat. What happens is that as the cells divide, the DNA associated with the TCR gets rearranged. Some of these rearrangements result in recognition of the specific immunological threat. Once this recognition occurs this sub-population of T cells expands, destroys the invader (viral, bacterial, or cancer), forms a memory pool, and then contracts back to a minor sub-population.

The reason this process is vitally important is that it can also work against the body in the form of autoimmune responses. These TCR genetic rearrangements or somatic mutations can lead to the recognition of self-peptides. This recognition in combination with the expression of CD80/86 by the target cell can result in the development of autoimmune diseases that have been mentioned in this section. The events that lead to this type a abhorrent T cell behavior are collectively called TCR ‘promiscuity.’ These types of T cell responses have to do with the fact that the TCR can have and sometimes must have, dual specificity. So in other words, there are clones of T cells that are specific for several antigens. Some of these antigenic peptides are structurally related on the amino acid level, but some are not. An example of this TCR duality is related to the autoimmune response to β-cell specific T cell responses. There are two peptide antigens recognized by a single clone of T cells and this recognition results in the destruction of β–islet cells and the pathology of type-1 diabetes (Li Li 2008). With this in mind it is now possible to understand how T cell anergy, either induced by autoantigens, or tumor cells can reduce responses to unrelated antigens. This is one of the reasons why many cancer patients are prone to simple bacteria or viral infections. Latent viruses such as herpes zoster (shingles) and other are a particular problem because they lay dormant and are held at bay by the T cell immune system. Once that system suffers from anergy there is more of a 'global' problem as far as the body is concerned.

So, here we are with these anergic T cells that now cannot respond to their specific peptide antigen and languish helplessly in the peripheral blood system. The question is why do they stay helpless for so long and what is their fate? The why has been determined because there are molecular pathways that basically sustain their non-responsiveness, but their fate in the long-term is uncertain. There are a series of transcriptional factors associated with the maintenance of the T cell anergy. These T cells have succumbed to either single-signal contact with autoantigens or have had contact with altered tumor cells. There is a family of transcription factors called E3 ligases such as GRAIL, Cb1-b, and Itch. These ligases have the ability to unbiquinate or destroy phospholipases that are essential for T cell activation. The gene related to anergy in lymphocytes or GRAIL is one of these E3 ligases that can degrade (unbiquinate) the TCR-CD3 complex and thereby promotes continued T cell anergy. However, it was determined that deletion of the gene that encoded for GRAIL resulted in wide spread T cell activation and a complete inability of Tregs to control it. In other words, GRAIL contributes to normal T cell functions by controlling T cell expression of the TCR-CD3 complex on a constant basis (Nurieva 2010). This is only one of the transcriptional regulators of the T cell anergy. Another important addition would be the transcriptional factors derived from the early growth response or Egr gene complex.

These are zinc finger transcription factors called Erg-2 and Egr-3. They are involved with several pathways discussed such as mTOR, MAP kinases, and most importantly NFAT. These two transcription factors are important as far the anti-tumor T cell response is concerned. Their detection in tumor-induced anergic T cell populations demonstrates that Erg-2 and Egr-3 play a role not only in the maintenance of anergy, but also the appearance of an autoimmune response (Safford 2005). However, there's an interesting interaction with Erg-2 and diacylglycerol kinases or DGK's, which as previously mentioned are important. DGKs control the induction of anergy by converting DAG into PA and thereby prevent DAG from activating RasGRP1, which leads to the activation of AP-1 that promotes T cell activation. There are two DGK isoforms (alpha and zeta) that can perform this function. Recently it was determined that there was a binding site for Erg-2 within the promoter of the alpha isoform of DGK. During TCR engagement in the absence of co-stimulation (one-signal) Erg-2 bound to the DGK promoter and increased its transcription and thereby allowing this isoform to prevent DAG from activating RasGRP1. If Erg-2 was deleted from T cells it was found that DGK levels were decreased as well as the ability of these T cells to become anergic in the absence of co-stimulation (Zheng 2012).

These translational events that perpetuate the anergic state of T cells, at first glance seem to be harmful to the normal functioning of the T cell immune system. As mentioned above, anergy-induction and maintenance can make the body susceptible to continued infection by not only pathogens (bacteria and viruses) that are introduced from outside of the body, but also latent viruses that were held at bay by the T cell immune system that is now compromised. However, despite this apparent disadvantage, the induction of a state of anergy in T cells is a vital function of the immune system because without it many of the T cells that would have become anergic due to contact with self-antigens would respond to those antigens and become autoimmune T cells. As mentioned in the beginning of this section, another vital aspect of the induction of anergy has to do with Treg immunobiology and how Tregs themselves are anergic T cells. One of the most fascinating aspects of this situation is that Tregs can induce T cell anergy in autoimmune T cells. This is related to Treg effector mechanisms, which is a separate topic that will be covered in the next chapter. Now the focus will be on the nature of the type of T cell anergic state Tregs are in because there are some differences between the normal T cell anergic state and the one that Tregs are in.

First of all there is a constant and continual transcription of cyclin-dependent kinase inhibitors or CDKIs. These inhibitors restrain cyclin-dependent kinase (CDK) complexes such as cyclin A and cyclin E. These CDK complexes control the entry of T cells into the S and G2/M phase of the cell cycle. As previously mentioned, one of those CDKIs is called p27Kip1 (Sherr 1999). It was determined the one of the characteristics of Tregs is constant presence of p27Kip1 throughout the life cycle of these cells (Li 2005). This process inhibits one of the familiar pathways to T cell activation, which is DAG to RasGRP1 that leads to AP1/NFAT activation. However, this inhibition of Treg activation, can be overcome by IL-2 because of how the activation of the high-affinity IL-2 receptor, which can diminish p13K expression (Simoncic 2002) and allow a limited amount of Akt to activate mTORC1. mTORC1 in turn overcomes the action of p27Kip1 and initiates Treg proliferation (Laplante 2012) by virtue if the fact that it is an upstream event. However, without the presence of IL-2, Tregs are prone to apoptosis (Li 2005).

Earlier, when the transcriptional regulation of T cells was discussed it was disclosed the NFAT that was not associated with AP1 was translocated to the nucleus where it activated multiple genes that regulated and sustained anergy (Baine 2009). NFAT association with AP1 and the subsequent induction of T cell proliferation is a part of the development of natural Tregs in the thymus because this process involves a burst of T cell proliferation in order to mobilize transcription factors such a cRel, which was discussed earlier, and its ability to bind to the promoter region of FOXP3 there-by inducing its expression in T cells in the thymus (Hori 2010b). However, the role of NFAT plays in the induction of adaptive Tregs is a complex one that involves the expression of FOXP3. Previously, during the discussion of the development of TH17 helper T cells and their ability to secrete IL-17A, it was determined that FOXP3 proteins and DNA interacted with protein products and DNA of the RORgt gene (Ichiyama 2008). It turns out that the FOXP3 transcription factors (gene products) function as DNA binding proteins that bind to specific DNA elements during the process of Treg development (thymus) and creation (adaptive). These DNA elements are called "enhancers" and their occupancy by FOXP3 transcription factors causes Treg-specific expression of proteins necessary to re-model a CD4+CD25- T cell into a CD4+CD25+ Treg cell. The binding of FOXP3 to these enhancers can also activate other transcription factors that bind to enhancer/promoter regions of genes specifically needed to construct the Treg phenotype. The enhancer elements that FOXP3 binds to pre-exist in CD4 T cells, but until called upon are occupied by FOXO1, which was mentioned earlier as playing a major role in the expression of FOXP3. ChIP-seq analysis revealed that in CD4+FOXP3- T cells FOXO1 was occupying the very sites that FOXP3 bound in Tregs and that FOXO1 binding to these sites in Tregs was diminished. The occupancy of these sites by FOXO1 is referred to as a "placeholder" effect. Both NFAT and AP1 contribute to FOXP3 during T cell proliferation prior to Treg development or creation by remodeling DNA in such a way as to allow FOXP3 transcription factors to bind with ease (Samstein 2012). However, there is another aspect of the role that NFAT plays in the establishment of the Treg phenotype and it has to do with the FOXP3 gene itself.

In Chapter I there was a discussion of how, during innate (thymic developed) Treg development, there was extensive remodeling (demethylation and acetylation) of a coding region within the FOXP3 gene called the Treg-specific demethylation region or TSDR (Huehn 2009). It was also mentioned that within the FOXP3 gene there was a promoter and two enhancer regions. The transcription factors that bind in this region are the TCR activation induced factors NFAT, AP1, Sp1, and STAT5 (FOXP3 promoter region), NFAT (TCR activation) and the TGF-β-induced SMAD complex (Enhancer 1). Proximal to the FOXP3 gene itself is Enhancer 2 where STAT5 and CREB-ATF bind (Boehmer 2008). CREB-ATF is a transcriptional activator that binds to a TGF-β-induced demethylated site in this enhancer region and actually drives the expression of the FOXP3 gene (Kim 2007). However, during the development of adaptive Tregs there is a characteristic histone acetylation pattern with in the enhancer 1 region, which is due to the specific binding of SMAD3 and NFAT. This process is essential as far as expression FOXP3 is concerned because inhibitors of SMAD3 and deletion of the NFAT gene in mice prevent its expression (Tone 2008). In addition, it was determined that a threshold level of NFAT is necessary for the induction of adaptive Tregs regardless of which of the four NFAT family members was present. Decreased NFAT activity did impair the TCG-B induction of FOXP3, but in mice that were deficient, but not devoid of NFAT were able to produce functional adaptive Tregs (Vaeth 2012). In a mouse model of melanoma it was determined that NFAT-deficient mice were not susceptible to tumor-induce CD4 T cell anergy (Abe 2012). Therefore, it is apparent that NFAT plays a role in not only the thymic development of Tregs by inducing T cell activation to self-antigens through the NFAT/AP1 pathway, but also NFAT actively induces FOXP3 gene expression. In addition, and as previously mentioned, NFAT has the ability to activate T cell anergy-related transcription factors such as DGK, which inhibits the RasGRP1 pathway to the activation of AP1. All of the translational pathways mentioned above contribute to the "anergic state" of the Treg. This is the condition where Tregs perform their primary function, which is to control autoimmune T cells. Obviously, during their proliferative phase Treg inhibition of T cell responses is momentarily decreased because during Treg activation both the calcineurin activation of NFAT is occurring, as well as the DAR induction of the RasGRp1, which leads to the activation of AP1. FOXP3 expression still exists, but during this burst of proliferation Tregs are momentarily non-functional. In fact, there is an inverse relationship between Treg proliferation and function (Singh 2012).

Importance of T Cell Regulation of Autoimmunity, the Anti-Tumor T Cell Response, and the Associated Translational Pathways

There are some very obvious observations one could make given the information provided during this chapter regarding autoimmunity, Tregs, and the anti-tumor T cell response. The first one is that during the formation of a tumor a series of complex biological events occur within the tumor that challenge the T cell immune system such as the appearance of neoantigens, which the system perceives as temporary inflammation. Tregs are called in to protect these cells under the expectation that at some point in time they will return to a normal state. Meanwhile, the surveillance arm of the cellular immune response, which includes NK cells as well as T cells, is held at bay by Tregs. Another aspect of autoimmunity has to do with inflammation and how inflammation can lead to the development of cancerous cells. Because of the natural ability of Tregs to protect inflamed cells from destruction by the T cell immune system, many times a cancer is formed through inflammation while being protected by Tregs. If left unprotected either NK cells or T cells would immediately destroy these inflamed cells. This is the function of the immunosurveillance arm of the cellular immune system. However, there has to be a balance. That balance being the difference between eliminating precancerous cells or the destruction of normal cells that have been insulted and become inflamed.

So there is this tenuous balance related to the recognition of self and non-self that the immune system must grapple with on a daily basis. However, there is an undeniable fact and that is autoimmune diseases are related in terms of susceptibility. For instance the situation with people who have generalized vitiligo and the fact that they are 20 times more predisposed to having separate autoimmune disease. These same people may develop SLE, IBD, or hyperthyroidism (Alkhateeb 2003). These seem to be totally separate autoimmune disorders that have no relation to one another. However, there is one commonality and that is the genetic basis of the development and function of Tregs. How Tregs function to inhibit the T cell response will be the topic of the next chapter, but up to this point it is apparent that the development of the Treg 'phenotype' involves a complex series of events. Each one of these events such as the conversion phase from naive CD4 T cells caused by TGF-β and IL-6 and the ability of the high-affinity IL-2 receptor to induce FOXP3 and other events associated with Treg development are based the genetic expression of the proteins involved in this process. Any mutations or genetic variations in these genes can result in the development of various forms of autoimmunity, which as above, seem to be totally unrelated. This is evidence that Tregs are apart of a generalized system of immune control and that they have the ability to induce homeostatic conditions within the entire immune system. Any slight genetic variations in the development or functional capabilities of Tregs can be disastrous for the body. This concept has been addressed previously during the discussions about the role Tregs play in pregnancy, diabetes, and cancer-induced autoimmunity.

It is now apparent that autoimmune diseases, cancer, inflammation, Tregs, anti-tumor T cells and the rest of the T cell immune system are related. As mentioned at the beginning of this section much of this 'relatedness' is reflected in the use of many of the same translational pathways in the cells mentioned above. For instance the cyclin-dependent kinase inhibitor (CDKI) p27kip1 is not only involved in the development of T cell memory (Jatzek 2012) and the 'anergic' state of the Treg (Adler 2008), but also IL-6-induced G1 arrest of tumor cells (Mori 1999). Another example of common translational pathways used in disparate cellular activity would be the activation of the P13/Akt pathway. This pathway is activated during increased tumor cell growth (Lopez-Bergami 2010), induction of tumor cell metastasis (Liu 2012), inhibition of DC maturation, which leads to adaptive Treg formation (Liang 2008), and CD8 T cell memory formation (Kim 2013a). There are but two examples of common translational pathways used by not immune cells, but also tumor cells. Regulation of autoimmunity by the Treg system (innate and adaptive) is the cornerstone of the immune system. Understanding the various translational pathways involved with the process of regulation can increase our ability regulate the Treg system and the entire immune system to treat cancer and autoimmune diseases. It was mentioned during the introduction that there was some redundancies in the transcriptional pathways in T cells, which means that if a particular pathway is not activated there is another that can be activated, which results in exactly the same cellular behavior.

Redundancy is a characteristic that complex biological systems have developed in order to deal with evolution or changes in the real-time environment. Since Tregs are the cornerstone of the entire immune system, the redundancy related to their development and function are far more sophisticated than any other immune cell, including the cells that Tregs target, which are antigen specific CD4, CD8, and immunosurveillance NK cells. From the data presented, it is obvious that the development and function of both types (innate and adaptive) of Tregs is complex. This complexity not only involves the signals in the thymus (innate) or the periphery (adaptive) that induce their development, but also the translational pathways that lead to the Treg 'phenotype.' Using computational analysis of the various transcriptional pathways that lead to the Treg phenotype, researchers discovered that these pathways, which were previously discussed, are layered upon themselves and if one was removed another would take is place. Amongst the multitudes of pathways that lead to Treg development the only genetic products that were essential to the establishment of the Treg 'signature' were the pathways induced by the expression of the FOXP3 gene and to a lesser extent NFAT because of its role in the induction of the 'anergy state' needed to maintain the Treg phenotype. Here, the main finding was that redundant pathways, which led to the development and function of Tregs were the result of a 'genetic switch' that was turned on as a result of the response to biological conditions that create Tregs (Fu 2012).

The next chapter will detail the effector function of Tregs. In order demonstrate how this redundancy in Treg immunobiology works, the next data that will be presented represents not only a preview of what's to come, but also show evidence of Treg redundancy in biological terms. For some time now it has been known that T cells and particularly CD8 CTL, use a series of redundant pathways that lead to INF-γ secretion. Many of these signal pathways are dependent on the strength of the TCR/CD28 signal that induces CD8 CTL precursors to become effector T cells (Nembrini 2006). It's now time to look at real-time evidence of Treg system redundancy. The effector CD4 and CD8 T cells that Tregs inhibit from functioning during either an autoimmune response or an anti-tumor response not only elaborate a plethora of cytokines, but also have the capability to kill target cells using the granulocytic system, which involves injecting perforins into their target. There will be detail about this later, but now it was found that Tregs have a more extensive arsenal of weapons than your average effector T cell. Effector T cells are susceptible to inhibition by inhibitors of the P13K/Akt pathway, which makes sense because this pathway controls multiple T cell functions such as activation, memory formation, and CD4 and CD8 precursor maturation. The inhibitors of translational pathways in T cells and especially Tregs are the topic of the last chapter of this book. Some of the inhibitory capabilities of Tregs are still unknown. One of them is quite amazing because when Tregs are activated they can be formalized, which renders the cell metabolically inactive. It was found that these 'inactive' Tregs could still inhibit T cell responses (Hagness 2012). Obviously, this is a cell-to-cell contact phenomenon, but the fact these cells, which are for all intents and purposes are dead, can still function as anti-T cell effectors is amazing. The redundancy part of this has to do with the fact that Tregs are impervious to CTL inhibitors because they have multiple effector mechanisms that allow them to control T cell responses in a way that completely shuts them down.

It is apparent from examining the information in this second chapter about autoimmunity, Tregs, and the anti-tumor T cell immune system that these three elements work together as far as the T cell response to self and cancer is concerned. However, one of the most interesting and encompassing activities is inflammation. If one thinks about how those three elements are related, inflammation is a unifying force. Many of the autoimmune responses in the body where the T cell immune system responds and also engenders the involvement of Tregs are a result of inflammation. A familiar example would be the response to inflamed pancreatic islet cells after steroid treatments and the subsequent inability of Tregs to prevent their destruction by autoimmune T cells and in some cases immunosurveillance NK cells. In this chapter and the previous one, there were discussions of how inflammation could lead to cancer formation, and how cancer cells created inflammatory conditions at the tumor site, respectively. Tregs are actually intimately involved in these two situations. In the first case where inflammation leads to cancer, the inflamed cells escape destruction via the T cell immune system by Tregs prior to and during the tumorgenesis process. This stands to reason because this is the job of Tregs, which is to protect inflamed cells until they return back to a normal state. Unfortunately, Tregs do not know the cells are becoming cancerous because they are not designed to do so. The second situation where cancer induces inflammatory conditions at the tumor site, Tregs are actually drawn to the site by inflammatory cytokines released by inflammatory cells such as neutrophils and mast cells and in some cases normal surrounding tissue. Each cell mentioned in this paragraph has a distinct function in the cellular immune system. However, within those specific functions and the cells that perform them, lies a series of complex intercellular pathways that have the ability alter the functional capabilities of the cells involved in these processes.

This is the domain of intercellular translational pathways. As mentioned in both Chapter 1 and Chapter 2, these pathways control a cells behavior as it responds to its environment. Some of these pathways and the genes that produce their transduction elements (proteins) can define the character (phenotype) of the cell itself such as the case with Tregs and the FOXP3 gene's translational products. However, many of these pathways exist to provide specific functional information based on the cells interactions with other cells and soluble mediators such as cytokines and antibodies. Knowing how theses pathways control cellular behavior and particularly Treg cell behavior can be the basis of successful treatments for conditions such as autoimmune disease, graft vs. host disease (GVHD) recurrent pregnancy loss (RPL) and of course Treg interference with the anti-tumor T cell response. This knowledge can lead to immune manipulation by using agents that either enhance the effectiveness of translational pathways in Tregs or inhibit them. This will be the topic discussed in Chapter 4, but next in order fully understand how Tregs can be manipulated, their functional capabilities (ability to inhibit T cell responses) must be examined. The information and examination of Treg effector mechanisms in the next chapter will unfold exactly like the topics discussed in the previous chapters. An initial introduction will be followed by detailed descriptions of the cellular behaviors involved and then translational pathways related to these behaviors will be examined. The hope is that these three chapters will set the stage for an effective discussion of the clinical aspects of Treg manipulation.

Chapter 3

Treg Effector Mechanisms

Introduction

One of the reasons why this topic is important to this book called, *The Functional and Translational Immunology of Regulatory T cells (Tregs), the Anti-tumor T cell Response, and Cancer* is the fact Tregs can create balance in the cellular immune system by regulating T cell responses. However, they can cause immune imbalance in the form of autoimmune diseases such as diabetes and arthritis through defective Treg function. Of course another type of immune imbalance, which is due to the normal function of Tregs and is their positive involvement with not only tumor development during inflammation, but also protecting established tumors that have created inflammatory conditions at the tumor site. In Chapter 1 it was quite clear that without functioning Tregs (FOXP3 gene expression) the immune system is completely deregulated and the condition called IPEX or polyendocrinopathy enteropathy X-linked syndrome leads to rampant T cell-based autoimmunity in the form of lymphoid proliferation (enlarged lymphoid organs), organ-tissue destruction, infections, and ultimately death (Bennett 2001). In addition, without Tregs all pregnancies would result in a condition called, "spontaneous abortion" where the fetus is rejected by the T cell immune system that recognizes male and fetal antigens as foreign (Yin 2012). Tregs play an essential part in controlling (by Treg effector mechanisms) these harmful T cell responses. The importance of Tregs to the normal and sometimes abnormal functioning of the immune system depends on a wide variety of Treg effector mechanisms. Tregs have a much wider and sophisticated spectrum inhibitory mechanisms compared to the most advanced "killing machine" the immune system possesses, which is the CD8 CTL. Tregs cannot only kill other T cells and DC using several cell-to-cell contact mechanisms, but also can starve or paralyze their targets using multiple effector mechanisms at a distance. The reasons why Tregs have this wide spectrum of effector mechanisms is because the T cell immune responses that they have to control are composed of complex interactions between T cells, NK cells, and B-cells with a wide variety of abnormal (inflamed), cancerous, and pathogen/virus-infected cells. In addition, there are the pathogen/gut mucosal immune responses and most importantly the complex tolerance state of pregnancy.

The immune system is totally dependent on Tregs to control the T/NK cell immune system because that system is designed to defend the body from 'non-self' in the form of viruses, bacteria, other pathogenic organisms, and of course cancer. The T/NK immune system does this through immunosurveillance by the recognition of cellular membrane irregularities, which were discuss earlier. The main problem with this system is that it is very efficient at what it does and cannot differentiate between cell membrane irregularities caused either by simple inflammation, virus-infection or precancerous proteins. Once the T/NK system detects what it views as non-self, the results are swift and deadly. If left unregulated, T/NK cell responses like this result in not only cellular destruction, but also the secretion of massive amounts of cytokines, which as mentioned earlier is called a "cytokine storm." This event occurs when there is unbridled activation of T cells during septic shock, acute respiratory distress (ARD), GVHD, and influenza infection. However, there are only nine out of the scores of cytokines produced by T cells that induce this condition such as IL-1, IL-2, IL-10, INF-γ, and others that participate in the creation of the cytokine storm (Hao 2012). T and NK cells can kill target cells at an alarming rate and the results not only at a cellular level, but also at the population level, can be devastating. An example of this type of immune devastation of entire populations would be the 1918 flu pandemic.

In 1996 the Nobel Prize in Physiology or Medicine was awarded to two scientists (Peter Doherty and Rolf Zingernagel) from Australia for the discovery of how human leukocyte histocompatability antigens (HLA) play a major role in immunity. They described how cytotoxic T cells (CTLs) attacked and killed flu virus infected cells through the recognition of viral peptide antigen-HLA complexes on the surface of infected cells. However, there was also a suggestion that the millions of deaths during the 1918-1920 flu pandemic were not actually caused by the virus itself, but were the result of T cells attacking normal cells. The virus induced such a strong immune response that the T cells lost the ability to distinguish between self (HLA) and non-self (flu virus). Therefore, influenza activated T cells were attacking normal tissues, which resulted in over 100 million deaths. This reaction was very serious because at that time there were no effective vaccines (Doherty 2008). An autoimmune response of this type is supposed to be stopped Tregs, but because of the secretion of IL-6 during the infection many of them were probably reprogrammed into IL-17 effector cells, which contributed to this type of autoimmunity (Longhi 2008). Apparently, Tregs were either absent due to dwindling numbers, reprogramming, or genetically defective in the 100 million or so people who died during this pandemic. So in a sense, there was a genetic "hole" (no Treg resistance to Th17 reprogramming, an autoimmune T cell-generating genetic mutation in TCR, or defective Treg genes) in the T cell immune system that allowed this type of autoimmune reaction to occur. It is apparent that this "hole" was a genetic anomaly because millions of other people got the same flu virus during that period yet survived with the usual flu symptoms. The survivors did not have this hole or absence of a critical T cell population. It is feared that one day such an epidemic will happen again. Recently, immunologists have discovered that Tregs do indeed play an active role in the development of these "holes" that occur in the T cell immune system. What they found was that Tregs were responsible for keeping these "holes" from forming during periods of rapid T cell division because their role is to kill autoreactive T cells, which they were unable to do in this case. Without the presence of Tregs these holes are formed and the T cell immune system is uncontrolled leaving normal cells vulnerable to attack (Winstead 2010).

The reason why so much time was spent on the effects of an unregulated T cell immune system has to do with understanding why Tregs, unlike other effector T cells, have an extensive arsenal of effector mechanisms to control not only T cells, but also B cells, DC, and

NK cells. To a certain extent, the effector mechanisms chosen by Tregs to attack these cells is dictated by the situation they find themselves in. A Treg cell that comes upon T cells in the process of attacking normal cells will use an effector mechanism that is different from the one used when the Treg is guarding or attached to the target cell. In the first case, where Tregs arrive at an active T cell-based autoimmune attack, their tendency is to kill the autoreactive T cells using cell-to-cell contact effector mechanisms. However, in the second case where Tregs are already present, they tend to use soluble effector mechanisms that do not require cell-to-cell contact. The possible reason for this is if the Treg were attached to the target cell by its TCR, it would have to relinquish that contact to physically interact with the autoreactive T cell leaving the target cell vulnerable. In addition, and as previously discussed, in a tumor microenvironment Tregs have the ability to direct DC's to convert anti-tumor T cells into Tregs. This issue and several others related to Treg effector mechanisms will be discussed during this chapter. However, initially it would be pertinent to this discussion to have a somewhat detailed look at the two major effector mechanisms possessed by CD4 and CD8 effectors, which are the perforin/granzyme system and the FAS/FASL system. Tregs can activate not only these effector mechanisms, but also many others that allow them to control multiple immune responses. At the end of this section a discussion of the significance and importance of these two effector mechanisms to Treg immunobiology will be presented as an introduction to the next major topic that will directly examine Treg-only effector mechanisms. These mechanisms will be separated into two sections because of their mode of action. These sections will discuss: 1) the use or induction of non-cell-to-cell mechanisms, which make use of soluble mediators to inhibit T cell responses and 2) cell-to-cell contact mechanisms. An effort will be made during this discussion to relate a specific Treg effector mechanism with a particular type of immune response in order to address the reasons why a particular effector mechanism is used under those circumstances. As per usual, this half of the chapter will be followed by the descriptions of translational pathways that relate to these Treg effector mechanisms. Many of these transcriptional pathways will be similar to previously discussed pathways because they involve events that occur near or in the inner cell membrane of both the effector and the target. However, many will be unique and to some extent unknown because this area of translational immunology is still developing. Every effort will be made to explain as much as possible based on current information about these intercellular translational pathways that lead to Treg effector function.

Immune Cellular Interactions

The Two Major Effector Mechanisms

The T cell effectors CD4, CD8, and Treg, as well as NK cells poses these two effector mechanisms, which are the perforin/granzyme system and the FAS/FASL system. These are the two most prevalent ways used to destroy target cells by the cells mentioned above, except for Tregs that use additional effector systems. Without the ability of these effector cells to execute these effector functions, the immune system would be useless, and the body defenseless against pathogenic attack, viral infection, and cancer. Of these two effector systems the FAS/FASL system, which will be discussed first is more of a global killing system used by the body to eliminate unnecessary and left-over cells such as normal cells that continue to grow in situations like the regeneration of liver cells (Nagata 1996) or T cells that remain after an immune response. The expression or induction of the FAS receptor (R) on the surface of any cell whether it be normal, malignant, or immune renders that cell susceptible to being killed by coming in contact with a cell that expresses the FAS ligand (L). The perforin/granzyme system is more sophisticated and is strictly associated with the immune cells mentioned above. The perforin/granzyme system, just like with the FAS/FASL system, requires cell-to-cell contact, but as will be explained shortly, in this case there is intimate contact between the effector and target in such a way that allows the effector to remodel the targets outer cell membrane. In some cases T cells and NK cells can use both of these systems simultaneously to ensure the death of the target. Therefore, when contact is made between the effector and the target there is a very high probability that the target will die immediately. This is one of the reasons why Tregs are so important because in the wrong circumstances (autoimmune response) Tregs can stop the almost certain death of normal cells and tissue systems. However, there is something called "target cell resistance" where the target cell has developed the ability to resist cell death administered by effector T cells. This will be discussed in this section because it directly relates to how T cells escape or survive Treg effector mechanisms in certain situations, which allows these "Treg resistant" T cells to kill normal cells.

The FAS/FASL System

The FAS receptor (R) called CD95 or APO-1 is a 36-kD cell surface protein that is a member of the tumor necrosis factor (TNF) and nerve growth factor (NGF) receptor supergene families (Nagata 1995). The FAS ligand (L) or CD178 is a type II 40-kD membrane protein. Both of these proteins are expressed or can be induced on a wide variety of cells in the body. The initial interaction between the FASL and the FASR results in the clustering (aggregation) of this complex at the membrane synapse of both cells. Inside the target cell (FASR) this complex is called the FAS associated death domain or FADD. A precursor enzyme called procaspase binds to this complex and activates effector caspases (caspases 2, 3, 6, 7, 8, 9, and others). These caspases begin the process of dismantling the cell by cleavage of essential proteins and the activation of transcription factor proteins that bind to specific DNA promoters. These promoters activate genes that regulate pro-apoptotic factors such as the BCL-2 family of proteins that suppress survival-promoting proteins. This cascade of biochemical events eventually leads to the fragmentation of DNA within the target cell and death (Afford 2000).

As previously mentioned, the FAS/FASL system is a way for the immune system to modulate immune responses that have ended. Activated T cells express FASR and after removal of the antigenic threat, the cells are eliminated by FASL expressing cells such as APC, but also in other circumstances, the reverse happens where the APC expresses FASR and are killed by FASL expressing CTL. In addition, the FAS/FASL system is also involved in the previously discussed "immune privileged" sites that are not apart of the immune surveillance circuit. It was found that in sites such as the nervous system, the eye, and testis contain cells that express FASL and any FASR expressing cells (activated T cells) are killed upon contact. However, another major problem is the fact that many tumors also express

FASL and effectively delete clones of activated anti-tumor T cells in the same manner (Waring 1999). Finally, there is the two-way dilemma where both the tumor and the anti-tumor T cell express FASR and FASL. It was found that in this situation, both the effector T cell and the tumor died to some extent. However, factors such as the stage of activation of the T cell and the expression of FASR transcriptional factors in the tumor cell determines which cell suffers more death by apoptosis (Zeytun 1997). One clear fact is that many tumors such as gastric and colon cancers constitutively express FASL regardless of their developmental stage and this expression of FASL is the main mediator of tumor immune escape. FASL expression by tumors gives these tumor sites "immune privilege" as described for normal tissues (Bennett 1999). Expression of FASL by tumor cells derived from normal "immune privilege" tissues such as melanomas and gliomas contribute to the inability of the T cell immune system to eliminate them.

Another interesting aspect of the FAS/FASL system is its role in immune-modulation and control of the T cell response. As previously mentioned, this system is in place to essentially "cull" or trim the T cell immune system after an immune response has occurred and the effector cells are no longer needed. Both CD4 and CD8 effector T cells use both the perforin/granzyme and FAS/FASL systems to kill cells, but as far as the FAS/FASL system is concerned the question is which cells are targeted and when? In order to understand this one must separately focus on each T cell phenotype. For both CD4 and CD8 effectors the FAS/FASL system is used to attack the primary target such as virus infected cells or tumor cells. However, beyond this straightforward usage of the system by both phenotypes, there are separate and distinct purposes to use of this system that has to do with this "trimming" of the T cell response. CD8 effectors can actually make a change in these two effector mechanisms within a given population or clonotype of effectors. As an immune response occurs, CD8 effectors primarily use the perforin/granzyme system to dispatch MHC class I/antigen targets. However, as the response wanes these very same CD8 effectors decrease the amount of perforin RNA leaving only the expression of FASL. This begins the process of "targeted cellular suicide" directed at the remaining perforin expressing CD8 effectors in order to prevent them from attacking normal tissues (Meiraz 2009). It was also determined that FASL production in CD8 effectors appears in two distinct waves. The first wave comes from stored FASL within the cell and is released upon high antigenic stimulation. The second wave of FASL production is from newly synthesized FASL and appears on the CD8 effector cell surface after the detection of weak antigenic signals. This type of FASL expression is also contributes to bystander killing of related and non-related target cells (Jin-Shu 2010). Therefore, the CD8 effector suicide phase is an intercellular program, no doubt controlled by transcriptional pathways, which will be discussed in the second half of this chapter.

As mentioned above, CD4 effector T cells utilize both of these effector systems to attack target cells, but unlike CD8 FASL effectors that initiate destruction of perforin/granzyme CD8 effectors, CD4 FASL effectors target MHC class II expressing cells possessing FASR such as activated macrophages, dendritic cells, T cells, and B-cells. Because of the wider specificity of these CD4 FASL effectors, these cells can cause more bystander cell death than their CD8 counterparts. To a certain extent this activity can be viewed as a pretext to autoimmunity (Hahn 1995). As mentioned above, the FAS/FASL system is responsible for considerable bystander cell death or put in another way, "collateral damage." Jin-Shu and co-workers demonstrated that FASL was synthesized after the utilization of stored FASL and that this FASL was responsible for bystander killing. The issue here is the identity of the cells being killed during this "bystander effect" mediated by FASL expression on CTL. As previously mentioned, the TCR is specific for the antigen presented in the context of the MHC molecule expressed on the antigen presenting cell surface. The full activation of the T cell requires not only the recognition of MHC molecules by is ligands (CD4 and CD 8 molecules), but also the interaction of the CD28 receptor on the T cell with its ligands CD80/86. However, T cells can interact with a target cells via antigen alone or MHC alone as in cases where T cell anergy is induced during an anti-tumor T cell response where contact was made in a "one-signal" setting. The reason why this information has to do with FASL bystander killing is that the CTL can make contact with the target in a "single signal" setting long enough for the initiation of FASL apoptosis to begin. Therefore, the killing of bystander cells can either be based on MHC alone or antigen alone. During islet cell graft transplantation CD8 effectors and CD4 effectors caused significant bystander damage through FASL to the point that engraftment failed. However, it was determined that the capacity of CD8 effectors to impede engraftment was dwarfed by the damage caused by CD4 CTL using solely MHC-class II molecules as its target. In addition, PD-1, which is a member of the CD28/CTLA-4 family and regulator of TCR signals, restrained bystander killing (Thangavelu 2013). Despite its non-specific nature, the FAS/FASL system is a very important component of immune homeostasis, but its most important role is being an integral component of the T cell effector arsenal.

The Perforin/Granzyme System

Perforin

This system is the main effector mechanism used by CTL and NK cells because it induces target cell death in a rapid and efficient manner. Unlike the FAS/FASL system, which can take up to 3hr to kill the target, the perforin/granzyme system kills target cells within 10 minutes. Despite this difference in time frames for killing the target, CTL and NK cells often use both systems on a single target. First of all, the time difference between FAS and perforin killing can be explained by the extensive mobilization of downstream transcription factors such as the caspases in the FAS system described above. In addition, and as will be described below, the perforin/granzyme system is a direct assault on the cell membrane and cytoplasm of the target cell (Hassin 2011). There is another aspect to perforin/granzyme vs. FAS killing that will be discussed at length and that is how dead target cells killed by either or both of these mechanisms are processed by APC. This has to do with presentation of peptide that either induces antigen specific immunity or autoimmune responses. However, now it is important to understand the components of this system and how they work together to achieve the target cell death. The system is contained in what are called "cytotoxic granules" found in the cytoplasm of effector cells. These cytotoxic granules contain perforin and granzymes.

Perforin is a 67-kilodalton compartmentalized protein that oligomerizes to form pores in the target cell membrane. The perforin molecule is "key-shaped" and at its end has an amino-terminal membrane attack complex or MACPF, which is attached to an epidermal growth factor (EGF) domain that, in combination with a carboxy-terminal sequence, forms a multi-tiered structure. Some of the perforin DNA sequence is similar to the compliment sequences coding for the C6-C9 complex, which is apart of the compliment attack unit (Law 2010). This protein has the ability to insert itself into the target cell membrane during the synapse process.

Genetic mutations in the perforin genome have been associated with a rare, but fatal disease called, familial hemophagocytic lymphohistiocytosis type 2 or FHL2 (An 2010). Other genetic mutations of the perforin gene have been associated with the development of early primary cancer because of perforin's role in immunosurveillance conducted by T and NK cells (Trapani 2013). The perforin part of the target cell lysis is quite elegant and efficient. Once the target cell and the effector membranes make contact (immunological synapse) cytotoxic granules begin their formation on the inner membrane of the effector. Inside these granules, the perforin is assembled like a scaffold and once against the effector inner membrane, it mobilizes intercellular calcium and begins to bore into the targets outer membrane. The molecule actually turns itself inside out and forms a pore or tunnel in the target cell membrane (Law 2010). The elegant part of this is when the target cell detects this it tries to repair itself by forming an internal vacuole. Essentially what happens is that by the time the vacuole is formed, the entire contents of the cytotoxic granule are deposited inside it as the perforin continues to form pores. Once this happens, granzymes are released and basically dissolve the cytoplasm of the target (Thiery 2011).

Granzymes

The other participants of this deadly effector mechanism are the granzymes. Granzymes (Grs) are a part of a related family of serine proteases. Humans have 10 Grs (A, B, C, D, E, F, G, K, M, and N). The genes associated with these Grs are found on 3 separate chromosomes. These proteases cleave proteins in specific ways. For instance GrB cleaves proteins at aspartic acid residues and GrA and GrK are tryptases and cleave basic amino acid residues called P1 residues. In fact, cleavage by GrB results in the activation of caspases 3, which in turn begins a process similar to the FAS/FASL system where rapid DNA fragmentation and chromatin condensation occur. The granzyme proteases are extremely important to the proper functioning of effector cells throughout the body. In mouse models where the Gr genes were deleted, the mice were highly susceptible to several strains of viruses such as cytomegalovirus, had an inability to mount a graft vs. host response and respond to allogeneic tumors. To a certain extent, each of the Grs can activate unique intercellular transduction pathways that lead to the death of the target cell. Some like GrB initiate the caspases system of apoptosis, but others like GrH target mitochondria through an as of yet unknown mechanism that causes DNA damage in the target cell nucleus.

Granzyme immunobiology has been the subject of study for some 25 years and there are still aspects related to their function that are not fully understood (Ewen 2012). As mentioned above, perforin has the ability to initiate not only pore formation on the target cell membrane, but also endocytosis of the cytotoxic granules of the effector prior to pore formation caused by the target cell trying to repair its outer cell membrane by forming an internal vacuole. This target cell vacuole or endosome is called a "gigantosome," and it enters the target cell cytoplasm as perforin continues to form pores in its membrane (Thiery 2011). It was found that this process happens very quickly (30 seconds). However, the target cell initiates membrane repair in 20 seconds and completes these repairs in about 80 seconds. It was also mentioned that GrB initiated the caspase death sequence similar to the FAS/FASL system that takes a much longer time to kill target cells. Here, once perforin opens pores in the gigantosome membrane, the caspase 3 begins to induce apoptosis in about 2 minutes, which is evidenced by membrane contraction of the target cell (Lopez 2013). Once this process is initiated, the target cell is destined to die, by not only the DNA fragmentation death of apoptosis, but also by granzyme-mediated proteolytic cleavage of cytoplasmic proteins. During a T cell-mediated autoimmune response, the quickness of this process necessitates a rapid response from Tregs. In fact, because of their increased expression of LFA-1, Tregs can appear very quickly at the response site to instruct DCs to secrete inhibitory cytokines and convert those anti-self effector T cells into Tregs (Onishi 2008).

It is obvious that granzymes play a major role in the destruction of CTL-recognized targets, but there is another role that granzymes play, which until lately (5-years or so) was not so obvious. It turns out that granzymes can be found in an extracellular form, not only between cells, but also in the circulatory systems of normal individuals (Bade 2005), virus infected (Rowshani 2005), and autoimmune disease (arthritis) patients (Tak 1999). Some of the extracellular granzymes that have been detected and associated with brisk CTL activity could be the result of it escaping from CTL during synapse formation between CTL and target cells. However, in situations where an inflammatory response is occurring, this is not the case because many times inflammatory cells such as mast cells, neutrophils, and macrophages constitute cellular milieu at these sites of inflammation. It was determined that macrophages found in rheumatoid arthritic-joint fluid expressed GrB and it dissolved the intercellular contacts between endothelial cells making blood vessels permeable to other cells and lymphokines (Kim 2007). This is part of the inflammatory process of which mast cells participate because they too secrete GrB, which again contributes to blood vessel permeability due the cleavage of fibronectin, collagen, and laminin, which are all extracellular proteins. This secretion of GrB by mast cell was found to be independent of perforin and is released by the activation of mast cells via cross linking of its Fc receptor. This can be archived by the attachment of IgE, which releases the contents of mast cell lysosomal compartments allowing these cells to control bacterial and viral infections (Pardo 2007).

The proinflammatory properties of granzymes go far beyond the initiation of this process by mast cells, neutrophils, and macrophages. When GrB is released during an inflammatory response it is responsible for producing the basic conditions of the inflammatory site. Because of GrB ability to remodel the extracellular matrix (ECM) by cleaving fibronectin, collagen, and laminin, the cells of the immune system gain easily gain access to the tissues involved (Buzza 2005). Setting up these basic conditions goes even further because the products of the proteolysis of fibrinogen by GrB creates what is called, "danger signals," which are the result of trauma-induced cell lysis (Matzinger 2002). As far as the proteolysis of fibrinogen is concerned, it can activate monocytes to secrete inflammatory cytokines such as IL-6, IL-8, TNF-α (Kuhns 2007). In addition, once cleaved the extracellular domain of fibronectin can induce IL-10 secretion from DCs (Okamura 2001). The interesting thing about the secretion of both IL-6 and IL-10 is that both of these lymphokines in concert with TGF-ß not only create Tregs, but also facilitate the reprogramming of Tregs into proinflammatory IL-17 effector T cells

Another consequence of GrB proteolytic activity operates on normal T cells that become activated and enter or are already present at inflammatory sites. The glutamate receptor (GluR3) and its ligand glutamate, which is a major neurotransmitter of the central nervous system (CNS) and plays a significant role in not only the development of the CNS, but also normal brain functions that depend on the interaction between this ligand and receptor (Danbolt 2001). However, it turns out that GluR3 receptor has immunological properties related to basic T cell functions. It is expressed on naive T cells, but is cleaved by GrB that is secreted by T cells upon activation. GrB is released to the cell surface by such cells as NK cells, CTL, and Tregs in an autocrine fashion. The reason why GrB is secreted under these circumstances has to do with the ability of non-activated T cells, which express high levels of GluR3 to adhere to laminin and fibronectin (Ganor 2007). Fibronectin is a part of the ECM and its presence allows normal T cells to momentarily "dock" at any given site within the body. Once the GluR3 receptor is removed from the T cell, it can move about the body freely and allows these T cells to follow any chemo attractant signals available. Therefore, secreted GrB is responsible for the unabated movement of T cells in an inflammatory situation. It is clear that secreted GrB has the ability to not only establish inflammatory conditions such as remodeling the ECM, but also induce immune cells to secrete inflammatory cytokines, which is the foundation of an inflammatory response. This granzyme plays an important role in the normal function of the immune system not only because of its ability to initiate an inflammatory response through proteolytic cleavage of ECM proteins, but also because it allows activated T cells to move about freely during an immune response.

Granulysin

There is another proteolytic enzyme/protein that is found not only in the lysosomal granules of effector cells, but is also secreted from these cells. It is called granulysin and was discovered by subtractive hybridization of antigen activated T cell lines. Granulysin or the designated gene "519" was among a series of genes that were activated in the "late phase" of T cell activation, much like the genes for perforin and the granzymes (Jongstra 1987). The granulysin protein belongs to a family of proteins that share homology with small granule-associated proteins called, saposin-like proteins or SAPLIP. What's unique about this protein family is that they have the ability to interact with target membrane lipids. There are two protein products of 15 and 9kDa in sizes. The 9kDa form is found in the cytotoxic granules of effector cell and has been shown to be able to kill tumor cells (Pena 1997). Just like many of the granzyme proteins, granulysin is a proinflammatory molecule and it was found that the 9kDa form of the protein that is cytotoxic to tumor cells, microbes, gram-positive and gram-negative bacteria, fungi, yeast, and parasites is a cleavage product of the 15kDa protein. The 15kDa form is a secreted from effector cells on a constant basis. In addition, granulysin is chemo-attractant for T cells, monocytes, and other inflammatory cells such as mast cells. Granulysin can induce the secretion of several inflammatory cytokines such as macrophage inflammatory protein MIP-a1, monocyte chemo-attractants MCP-1 and MCP-3, as well as T cell secreted IL-1, IL-6, IL-10, and INF-A (Krensky 2009).

As mentioned above, the 15kDa protein is unlike GrB, which is secreted in a purposeful way by effector cells. It is stored in separate cytotoxic granules that release their contents upon precursor CTL or precursor NK cell activation. These granules are different from the cytotoxic granules that contain the 9kDa form of granulysin because they are devoid of perforin and GrB and as mentioned above, are released during the cell's activation phase and not during effector-target contact. In addition to these differences, the 15kDa form of granulysin has no cytotoxicity for tumors or bacteria as the 9kDa form has. However, unlike the 9kDa form, the 15kDa form has the ability to directly activate monocytes and immature DC in a way that is genetically different from the activation pathway induced by GM-CSF (Clayberger 2012). As previously mentioned in chapter 1, mature DCs have the ability to activate TH-1 T cell responses, which in the situation of a growing tumor can be inhibited by Treg contact. This contact between the DC and Tregs occur at a rapid rate and is believed to be why the response rate of using DCs matured by GM-CSF as an anti-cancer therapeutic toll is less than ten percent. However, unlike DC maturation mediated by GM-CSF, 15kDa granulysin does not inhibit either co-stimulatory molecule expression or secretion of chemo-attractants for cells such as neutrophils, memory and activated T cells, as well as macrophage/dendritic cells (Castiello 2011). In fact, in granulysin transgenic mice had an enhanced anti-tumor response that was not due to the presence of the 9kDa tumorcidal form, but directly related to the increased expression of the DC co-stimulatory molecules CD40 and CD86 (Clayberger 2012). The use of 15kDa form of granulysin to activate therapeutic DCs for cancer therapy may be an important step in overriding Treg control of these cells in a clinical situation.

The Significance of Perforin/Granzyme and FAS/FASL Mechanisms to Treg Immunobiology

These two effector mechanisms (perforin/granzyme and FAS/FASL) represent the most effective ways the T cell immune system has to not only attack and kill target cells (tumor, virus infected, bacteria, and pathogens), but to also maintain immunological homeostasis and in some instances, thwart unwanted autoimmune reactions initiated by left-over antigen specific effector T cells. As shown above, these two systems are complex and have multiple purposes that relate to almost all areas (autoimmunity, anti-tumor, and anti-microbial immunity) of cellular immunity. However, just like in many areas of T cell immunity, a higher order of complexity is involved when Tregs are included in the discussion. The reason for this has to do with the fact that the Treg is probably the most advanced T cell in the body. The Treg is not just another T cell such as a CD4 or CD8 T cell, but it is in a sense, a conceptual T cell that not only originates in the thymus like other T cells, but can also be created, reprogrammed, and de-programmed depending on the environment it finds itself in. This type of cellular "plasticity" that was mentioned earlier, can induce an extra layer of complexity to standard T cell functions and this situation with these two effector mechanisms is no exception. As mentioned earlier, Tregs certainly use these two mechanisms, but which one or ones do they use for which specific purposes?

For instance, earlier it was mentioned that FASL production in CD8 effectors appears in two distinct waves. The first wave comes from stored FASL within the cell and is released upon high antigenic stimulation. The second wave of FASL production is from newly synthesized FASL and appears on the CD8 effector cell surface after the detection of weak antigenic signals. This type of FASL expression is also contributes to bystander killing of related and non-related target cells (Jin-Shu 2010). It's thought that the purpose of newly synthesized FASL was to eliminate CD8 effector T cells that were not needed after the immune response had waned. This is the process of "targeted cellular suicide," which is directed at the remaining perforin expressing CD8 effectors is initiated in order to prevent them from attacking normal tissues (Meiraz 2009). This is an example of effector mechanism use that is designed for a specific purpose and induced by the changing environment of the immune response. These are the types of situations that will be addressed throughout this chapter as far as Tregs are concerned. This is especially important in the second half of the chapter where analysis of intercellular translational pathways of these effector mechanisms should reveal the molecular cue or signals that lead to the use of a particular mechanism based the changing environment of the immune response.

Functional Use, Sensitivity, and Resistance of Tregs and Accessory Cells to Perforin/Granzyme and FAS/FASL Effector Mechanisms

Despite the fact that Tregs are the most "advanced" T cell in the T cell immune system, they are nonetheless T cells and to a certain extent, adhere to T cell immunobiological rules. One of those rules is that as long as an effector T cell is needed it is allowed to survive in the body. However, when its usefulness comes to an end, it is promptly eliminated or deleted by the immune system. The example above concerning "targeted suicide" of CD8 effectors is a natural built-in immunological mechanism to eliminate unwanted CTL. As far as the functional use of these mechanisms by Tregs is concerned, there are some interesting ways Tregs use them to attack other T cells. It was mentioned earlier that other inflammatory cells of the immune system such as mast cells had the ability to secrete GrB upon activation through the cell's Fc receptor in a perforin independent fashion (Pardo 2007). This secreted GrB facilitated permeability of blood vessels and the remodeling of the ECM (Buzza 2005), which are two very important stages of the inflammatory process. However, the use of granzymes to induce target cell death by CTLs and NK cells is normally associated with pore formation by perforin. It turns out the Tregs can secrete GrB in a perforin-independent way during their attack of CTL. The GrB is secreted during cell-to-cell contact (immunological synapse) directly onto the target cell membrane. This secreted GrB can initiate apoptosis like it does during perforin-mediated pore formation, but it also severely damages the target cell membrane due to the proteolytic action of GrB (Gondek 2005). As mentioned above, this method of attack by Tregs is not the usual way CTL dispatch target cells by the use of granzymes. However, the secretion of GrB by Tregs is a normal function of these cells because of their role in regulating the inflammatory "state."

Functional Use of Perforin/Granzyme and FAS/FASL by Tregs

In chapter 2 it was apparent that Tregs are attracted to sites of inflammation not only from the chemo attractant trail secreted by immune cells at the site, but also by the massive amounts of IL-2 that are released by responding T cells. Coincidently, these responding T cells were able to enter the inflammatory site because of the conditions (vascular permeability and ECM remodeling) created by inflammatory cells (mast cells, neutrophils, eosinophils) through the secretion of GrB. Once at the site, Tregs go about the business of controlling the inflammatory response by attacking and inhibiting CTL and NK cells, de-differentiating DCs to an immature Treg-inducing state, and basically setting up a perimeter around the inflammatory site. The elaboration of GrB by Tregs is a trap these cells set for responding T cells. As Tregs secrete more GrB there is even more vascular permeability and more ECM remodeling, which really amounts to creating gap junctions between cells so that more lymphocytes (T cells) can enter. Once these additional T cells enter the site they are immediately converted into Tregs by immature DCs and from that point on, either join the other Tregs that control the inflammatory site or get reprogrammed into TH17 inflammatory effector cells. As mentioned in the previous chapters, TH17 effector cells not only contribute to the inflammatory process by the release of IL-17, but also contribute to the eradication of pathogens, which often cause inflammatory immune reactions (Bettelli 2008). In addition to the increased permeability of blood vessels caused by Treg secreted GrB, it has recently been discovered that Tregs also secrete vascular endothelial growth factor (VEGF), which was mentioned in chapter 2 as the main signal protein that promotes angiogenesis. The secretion of VEGF by Tregs has implications related to tumor cell escape from the primary tumor site via an increased blood supply (Facciabene 2012), but also relates to role of Tregs during an inflammatory response. Again, this is another way Tregs gain control of an inflammatory response by allowing specific inflammatory effector cells into the site long enough to have an impact on what ever is causing the inflammation, but eventually those effectors are inhibited, killed or converted into Tregs.

As mentioned earlier, Tregs being the T cells that they are just like normal effector T cells that become obsolete after their role in the immune response has ended. There is an example of this targeted obsolescence and the functional use GrB secretion by Tregs. This example also introduces the topic of T cell resistance to apoptosis. As discussed in the first chapter, Tregs are a heterogeneous population of T cells comprised of innate or 'natural' Tregs and adaptive 'created' Tregs. There are also subpopulations within these two major categories such as the subpopulation that was previously discussed, which express LAG-3 (Camisaschi 2010). However, there is another subpopulation of innate Tregs that express MHC-class II (human HLA-DR), are highly suppressive, and express higher than normal levels of FOX-P3. These Tregs represent a full one-third of the circulating population of Tregs. HLA-DR+ Tregs were shown to suppress effector T cell proliferation and cytokine production in the early stages of an immune response through a cell contact mechanism that accompanied increased expression of FOXP3 mRNA. In contrast to this, HLA-DR- Tregs initially secrete IL-10 and IL-4, and then later suppress effector function by cell contact, followed by increased expression of FOXP3 mRNA. These studies demonstrated that this was a separate subpopulation of innate Tregs and not a lineage variation of the total Treg population (Baecher-Allen 2006).

Sensitivity of Tregs to Perforin/Granzyme and FAS/FASL Apoptosis

Highly suppressive HLA-DR+ Tregs become vulnerable to responding CD4 T cell under conditions that cause strong TCR signals in the responding T cell. These CD4 responders exert control over HLA-DR+ Tregs by the secretion of GrB. However, during weak antigenic signals DR+ Tregs efficiently suppressed CD4 responders. As the strength of the TCR signal increases more GrB is secreted by the CD4 responders. The type of death suffered by DR+ Tregs in this situation is apoptosis via the activation of caspase 3. Part of caspase 3's ability to induce apoptosis is its ability to affect the ratio of proteins from the pro-survival and pro-apoptotic BCL genes. If pro-survival proteins like BCL-xl or BCL-2 outnumber pro-apoptotic proteins such as BIM and BAX the cell survives. If the reverse is true apoptosis occurs. The positive survival ratio of the BCL proteins in activated T cells is controlled by the interaction of CD28 with its ligands CD80/86 on APCs and the upregulation of cytokine receptors such as IL-2RA or CD25 (Kouchkovsky 2013). However, here it was found that unlike DR- Tregs, DR+ Tregs expressed a lower level of the pro-survival protein BCL-xl compared to level of the pro-apoptotic BAX protein. In essence, DR+ Tregs are more sensitive to apoptosis than other innate Tregs. Therefore, CD4 T cells under conditions of strong TCR stimulation can resist the inhibitory effects of DR+ Tregs by secreting GrB and inducing apoptotic cell death of these Tregs (Ashley 2009).

As mentioned previously, this reciprocal death between cell types occurs in the FAS/FASL system. That example had to do with anti-tumor effector T cells and tumor cells (Zeytun 1997). There is a similar example with Tregs and CD4 responders. During an examination of Tregs and CD4 responders from cancer patients it was determined that when these Tregs were activated by TCR stimulation they upregulated both FAS and FASL expression and were able to suppress CD8 proliferation by FAS-mediated apoptosis. However, Tregs eliminated CD4 responding T cells through a cell contact mechanism at high IL-2 concentrations. Conversely, at lower IL-2 concentrations Tregs were sensitive to responding T cell mediated apoptosis. In addition, both cell types upregulated FAS and FASL under high IL-2 concentrations. At these IL-2 concentrations (1000 IU/ml) Tregs became resistant to FAS-mediated apoptosis, but responding T cells were not, leaving them vulnerable to this effector mechanism (Strauss 2009). Later, it was determined that cell contact mechanism used in the 'reciprocal apoptosis' was unlike the situation above with DR+ Tregs, a perforin-dependent delivery of GrB by both cell types under different (IL-2 concentration) physiological conditions (Czystowska 2010). Despite the differences between the delivery method used in the GrB-induced apoptosis in both of these examples is was clear that two elements were in operation that dictated which T cell type (Treg or CD4 responding T cell) could inflict apoptotic death upon the other. Those elements were environment (strong or weak TCR signals and increasing IL-2 levels) and the ability of either cell type to become resistant to FAS or GrB-mediated apoptosis.

Resistance to Perforin/Granzyme and FAS/FASL Apoptosis by Tregs and DC Mechanism of Treg Apoptosis

In many instances resistance to apoptosis by a cell can determine the outcome of an immune response or inflammatory reaction. There are two basic mechanisms that targeted cells use to become resistant to perforin/granzyme and FAS/FASL-induced apoptosis. Both of these effector mechanisms activate the caspase cascade of apoptosis. One of those mechanisms was mentioned earlier and has to do with the ratio of pro-survival and pro-apoptotic proteins from the Bcl-2 gene family. This is related to how the serine protease granzyme GrB induces cell apoptosis. The other method of target cell resistance to apoptosis involves several natural serine protease inhibitors. As mentioned previously, this apoptotic pathway will be discussed in detail in the second half of this chapter. However, now it is important to summarize these mechanisms because they play an important part in the resistance or susceptibility to apoptotic death by Tregs. There are two pathways associated with GrB activation of apoptosis. The main pathway results in the release of cell death factors from mitochondria and the other minor pathway involves GrB activation of caspases downstream of mitochondrial involvement. The major pathway leads to mitochondrial-induced apoptosis and is the result of multiple pro-apoptotic factors that are released from the mitochondrial membrane such as Smac/Diablo, Omi/HtrA2, and cytochrome *c*. These factors then activate executioner caspases that begin to dismantle the target cell cytoplasmic proteins (Bao 2007).

However, the expression of the pro-survival protein Bcl-2 can block the ability of GrB to initiate this process. The major pathway towards the release of cytochrome *c* induced by GrB involves the proteolysis of BID, which is a "death agonist" and part of the BCL-2 family of death regulators (Wang 1998). These death regulators (BID, BAX, BAK, BIM, and BAD) and how they function not only control mitochondrial apoptosis, but also these proteins can 'sense' cell damage as they transit through the cytoplasm of a cell (Gross 1999). GrB has the ability to degrade BID by proteolysis. Once proteolysis of Bid occurs it activates BAX. This activation leads to permeabilization of the mitochondrial membrane and release of pro-apoptotic factors (Moldoveau 2013). As a result of the release of these factors, executioner caspases are activated. This process can be can be thwarted by the upregulation of BCL-2 and as previously mentioned, CD28 activation initiates the process of increasing the ratio of pro-survival proteins BCLxl and BCL to the pro-apoptotic proteins BIM and in this case BID. In addition, this process of increasing pro-survival proteins while decreasing pro-apoptotic proteins also occurs when the high-affinity IL-2 receptor (IL-2RA or CD25) is upregulated in Tregs (Kouchkovsky 2013). This apoptotic GrB pathway is not dependent on the activation of caspase 3 or 8. However, the alternative pathway driven by GrB does involve the direct activation of executioner caspases because it was determined that a small percentage of BCL-2 expressing cells did undergo GrB apoptosis. This led to the hypothesis that GrB could activate executioner caspases on its own, but in a less efficient manner than the proteolysis of BID by GrB. (Pinkoski 2001). The ability of GrB to by-pass the involvement of mitochondrial release of pro-apoptotic factors that lead to caspase activation is a built-in redundancy that guarantees the death of the target cell. However, many cells in the body deploy a method of resisting apoptosis at the immunological synapse, which is the target cell membrane that literally voids the proteolytic action of GrB.

Serine Protease Inhibitor Resistance to Treg Apoptosis

Serine protease inhibitors or serpins secreted by cells (immune and normal cells) act as serine protease substrates and take the place of naturally occurring serine expressed in the membranes of almost all cells. These inhibitors act as "pseudo- or suicide substrates that absorb the proteolytic effects of granzymes A and B as well as procaspases used by the FAS/FASL system. The most important of these serpins is PI-9 (PI-6 is the mouse analogue), which is a part of a supergene family associated with ovalbumin serpins. PI-9 is particularly active as far as GrB is concerned and protects effector CTL from the proteolytic damage caused by the GrB they secrete to kill target cells (Sun 1996). PI-9 is expressed on a wide variety of cells in the body. Most of the cells that secrete GrB in the inflammatory arena such as activated mast cells, express PI-9 as well as mast cells associated with mastocytosis (Bladergroen 2005). PI-6 in mice has been shown to protect natural NK cells (Ansari 2010) and CTL (Zhang 2006) from the proteolytic effects of granzymes that as have been previously been shown to do more that superficial damage to target cell membranes. Recently, it was demonstrated that as both innate and adaptive Tregs become activated they not only increase their intracellular levels of GrB, but also at the same time express higher levels of PI-6. By using transgenic mice that lacked the PI-6 gene it was found that these Tregs demonstrated a higher level of GrB-mediated apoptosis in target cells, but also had a higher rate of apoptosis themselves. In other words, the GrB they were secreting was killing them evidenced by the fact that these PI-6-deficient mice rejected heart allografts at a much faster rate when compared to wild-type mice because dwindling numbers of Treg through apoptosis (Azzi 2013). Therefore, secretion of serine protease inhibitors by Tregs is an essential function associated with their use of the perforin/granzyme or granzyme secretion effector mechanism.

Mechanisms and Resistance to Apoptosis by DC

In addition to its role in naturally protecting not only immune effectors, but also in many cases normal cells as well, the expression of serine protease inhibitors can contribute to disease states. For instance, when alveolar monocytes or peripheral monocytes are infected by phagocytosis of *Mycobacterium tuberculosis*, this bacterium has the ability to induce PI-9 expression and inhibit apoptosis by increasing BCL-2 expression. This is a mechanism the bacteria use to protect infected cells (Toossi 2011). Another disease-related expression of serine protease inhibitors is the increasing expression of PI-9 in lung cancer cells as the disease progresses (Soriano 2012). One of the most interesting aspects of Treg control of either an inflammatory reaction site or a precancerous tumor site is the relationship between the Treg and DCs. These two immune cells often find themselves called to both types of sites. The relationship between Tregs and DCs in both of these situations has been discussed in the previous two chapters. Tregs immediately take control of DC's that are differentiated from monocytes at an inflammatory site and they command these cells to do several things. The first thing Tregs do is to retard the maturation of these cells because a mature DC can induce a TH-1 CD4 T cell response by the release of IL-12. Once the de-maturation of the DC is accomplished, these immature DCs begin to secrete the IL-6 and TGF-ß. This cytokine milieu can convert antigen-specific CD4 effector cells into antigen-specific Tregs. The next command, which occurs as the de-maturation process proceeds, is the secretion of IL-1a by these immature DCs. The secretion of IL-1a results in the conversion of Tregs into pro-inflammatory CD4 TH17 cells that contribute to the inflammatory process.

However, Tregs can go one step further in their control of either of these sites and that is to kill mature DCs before they have an opportunity to activate CD4 or CD8 antigen-specific CTLs. DCs have a finite lifespan because of the powerful T cell activation functions they possess. As mentioned earlier when discussing mitochondrial-induced apoptosis, members of the BCL-2 family also control the lifespan of DC because signals from BCL-2 can block the activation of the death regulator BIM (Nopora 2001). The type of apoptosis experienced by DCs is a natural process (Hou 2004) that must occur after these cells have induced a productive CD4/8 T cell response. Therefore, DCs are designed to "auto self-destruct," which is dependent upon immunological environmental conditions such as priming naïve CD4 T cells. This is where CTL and Tregs come into play. Studies looking at BAX and BAK gene negative mice have determined that Tregs use LAG ligation of DC MHC class II (see below) induce DC apoptosis in a mitochondrial-induced fashion (Chen 2011). If BIM genes are deficient in mice autoimmune reactions occur due to the continued stimulation and rampant proliferation of antigen-specific T cells, which leads to the induction of autoantibodies (Chen 2007).

As mentioned above, during an immune response Tregs have the ability to de-differentiate mature DCs into immature DCs that can convert antigen specific responding CD4 and CD8 T cells into Tregs. Once newly converted antigen specific Tregs encounter DCs presenting that antigen, they are killed to prevent any further activation of responding T cells. At inflammatory or tumor sites Tregs may kill DC using two separate or coordinated effector mechanisms. The first mechanism Tregs use is the standard perforin/granzyme form of apoptosis, which involves the release of pro-apoptotic factors from mitochondria as described above (Boissonnas 2010). However, there is another effector mechanism used by Tregs to induce or add to BIM/mitochondrial-induced apoptosis in DC. In Chapter 1 there was a discussion of how Treg expressed lymphocyte activation gene-3 or LAG-3 engagement of the MHC class II molecules on the DC inhibited its ability to become activated and thereby present antigen (Liang 2008). However, it turns out that the interaction between LAG and MHC class II molecules can do more than inhibit DC function; it can cause apoptosis. It has been known for some time now that ligation of MHC class II molecules can cause apoptosis in immune cells. This type of apoptosis is independent of FAS/FASL and perforin/granzyme activity because it is similar to the direct activation of BIM in mitochondrial-induced apoptosis (Drenou 1999). Later it was determined that anti-MHC class II antibodies could induce apoptosis in mature DC that led to mitochondrial-induced apoptosis, which was independent of BIM activation and caspase involvement. It was thought that this was a "built-in" proapoptotic pathway possessed by mature DC to guarantee their removal after an immune response (Leverkus 2003). However, the induction of DC apoptosis by Treg expressed LAG-3 does involve the activation (cleavage) of BIM and the subsequent activation of BAK that leads to mitochondrial-induced apoptosis. As previously discussed, expression of LAG on Tregs is a result of Treg activation and in this case only activated, but not un-stimulated Tregs were able to induce DC apoptosis (Chen 2011).

DCs do have the ability to resist both FAS/FASL and perforin/granzyme apoptosis as the mature by the expression PI-9. In addition, it was determined that PI-9 had not only the ability to inhibit GrB proteolysis, but also the proteolytic activities of caspases that are activated by FAS/FASL apoptosis (Cunningham 2007). The expression of PI-9 is tightly linked to the maturation process of DCs because it is expressed in conjunction with the expression of CD86, but not with the secretion of IL-12. Its expression is also dependent on the p38 MAPK pathway, which is linked to DC activation (Bots 2007). Expression of PI-9 in mature DC serves a dual role. Its expression on DCs allows these cells to escape apoptosis induced by CTL that become activated during the antigen presentation process. Just as artificial survival (BIM deficiency or over expression of BCL-2) of DC leads to increased T cell proliferation and autoimmunity, loss of DC can through apoptosis can lead to either disease progression or the development of tolerance. The expression of PI-9 by DC augments the ability of CTL to kill specific targets because of the continual stimulation provided by antigen presenting DCs. In addition, the expression of PI-9 in DC is type-specific because only DC that participate in thymic selection of T cells and present antigen during an immune response express high levels of this serine protease inhibitor (Hirst 2003). PI-9 expression prevents the development of immune tolerance by inhibiting DC apoptosis. When DC undergo apoptosis the dead cells are endocytosed by immature DC using an integrin called αv, β3 and CD36, which is a member of the class B scavenger receptor family that bind lipid-rich ligands such as collagen. These two molecules are unique to the CD14+ immature DC population and are involved in phagocytosis of apoptotic cells (Albert 1998). Antigen processing of apoptotic DC by immature DC may cause several things to happen that can directly result in immune tolerance. The first one of these things is called, "cross priming" and is the result of immature DC presenting autoantigens derived from the dead DC. The presentation of autoantigens leads directly to the induction of autoreactive T cell responses, but also activate innate Tregs via their autoimmune TCR. The second tolerance-inducing event that occurs is that the processing of apoptotic DC by immature DC causes them to secrete TGF-ß that, as previously mentioned induces the formation of adaptive Tregs (Kushwah 2010). Therefore, PI-9 expression does more than just protect DCs from apoptosis by CTL. It also prevents tolerance, thus allowing a productive immune response to occur. However, despite DC resistance to apoptosis by PI-9, Tregs still have the ability to kill them using the LAG/MHC class II method described above.

The Role That Perforin/Granzyme and FAS/FASL Effector Mechanisms Play in Treg Immunobiology and Lifespan

Mechanisms of Apoptosis in the Natural Treg Lifespan

Tregs are possessed with multiple functions in the immune system because they are supposed to control and normalize T cell-based immune responses. This is called homeostasis and has been discussed previously in regards to specific immunological responses that involve particular tissue systems and situations such as sites of inflammation and tumor growth as well as pregnancy. However, there is a global or system-wide aspect to homeostasis induced by Tregs. Since the immune system cannot function without them, Tregs and their immunobiology may be the key to the development of numerous diseases that previously had not been attributed to defects in the function of Tregs. It was mentioned earlier that almost any genetic anomaly that affected Tregs, even in the slightest way, could lead to disease development or exacerbation of an existing disease. Another, and possibly more important factor that affects the ability of Tregs to maintain immunological homeostasis is their death. As mentioned before, despite the fact that Tregs are an "advanced" version of a T cell, they are still governed by immunological rules that apply to all T cells, which is a limited lifespan.

The lifespan of Tregs, like other T cells is based two fundamental immunological factors. The first one of these factors is an inherent or innate genetic program that naturally induces apoptosis of the cell once its usefulness comes to an end. For Tregs there are two "conditions" that this population of T cells exists in. The first condition is senescence where innate Tregs exist in the circulation for prolonged periods of time (years) in the body. The second condition, also related to innate Tregs is where the cells exist for some time in a semi-activated state by exposure to self-antigens in the body, but once they become fully activated they have a limited lifespan (Fission 2003). This is a situation much like the previously discussed situation with memory T cells that needed exposure to antigens similar to their specific antigen (melanoma-specific) to survive, but in this case inadvertently caused vitiligo in melanoma patients (Byrne 2011). Fully activated Tregs, which include adaptive Tregs, are different from activated T cells in that their continued survival and function does not depend on IL-2 and antigen, but on IL-2 alone. This is based on the fact that Tregs do not produce this lymphokine and when activated, use it to attack responding T cells that secrete IL-2 during an immune response. Therefore, when all of the IL-2 is used up or disappears, Tregs undergo apoptosis (Pandiyan 2008). This is in stark contrast to activated responding T cells in that IL-2 they secrete induces conditions in these cells that promote apoptosis (expression of FAS), where the same IL-2 makes Tregs resistant to apoptosis (expression of FASL only). This difference allows Tregs to eliminate antigen-reactive responding T cells that are producing IL-2 (Yolcu 2008). This type of natural Treg apoptosis is regulated by the genes responsible for the Treg's expression of the high-affinity IL-2R (Malek 2010) and the translational pathways that control this activity will be detailed in the second half of this chapter. Here, the death of Tregs is based on genetic elements that are pre-programmed to induce apoptosis under the standard functioning conditions of the cell. However, there are immunological conditions in non-standard environments that lead to Treg death and subsequent autoimmunity.

Mechanisms of Apoptosis in the Unnatural Treg Lifespan That Can Lead to Autoimmunity

Often Tregs find themselves in specialized immunological environments such as the site of an organ transplant, lethal viral infection, or the inception of autoimmune diseases such as diabetes or arthritis. These situations present the Treg with conditions that are very much unlike the standard T cell responses to common viral infections or basic inflammatory responses. This variability in the Tregs environment affects the cell's sensitivity to apoptosis and in many cases results in the induction of autoimmune responses as a consequence of dwindling numbers of Tregs. As just mentioned, Tregs can exist in a semi-activated state for prolonged periods of time. This pertains to both "innate" and "adaptive" Tregs. In this state these cells are poised to be attracted to IL-2 sources and respond to minute concentrations of IL-2 because of their high-affinity IL-2R. Once Tregs are activated by high concentrations of IL-2 and the CD28 ligands CD80/86 they begin to secrete IL-10 and change the receptor pattern of migration. Prior to activation Tregs normally express CCR7 and not CCR5, which is a homing receptor pattern for lymph nodes. After activation they switch to a CCR7-CCR5+ pattern that allows them to home to sites of inflammation. Secretion of IL-10 by Tregs allows them to control inflammatory sites through the powerful suppressive activities of this lymphokine. However, once Tregs are activated to secrete IL-10 they become sensitive to FAS/FASL apoptosis because FAS is upregulated on the cells. In addition, it was also determined that there was an upregulation of pro-apoptotic proteins such as BIM and caspase 3. In conjunction with the increase expression of these proteins there was a reciprocal reduction in the expression of the anti-apoptotic protein BCL-2 (Langenhorst 2010). This example of Treg susceptibility to apoptosis is in the category of genetically programmed T cell death because it occurs following the resolution of a normal inflammatory event. However, the reason why it's important is because this process is accelerated during massive viral/bacterial infections and transplantation. Often these activated Tregs become depleted during these responses and pathogenic autoimmune CD4 effector cells take over the response and cause serious tissue damage.

Bronchiolitis obliterans syndrome (BOS) is a condition associated with lung allograft rejection during lung transplantation. This syndrome has a mortality rate of 50-70% in lung transplant patients after a 5-year period (Heng 1998). The induction of this syndrome is associated with several factors such as acute tissue rejection, respiratory viral infections, and autoimmunity (Snyder 2006). Often during the course of BOS Treg numbers dwindle to significantly lower numbers when the transplant rejection was accompanied by respiratory syncytial virus (RSV) infection. This reduction in Treg numbers during this process was related to the expression of FASL on RSV-infected epithelial cells (Bharat 2010). In this same system it was demonstrated that during transplant tolerance Tregs were able to induce CD4 T cells to secrete IL-10 through a cell-to-cell contact method that allowed these CD25-CD4 T cells to induce immune tolerance (Bharat 2006). It was determined that Treg cell-bound TGF-ß was responsible for the induction of this tolerance inducing capability of CD4 T cells (Jonuleit 2002). The situation with Tregs being susceptible to apoptosis is related to the "activation" state of Tregs mentioned above as related to their ability to secrete IL-10. Treg homeostasis is a critical factor in the transplantation process. However, as shown above, transplantation can accelerate the maturation process of Tregs and make them vulnerable to apoptosis. The reason why Treg function is so important during transplantation is that they have the ability to prevent graft vs. host disease or GVHD. This is particularly applicable during (HLA)-haploidentical hematopoietic stem cell transplantation (HSCT) treatment for leukemia, where Tregs not only prevent donor cells from damaging host tissue systems, but also allow the graft vs. leukemia reaction to proceed normally (Di lanni 2011). However, with treatments for leukemia that use allogeneic hematopoietic stem cell transplantation (HSC) and result in the development of lymphopenia (loss of white blood cells) as a result of myeloablative conditioning to remove host leukemia cells, Treg numbers dwindle as GVHD progresses in patients that remain lymphopenic. Again, this situation has to do with the acceleration of Treg maturation, but in this case because the patients were CD4 deficient, it is possible that activated Tregs had no source of IL-2 and became prone to FAS-mediated death (Matsuoka 2010). The result of this development means the donor T cells are allowed to destroy the recipients organ systems.

The loss of Tregs (Treg apoptosis) though this accelerated process of maturity is a serious problem when it comes to lethal or near lethal infections by pathogens or viruses. When the host becomes overwhelmed by infection several things happen that are last attempts of the T cell immune system to save life. Overwhelming infections by pathogens and viruses induce autoreactive CTL. These effectors are generated because almost every cell in the body displays infection. These target cells, which sometimes include uninfected cells, must be eliminated to rid the body of the infection. Tregs are supposed to control the autoreactive T cells, but at a certain point during the infection they suffer from T cell "exhaustion," evidenced above and caused by the acceleration of the maturation process. While all this is going on responder CD4 and CD8 T cells are maturing into effector cells and as a result, stop secreting IL-2. As discussed previously, the lack of an IL-2 source pushes Tregs down the apoptosis pathway initiating the down regulation of BCL-2 and upregulation of BIM. However, the Tregs that are left over are instructed by DC to secrete INF-Γ through the expression of T-BET. The expression of the transcriptional factor T-BET and the secretion of INF-Γ by Tregs under these conditions convert these cells from regulatory T cells into effector T cells (Oldenhove 2009). Recruitment of Tregs to serve as effectors is a process the T cell immune system uses to make a last-ditch effort to save the host from a potential lethal infection. The secretion of INF-γ by Tregs is a characteristic of what is called ex-Tregs, which are Tregs that have lost expression of FOXP3 (Bailey-Bucktrout 2011). INF-γ secretion has positive effects on the T cell immune response because of its ability to induce MHC-class II expression on APCs and thereby activating CD4 T cells that in turn secrete IL-2. This newly secreted IL-2, in conjunction with TGF-ß can induce the creation of new adaptive Tregs that control autoimmune CD4 T cell effectors. However, during the initial stages of this process Treg numbers are diminished as mentioned above and to a certain extent, this event fosters the induction of autoimmunity.

In this context, where you have a life-threatening infection facing the host, Tregs become vulnerable because the T cell responses that they are controlling are massive. Tregs only proliferate where there is the combined stimulus of IL-2, engagement of CD28 by APC, and TCR activation (not essential). Loss of the first two stimuli, but not the latter, moves Tregs down the path of apoptosis. An interesting anomaly that affects both humans and mammals is the fact that when the host ages, Tregs take on a new and unfortunate characteristic. That characteristic is that Tregs in aged individuals are resistant to apoptosis. This resistance seems like a good thing, but actually it's bad for senior humans and mammals. This is one of the reasons why infections and cancer become an issue with age. As youth progresses, bacteria and pathogens regularly induce T cell immune responses. These responses are a normal aspect of a healthy T cell immune system and result in the increase the repertoire of T cells in our bodies. Because of this, we have a steady-state level of IL-2 secretion until advanced age begins and our T cell repertoire is complete as the thymus begins to shrink. However, during this youthful process of secreting IL-2 another population of Tregs is developing. This population of Tregs develops a lower expression of BIM, which causes Tregs to accumulate throughout the body (Chougnet 2011). This has a major impact on the T cell immune system because as previously discussed; Tregs normally have a finite lifespan, which is dependent on environmental signals that activate BIM to induce mitochondrial apoptosis. The most interesting aspect of this resistance to death by Tregs in aged individuals is the fact that instead of Tregs depending on dwindling supplies of IL-2 as we age, these cells make use of another gamma-chain lymphokine called IL-15. Since IL-15 is a gamma-chain lymphokine, it operates through CD122 (IL-2/15Rβ) receptor. This is a common IL-2/IL-15 receptor that can activate both STAT5 and P13K/Akt pathways. Once Tregs in aged individuals become IL-15 dependent, there is a change in BIM expression that may be related to the phosphorylation of the molecule (Raynor 2013). Individuals of advanced age face a plethora of T cell immune abnormalities. The diminution of BIM expression in Tregs is one factor that allows Tregs to control or suppress inflammatory or anti-tumor responses. Again, suppression of inflammatory responses seems like a good thing, but in fact the 'aged' Tregs interfere with a T cell repertoire that has been developed over a lifetime and to a certain extent cannot be replaced by a shrinking thymus.

The information provided above not only demonstrates how Tregs exist as T cells, but also their fragility as effector T cells. Because Tregs basically control the T cell immune system they are endowed with extraordinary effector capabilities above and beyond what has been described so far. Aside from the perforin/granzyme and FAS/FASL mechanisms that Tregs are efficient at, these cells have effector mechanisms that go way beyond the standard T cell's ability to cause disability and death to target cells. First of all, Treg effector mechanisms are mostly, but not always targeted to T cells. Secondly, some of these mechanisms involve invasion the responding T cell's cytoplasm by small biochemical agents (nucleotides such as cAMP) that have the ability redirect translational pathways and cause that T cell to shutdown. It is important to remember that if Tregs are defective, the host usually doesn't survive well. In Chapter 1 there was a discussion of genetic mutations in the FOXP-3 gene and how those mutations led to IPEX syndrome (Bennett 2001). This particular disease is actually fatal, but there are more subtle defects in Treg immunobiology that lead to a host of other diseases. There are a series of diseases associated with primary immune deficiencies (PID) that are Treg-associated. These diseases involve defects in the function of Tregs because of their special requirements for survival. For instance a defect related to the IL-10 receptor can result in inflammatory bowl syndrome (IBS) because the elaboration and autocrine use of this lymphokine by Tregs controls the immune responses to gut bacteria, which are essential for proper digestion. However, the real issue here is that Tregs are the regulators of T cell immune responses that interface with the outside environment (Rubtsov 2008). An even more important aspect to the dysfunction of Tregs associated with PID, whether it be due to the failure of T cells to produce IL-2, or Tregs to respond to IL-10 is the fact that almost all of these disorders such as Wiskott-Aldrich syndrome, Stim1/Oral deficiency, and Omenn syndrome are characterized by debilitating autoimmune responses (Verbsky 2011). Almost all of the problems (IL-2 deprivation, loss of FOXP3 expression, unnatural apoptosis, etc.) associated with Treg control of T cell responses affect the execution of the remaining Treg effector mechanisms that will be described next. Not only will an effort be made to link the use of these mechanisms to particular immunological environments, but also how these environments can inhibit the actions of these Treg-only effector mechanisms.

Treg-Only Effector Mechanisms

The following effector mechanisms described below are for the most part only used by regulatory T cells to not only control other immune cells such as T, B, and NK cells, but also the immunological environment that these cells operate in. There were two instances of this discussed in the previous section. The first was the secretion of GrB by Tregs at an inflammatory site, which contributed to increased permeability of blood vessels and the remodeling of the extracellular matrix to allow for an influx of immune cells and bioactive proteins to enter the site (Buzza 2005). The second instance of Treg control of the immunological environment was related to their presence at the site of a growing tumor where Tregs have the ability to secrete VEGF, which induces angiogenesis and can aid in the escape of tumor cells from the site (Facciabene 2012). Control of these sites (inflammatory and tumor) by Tregs is of paramount importance when it comes to preventing tissue damage by autoreactive T cells. This control by Tregs was mentioned in the previous section during the discussion of the two main effector mechanisms (perforin/granzyme and FAS/FASL) used by T cells, NK cells, and Tregs. This form of control enacted by the use of the perforin/granzyme and FAS/FASL systems was based on apoptosis of either target responding T cells or Tregs themselves. In other words, control of these sites and the autoimmune responses induced by them through the use of these effector mechanisms by Tregs was based on the deaths of immune cells. However, Tregs exert another type of control over these sites and it has to do with the inhibitory function of the non-cell-to-cell contact effector mechanisms. As shown above and will be detailed below, Tregs can secrete powerful immune regulators other than IL-10, VEGF, or GrB. These substances can sometimes permanently or transiently paralyze not only the functions of T cells, NK cells, and DC, but also alter the surrounding cellular milieu and normal tissues. If a massive Treg response occurs in multiple locations in the body it is possible that the host entire immune system may be compromised. As a result, the immune system itself would be unable to protect a body that would be susceptible to additional bacterial and viral infections as well as allowing the induction of cancerous cells or spread of an already established tumor. To a certain extent, this is similar to the "bystander" effect discussed earlier, but on a system-wide level. Therefore it is important to understand how these non-cell-to-cell contact effector mechanisms affect target cells because non-target cells may also be sensitive to their effects.

During this section, and as previously discussed in the prior one, there will be a concerted effort understand under what circumstances a particular Treg effector mechanism is used and why. This is important information because in the next chapter, which deals with Tregs in a clinical setting, the ability to either intervene or augment the function of Tregs during a developing tumor or pre-autoimmune setting may be dependent on which effector mechanism is in use in that particular situation. This will become clear as that chapter unfolds during the descriptions of real immune-based therapeutic clinical trials for the treatment of cancer. However, now it is time to address these varied and complex Treg-only effector mechanisms. Since this book has the unique design of describing the cellular interactions within a particular topic and then describing the translational pathways associated with those interactions in a separate section, some of the transduction pathway descriptions here will be brief. The reason why they are discussed at all has to do with the nature of many of these mechanisms. Many of them are totally based in the translational biology of both the Treg and the target cell. However, just like in the previous section that briefly described the translational pathways involved in mitochondrial apoptosis, it will be necessary to superficially mention pathways associated with these mechanisms because they are intimately related to how Tregs impair the function of its target cell. As described previously, Tregs exert their control over target cells by either making direct contact with the cell (cell-to-cell) or by secreting immunosuppressive substances (non-cell-to-cell) that can kill, inhibit, or paralyze a target cell. However, some of these mechanisms originate from a similar source, but the delivery and agent used to affect the target is different. Such is the case with the cell-to-cell contact mechanism of cAMP injection of effector cells and the non-cell-to-cell contact mechanism the secretion of adenosine. Both of these mechanisms, which will be discussed at length below, utilize ATP stores within and without Tregs to produce the inhibitory effector molecule cAMP. This is a preview of the complexity of these Treg-only effector mechanisms described below.

Non-Cell-to-Cell Contact Treg Effector Mechanisms

Adenosine

The release of adenosine is one of its most powerful immunosuppressive effector mechanisms possessed by Tregs because of the multiple effects induced in the many cells throughout the body that posses the adenosine receptors. The effects of Treg-secreted adenosine during inflammatory responses tend to be immunosuppressive in nature and add to the ability of Tregs to control inflammatory sites. Some of these activities are beneficial and some can be detrimental to the normal functioning of the immune system (Ernst 2010). Adenosine itself is the product of catabolism of ATP by extracellular ecto-5' –nuclease (CD73) and ecto-NTPDase-1 (CD39) and will be discussed in more detail later. The source of ATP is drawn from intercellular sources because cells release it during inflammation as they die and is utilized by Tregs to produce adenosine (Deaglio 2006). There are four types of adenosine receptors (A1, A2A, A2B, and A3) of which several are widely expressed on cells throughout the body and the resultant cellular activity depends upon which receptor receives the adenosine (Fredholm 2001). As far as the expression of adenosine receptors by activated helper CD4 and CD8 CTL is concerned, the adenosine receptors A2A, A2B, and A3 are expressed on CD4 cells, but only A2A and A2B on activated CD8 CTL (Mirabet 1999). Binding of adenosine to is receptor leads to an increase in target cell intracellular cAMP. There are multiple negative effects on not only responding T cells, but also on DC and macrophages.

Adenosine receptor ligation on activated T cells and the subsequent build-up of cAMP results in a significant reduction (80-90%) in the ability of T cells to produce two inflammatory cytokines (IL-12 and TNF-α) that initiate the inflammatory process (Hasko 2000). Another anti-inflammatory aspect of this interaction of adenosine with its receptors is the marked reduction in IL-2 secretion by responding T cells. Engagement of the A2A and A2B receptors by adenosine induces the accumulation of cAMP, which activates the cAMP-dependent protein kinase pathway (PKA) and leads to the phosphorylation of PKA substrates such as the cAMP response element binding protein (CREB), cAMP response element modulator (CREM), and activating transcription factor-1 (ATF-1), which are located in the nucleus (Taylor 2008 and Sands 2008). Once these substrates increase their transcriptional activity multiple lymphokine pathways are affected. The action of cAMP on cell processes is mediated by what is called cAMP "sensors," which the PKA pathway is one of. Another one of these cAMP sensors is an exchange protein called cAMP/cAMP-regulated guanine nucleotide exchange factors (EPAC/cAMP-GEF) or EPAC (Cheng 2008). EPAC, like PKA is activated by cAMP and is involved in cell proliferation, survival, and secretion/metabolism of Ca2+. EPAC (EPAC1 and EPAC2) also regulates integrin-mediated adhesion and cell-to-cell synaptic formation. This is an important function for Tregs because they have a unique ability to interface (synaptic formation) with target cells such as T cells and DC. Epac1 can signal either by itself or in concert with PKA to induce expression of the suppressor of cytokine signaling proteins (SOC1 and SOC2), which inhibit T cell responses by limiting lymphokine secretion (Dimitriou 2008). There are several other cAMP sensor translational pathways, but this one and the next are important because they directly impact the dependence on inflammatory lymphokines needed by responding T cells.

Adenosine and Lymphokine Secretion

The diminution of IL-2 secretion by Treg-secreted adenosine is an important factor in controlling T cell responses during an anti-tumor or inflammatory response. Initially, it would seem that the reduction of IL-2 production by responding T cells induced by Tregs would be detrimental to their existence since they are totally dependent on this lymphokine to not only induce tolerance, but also to survive. However, one must realize the magnitude of sensitivity to IL-2 that Tregs posses because of their high-affinity IL-2 receptor. Tregs can function and survive on amounts of IL-2 that are insufficient to support normal naïve T cell activation. As will be shown below, the simple secretion of adenosine endows Tregs with the ability to control T cell responses by controlling not only the inhibition of secretion of lymphokines by responding T cells, but also induce the positive secretion of lymphokines by responding T cells and DC that either redirect T cell differentiation or contribute to the control of the anti-inflammatory setting imposed by Tregs. As far as the inhibition of the most important lymphokine (IL-2) is concerned, a study of HIV infection and the resulting loss of CD4 T cells revealed that CD39/73 produced adenosine from Tregs and the resultant induction of adenyl cyclase activity (cAMP production) induces the inhibition of target T cells to demethylated the CpG site1 region of the IL-2 promoter, which halts IL-2 secretion (Jenabian 2013). Another model, which involves the cAMP PKA pathway, results in the activation of SHP-2 that causes the dephosphorylation of STAT5. If left unabated, phosphorylated STAT5 forms a complex with other STAT proteins in the nucleus (covered in Chapter 1) that results in the transcription of IL-2. The cAMP PKA pathway interferes with this process and it results in the inhibition of IL-2 secretion by responding T cells (Zhang 2004). The intracellular pathways that are responsible for the inhibition of IL-2 secretion will be detailed in the next section. However, here Treg control of these inflammatory sites induces a redirection of T cell differentiation into phenotype that only induces antibody production. Once antigen specific CD4 T cells arrive at a inflammatory or tumor site their task is to respond, secrete lymphokines (IL-2, INF-γ) and multiply, but most importantly to activate CD8 effector cells that go about the task of killing the invasive threat. This is a TH-1 CD4 activity that is induced by TCR and CD28 stimulation and is dependent upon IL-2 and IL-12 secretion at the site. Unfortunately, when CD4 T cell responders encounter adenosine and accumulate intercellular cAMP, the PKA pathway takes control. The result is a down-regulation of IL-2 and INF-γ secretion, but an up-regulation of the secretion IL-4. What this means is that as CD4 T cells arrive at these sites where Tregs dominate, they are redirected to produce antibodies via the activation of B-cells (Tokoyoda 2004). However, this is not the only way Treg-secreted adenosine controls the T cell response at these sites.

Adenosine and DC

Another way Treg-secreted adenosine can influence an inflammatory site is its effects on DC. Immature DC can actually use adenosine as a chemoattractant through the A1A receptor expressed by these cells. DCs will be attracted to inflammatory sites by adenosine, which in addition to being a chemo attractant can also inhibit IL-12 and TNF-A secretion. In addition, it was determined that both cAMP and adenosine itself cannot only cause the effects mentioned above, but could also induce these immature DC to secrete high levels of IL-10. As DC fully mature they lose the ability to express the A1A receptor yet retain the expression of both A2A and A2B receptors and this is thought to facilitate their homing to the regional lymph nodes (Panther 2013). Earlier in Chapter 1 it was stated that TH17 T cells secrete CCL20 or MIP-3α at inflammatory sites to attract Tregs and other inflammatory cells that express the CCL20 receptor CCR6 (Yamazaki 2008). It turns out that adenosine induces DCs to hypersecrete CCL17, which is a powerful chemo attractant for Tregs (Mizukami 2008). Binding of adenosine or adenosine agonist such as 5'-N –ethlcarboxamidoadenosine (NECA) to the A2B receptor has profound effects on newly generated immature DCs. Once this receptor is occupied by adenosine (agonist), the normal differentiation pathway into the standard mature myeloid DC phenotype is altered. This is a distinctly different population of DC totally unable to induce a TH-1 CD4 T cell response. Instead, these DC induce TH-2 responses (antibody production), which in itself is not a good thing because of the propensity of DC to induce the secretion autoantibodies as discussed previously. As mentioned above, these DC are unable to secrete IL-12 and TNF-α, but instead secrete proinflammatory cytokines such as IL-6, IL-8, and as also mentioned above, the immunosuppressive lymphokine IL-10 (Saraiva 2010), which inhibits INF-γ secretion by activated CD8 T cells. In addition to these cytokines, adenosine responsive DC secrete Treg-forming TGF-ß. Two other factors are secreted by these A2B receptor activated DC and those are indoleamine 2,3-dioxygenase (IDO) and VEGF (Ryzhov 2008). IDO, which was mentioned previously, induces T cell paralysis and VEGF secretion was just mentioned as a Treg secreted angiogenic factor that increases vascularization of a tumor site. Here, the purpose is to allow as many cells as possible to enter the inflammatory site. The main cells that enter inflammatory site of this type are CD4 T cells and they two are directly affected by adenosine altered DC.

Because adenosine redirects DC differentiation by inhibiting DC maturation, the ability of DC to present antigen is practically lost due to the minimal expression of CD80 and CD86 (B7.1 and B7.2) and MHC-class II. In fact, when studying bone marrow derived DC it was found that there was no adenosine agonist (NECA) effect on the cells until they were stimulated with LPS. Once stimulated by this adenosine analogue the DC took on the tolerance inducing phenotype described above (Wilson 2009). Therefore, it is not until resting DC/monocytes become activated that adenosine can redirect the phenotype of DC to induce a non-productive CD4 T cell response. Not only do these tolerogenic DC impede the development of a TH1 CD4 response by skewing CD4 T cell differentiation to the TH2 type of response, but they are also able to induce proinflammatory TH17 effector cells. In Chapter 1 there was a considerable amount of time spent on the "reprogramming" process of Tregs into inflammatory TH17 T cells. It was pointed out that a growing tumor had the ability to direct DCs to secrete IL-6 and TGF-ß in order to transform Tregs into TH-17 T cells (Bonnefoy 2011). It was determined that in order for DCs to accomplish this "reprogramming" event IL-1β had to be present (Li 2010). The source of the IL-1β comes from the interaction of systemic ATP released from "stressed" cells and TLR-2 activation in blood monocytes and as they enter the inflammatory site these cells begin to secrete IL-1β (Paustian 2013).

Adenosine is a modulator of the inflammatory site. Because of the wide array of cells and tissues that have adenosine receptors, the elaboration of adenosine by Tregs is a pivotal juncture in the control of the inflammatory process. Its involvement in sculpting inflammation based on the inflammatory agent is crucial to a successful outcome. Tregs facilitate control over the T cell response in many ways, but the secretion of adenosine has wide-ranging effects. Once DCs are altered by their encounter with adenosine they begin to alter the cellularity of an inflammatory site to suit the situation. When it comes to dealing with pathogens DCs, under the influence of Treg-secreted adenosine, begin to secrete massive amounts of IL-6 via adenosine activation through the A2B receptor. It was found that IL-6 secretion was not entirely dependent on elevated levels of cAMP as shown for the A2A receptors, but that the participation of MAPKs such as ERK played a major role. What this does is that when CD4 responders enter the site they are immediately transformed or "converted" into TH17 effectors mainly through the secretion of IL-6 by A2B receptor activated DC. However, TGF-ß is an important component because antibodies against it inhibited TH17 development. TH17 T cells are an important part of the anti-microbial immune response during the inflammatory response to pathogens (Bettelli 2008). Once this CD4 T cell to TH17 T cell conversion begins to occur there is a decrease in FOXP3 expression as if some of the TH17 T cells were derived from "reprogrammed" Tregs or that since TGF-ß was limiting in this system, the development of Tregs was also limited (Wilson 2011). In addition, the antigen presentation capabilities of DCs in this situation (systemic secretion of adenosine) favor the selection of TH17 T cells because the antigens are microbial in nature and not self, which would favor the creation of Tregs (Kushwah 2010) through the phagocytosis of apoptotic DC (Albert 1998). Nonetheless, the triggering of this process during an inflammatory response may induce tissue damage by these TH17 effectors. This process by which DC control the fate of T cells based on the secretion of adenosine by Tregs is primarily centered on the A2B adenosine receptor.

Adenosine and Responding T Cells

When addressing the effects of adenosine on T cells such as above with the adenosine-mediated inhibition of IL-2 secretion by responding T cells, the A2A adenosine receptor is the main focus. As mentioned above, the vast majority of T cell types express this receptor including Tregs. The effects of adenosine binding to the A2A receptor on CD4 and CD8 activated T cells resemble the anergic "state" mentioned in Chapter 2. How adenosine, through its interaction with the A2A receptor, induces T cell anergy starts with the accumulation of cAMP within the responding T cell and will be discussed at length shortly. However, now the similarities in the T cell functional characteristics of the classic "anergic state" such as that induced by the single-signal (TCR-only stimulation) method, and that induced by the adenosine A2A receptor will be examined. A2A receptor induced anergic T cells and "classic" anergic T cells share quite a few common features. One of these is the inability to respond to re-challenge with either specific antigen or activation by anti-TCR antibodies for an extended period of time. One of the main reasons for this inability to respond is that as a result of the induction of anergy either through classic methods (Jenkins 1990) or by A2A activation (Jenabian 2013 and Zhang 2004), responding anergic T cells lose the ability to secrete IL-2, which is the main lymphokine responsible for T cell proliferation. Despite the fact that exogenous IL-2 can reverse the anergy in both cases (Schwartz 1987 and Zarek 2008), these anergic effector T cells often find themselves in an IL-2-deprived environment due to the presence of Tregs, which absorb vast amounts of the lymphokine in order to function. IL-2 depravation of effector T cells by Tregs will be addressed shortly, but now it is important to know that this Treg effector mechanism has a purpose. The anergic state found in CD4 T cells induced by single-signal stimulation and by A2A activation have transcriptional characteristics in common, which will be discussed in detail during the next section concerning the translational pathways of Treg effector mechanisms. Now as an introduction, translational pathways involved in the initiation phase of anergy in both systems will be briefly mentioned.

During the discussion of single-signal T cell anergy induction in Chapter 2 it was shown how NFAT could play dual roles in induction of T cell proliferation or T cell anergy. During the two-signal (TCR and CD28 engagement) induction process NFAT has ability to form complexes with AP-1 and in cooperation with NFkB and induce T cell proliferation through IL-2 promoter binding to specific NFAT/AP-1 binding sites. However, during the single-signal process diacylglycerol (DAG), which controls the activation of pathways that lead to AP-1 and NFkB activation, which gets converted into phosphatidic acid (PA) by diacylglycerol kinases or DGKs results in calcineurin dephosphorylated NFAT that enters the nucleus (Zhong 2008). Once in the nucleus NFAT and its isoforms can activate over 100 anergy-inducing proteins such as E3 ubiquitin ligases (Itch, Cbl-b, and GRAIL) as well as the DGK genes that inhibit AP-1 activation through the DAG to PA conversion process (Baine 2009). As far as A2A activation by adenosine and the induction of T cell anergy is concerned, the clue to the involvement of NFAT was derived from the observation that Tregs, which constituently express high levels of cAMP, also expressed high levels of inducible cAMP early repressor (ICER) and cAMP response modulator (CREM). ICER is a transcriptional repressor protein derived from the 3' end of the CREM gene. ICER can form complexes with NFAT. These complexes can bind specifically to NFAT/AP-1 sites within the IL-2 promoter region, which effectively block the ability of NFAT/AP-1 complexes bind to the IL-2 promoter, which halts IL-2 secretion (Bodor 1998). Because Tregs naturally have a build-up of cytoplasmic cAMP, this is the primary reason why Tregs do not secrete IL-2.

However, it was found that responding T cells, which had been induced to become anergic by either increased cAMP build-up due to Treg-secreted adenosine or cAMP directly injected into these cells by Tregs, a very similar transcriptional pathway involving another member of the NFAT family called NFATc1 was involved. NFATc1 is one of five NFAT family members (NFAT, NFATc1, c2, c3, and c4), but unlike NFATs c2, c3, and c4 that induce T cell anergy, reduce T cell proliferation, and increase the sensitivity to activation-induced cell death (AICD), NFATc1 expression enhances T cell proliferation and resistance to AICD (Serfling 2013). When expression of NFATc1 is inhibited T cell proliferation ceases. This is exactly what happens when ICER alone or ICER/NFAT complexes bind to the NFATc1 P1 promoter, which results in the blockage of gene transcription (Vaeth 2011). It was also later determined that ICER could form complexes with NFATc1 and c2 with the same result (Bodor 2012). In addition to this, NFAT/AP-1 binding sites are present in the promoter regions of several important cytokines such as TNF-α, IL-4, IL13, and GM-CSF, which are all susceptible to transcriptional suppression by NFAT/ICER complexes (Hogan 2003). Therefore, the induction of cAMP in responding T cells can result in more than simple inhibition of IL-2 secretion, which is the induction of anergy as in the single-signal model. Moreover, the type of anergy induced by the Treg secreted adenosine-A2A interaction or Treg injection of cAMP is specifically immune-paralytic in nature, which renders active responding T cells unable to function as immune cells.

Adenosine and Treg Immunobiology

One of the most interesting aspects of the role adenosine plays in the regulation of cells that participate in the inflammatory process has to be how adenosine affects the cell that produces it; the Treg. In the beginning of this chapter, in the first section called, *The Two Main Effector Mechanisms* and under the sub-heading *Functional Use, Sensitivity, and Resistance of Tregs and Accessory Cells to Perforin/granzyme and FAS/FASL Effector Mechanisms* there was this sentence: "Despite the fact that Tregs are the most "advanced" T cell in the T cell immune system, they are nonetheless T cells and to a certain extent, adhere to T cell immunobiological rules." The operative words in that sentence are "to a certain extent." Yes, Tregs are the most advanced T cells in the T cell immune system and yes, Tregs are T cells and for most of they're existence follows the biological rules that govern all other T cells. However, their response to adenosine and the subsequent increase in cytoplasmic cAMP is one of the only exceptions to the statement made in that sentence extracted from the first section of this chapter. As will be shown below, not only is it a major exception in terms of T cell immunobiology, but also the description of the response to adenosine by Tregs will reveal the true nature of the biological functions that separate all other T cells from Tregs. One of the clues to the assertion that this response to adenosine by Tregs is a major exception to T cell "biological rules" is how the Treg response is completely opposite to the response to adenosine by its target cell, which are activated responding CD4 and CD8 T cells. The effects of Treg-created adenosine on DC are not relevant to this discussion because it has been previously demonstrated that adenosine-induced changes in DC target responding T cells. The description that is about to follow begins with the synthesis of adenosine by Tregs and ends not with Tregs suffering adenosine-induced anergy, but with Treg proliferation. As just mentioned, this is an opposite T cell response and for Tregs, a cycle necessary to establish immunological homeostasis.

In order to really appreciate this topic it would be good to start with adenosine synthesis by Tregs and specifically adenosine produced by the ecto-enzyme CD73 (CD73/ecto-5' – nuclease). This cell surface molecule expressed by Tregs and endothelial cells has the ability to de-phosphorylate extracellular ATP into adenosine through a hydrolization reaction. The reaction is as follows: ATP converted into ADP, then to AMP and conversion into adenosine is next, with inosine as a by-product. This is called the purinergic pathway and it enables Tregs to freely elaborate adenosine into the cellular matrix of an inflammatory site where dead and stressed cells are releasing ATP (Salmi 2012). When Tregs arrive at either a site of inflammation or cancer they begin to basically synthesize adenosine as a first response because of the prevalence of cell damage caused by the tumor. As Tregs establish themselves they proceed to do what has been described above, which is take control of the situation by altering immune cellular behavior in such a way as to dampen the T cell immune response. It was mentioned that Tregs, like the rest of the T cells express the receptors (A2A, A2B, and A3) that are characteristic adenosine receptors for responding T cells. The adenosine that they secrete does two things. The first is what has been mentioned in terms of shutting-down the T cell response in an active inflammatory situation, but the second thing that happens is that the Treg cell becomes activated. The Treg is actually a biological adenosine-synthesizing pump. During injury caused by viral, bacterial infection, transplantation or cancer, the release of ATP by the cells affected is a natural by-product of cellular damage as mentioned above. Tregs arrive, sense the presence of ATP and immediately begin to convert it into adenosine and this dampens the possibility of there being an autoimmune response based on the rampant proliferation of T cells responding to the above mentioned events.

As far as cancer is concerned the Treg, via its elaboration of adenosine into not only the tumor site itself, but also the draining lymph nodes, initiates a two-step inhibitory process directed at anti-tumor responding T cells and the escape of tumor cells from the site. The Treg-mediated escape of tumor cells from the site was mentioned earlier when it was determined that Tregs can secrete VEGF and induce angiogenesis thereby increasing the blood supply to the tumor mass and providing a means of escape to the periphery (Facciabene 2012). In addition, just previously there was a discussion on the effects of adenosine on monocytes and DCs and how adenosine induced these cells to create immunosuppressive conditions during inflammatory responses. It turns out that adenosine also has the ability to induce the secretion of VEGF by macrophages through all three (A2A, A2B, and A3) receptors (Hasko 2012). Again, by the secretion of adenosine, Tregs command control of the inflammatory site through the invitation of lymphocytes by the secretion of chemo attractant lymphokines and increased vascularization. Once at the site, the function and sometimes the phenotype (Treg conversion) of responding T cells are taken over by not only the effects of adenosine, but also by the directed secretion of immunosuppressive lymphokines such as IL-10. This two-step process (tumor escape and responding T cell suppression), which results in the inhibition of the anti-tumor T cell response by Tregs, represents one of the most complex problems to address concerning the immunotherapeutic treatment of cancer. The reason has to do with not only the multiple ways the Tregs directly suppress responding T cell function, but also the involvement of other immune cells in that process. This topic will be addressed in the next chapter concerning the clinical aspects of cancer immunotherapy as they relate to Treg immunobiology.

Adenosine and Treg Survival

As previously mentioned in the section above, the response to adenosine by Tregs is completely different from the response of Treg target cells (responding CD4 and CD8 T cells) to adenosine via the A2A receptors. The first aspect of this discussion regarding Treg survival and adenosine is actually related to how adenosine and activation of the A2A receptor by adenosine or adenosine agonist interfere with FAS/FASL activation-induced cell death or AICD in T cells. The role that the activation of the A2A receptor plays in T cell function is a complex one. It is highly dependent on the stage of development of the T cell in question and the immunological environment T cells find themselves in. For instance, activation through the A2A receptor does cause apoptosis in a variety of non-T cell types (Jacobson 1999) and in thymocytes (Apasov 2000) under adenosine deaminase deficiency (ADA) conditions. However, it was recently determined that A2A receptor activation in TCR activated T cells resulted in their resistance to cell death mediated by the FAS/FASL interaction by interfering with production of both FAS and FASL proteins. As mentioned earlier, once A2A receptor is activated adenyl cyclase production is increased and initiates the cAMP-dependent protein kinase pathway (PKA). Here, the A2A receptor mediated inhibition of FAS/FASL death is sensitive to PKA inhibitors. With just looking at the reduction of FASL expression caused by A2A activation in CD4 T cells it was apparent that the FASL promoter was one of those 100 T cell anergy-inducing promoters mentioned earlier that was controlled by NFAT and NFkB binding (Landinis 1997) as a result of inhibition of the API pathway that led to the 'state' of T cell anergy (Baine 2009). With respects to resistance to AICD in CD4 T cells mentioned here, it was determined that A2A stimulation not only diminished NFAT and NFkB activity, but also reduced the upregulation of ERG-1 and ERG-3, which also participate in FASL promoter activation of the FASL gene (Himer 2010). The ability of A2A receptor activation-mediated inhibition of AICD through the FAS/FASL system by the suppression of the activities of particularly NFAT is understandable considering what was previously discussed in regards to the affects of adenosine on T cell IL-2 secretion and proliferation. This was the activation of the A2A receptor and the subsequent build-up of inducible cAMP early repressor (ICER) and the ability of ICER to form complexes with NFAT, which results in the inhibition of IL-2 secretion (Bodor 1998). In addition, it was found that ICER alone or ICER/NFAT complexes could block the NFATc1 promoter effectively stopping T cell proliferation mediated by NFATc1 (Vaeth 2011). In light of this information it is clear that this action mediated by the activation of the A2A receptor by adenosine or adenosine agonist allows Tregs to avoid FAS/FASL AICD, which gives them a survival advantage during inflammatory situations where Tregs are producing adenosine.

For Tregs and other T cells this is just one stage of survival, which is to resist multiple forms of cell death and in this case the adenosine receptor provides protection from AICD. This advantage is an obvious one for Tregs because it allows them to operate in immunological environments full of cells expressing FASL without being killed. Indeed, the standard inflammatory environment induced by injury, infection, and cancer draw in FASL expressing cells such as activated T cells and APC. With regards to a growing tumor mass, it was discussed earlier that tumors derived from "immune privileged" FAS-expressing tissues protected themselves from destruction by anti-tumor T cells, but during cancer-induced inflammation where Tregs begin to elaborate adenosine, they are allowed to freely function in this environment because of this reduction of FAS expression. As far as activated anti-tumor CD4 and CD8 T cells are concerned in this situation, they too are allowed to be present in the tumor mass, but because of the immunosuppressive conditions induced by Tregs, these responding T cells are powerless to attack the tumor. The induction of FAS/FASL resistance in responding T cells is a way to temporarily paralyze responding T cells, but not kill them. If any of these paralyzed responding T cells does manage to escape the tumor site eventually they regain immunologic capabilities. Initially, this allows the T cell immune system to destroy metastasizing tumor cells that take-up residence in off-site tissues. However, it becomes a numbers game after that because each single tumor cell that escapes the initial tumor site begins to rapidly form another tumor site at a distant location. These new sites begin to initiate the cancer-induced inflammatory process and Tregs begin to appear as the cycle begins anew. Therefore, the resistance to ACID bestowed on responding T cells by A2A activation does give the host a second chance to defeat the tumor by allowing these cells to survive the inflammatory environment of the tumor mass. As mentioned above and with regards to Tregs, resistance to cell death is only the first step cell survival. The next step, also involving the A2A receptor is Treg proliferation.

Adenosine and Treg Proliferation

In general, Treg proliferation by itself is complex because essentially as outlined in this and the preceding chapters, Tregs exist in a state of T cell anergy. As will be shown, they do have the ability to proliferate in response to minute amounts of IL-2. However, Tregs use the high-affinity IL-2 receptor not only as a lymphokine sensor, but also an inducer of effector functions (Barron 2010), the proliferative capabilities of the Treg are limited and restricted to certain inflammatory conditions. On a transcriptional level the "anergic state" of Tregs closely resembles that of T cells that were induced to become anergic through the single-signal activation of T cells via the TCR. For the most part the anergic state of the Treg is focused on the expression of the FOXP3 gene. When FOXP3 gene expression is diminished Tregs can begin the process of cell proliferation. Even though there are other factors involved such as cAMP/PKA pathway, which will be discussed shortly, the expression of FOXP3 is an essential element in creating the Treg anergic state. As discussed in chapter 2, during normal T cell proliferation in response to antigen, cyclin-dependent kinases (CDKs) control the T cell's entry into the cell cycle and facilitate cell division (Sherr 1999). However, in Tregs proliferation is inhibited by the activation of the MAPK/P38 pathway, which leads to the upregulation of cyclin-dependent kinase inhibitors (CDKIs) such as P15, P19, P21 and the most important one, P27kip1 (Adler 2008). The expression of P27kip1 effectively halts T cell proliferation. It is constitutively produced in functional Tregs that express FOXP3 (Li 2005). As mentioned previously, FOXO3 transcriptional proteins that enter the nucleus control

CDKIs. These FOXO3 proteins have the ability to activate the genetic expression all of CDKIs mentioned above (Hendrick 2012). As previously discussed, high-level signals from the Tregs IL-2 receptor generally support the expression of FOXP3 and if these signals are diminished FOXP3 expression weakens. If at the same time, Tregs become stimulated through the TCR and CD28, the P13/Akt pathway is activated. Akt has the ability to phosphorylate FOXO3, which makes its entry into the nucleus impossible and therefore the activation of CDKIs does not occur and at the same time CDKs become active. It was recently determined that the FOXP3 gene posses several CDK motifs in its N-terminal repressor domain that become sites of phosphorylation by the activity of CDK2 and cyclin E. Once these sites on the FOXP3 gene are phosphorylated, genetic stability and function is lost (Morawski 2013). As far as Treg proliferation during an inflammatory response is concerned, there are other restrains contributing to the anergic state related to the activation of the A2A receptor by adenosine, yet under these conditions Tregs have the ability to proliferate. T cell proliferation is the mainstay of Treg cell survival because without it, their targets can quickly outnumber them.

Adenosine, Treg Proliferation, and GVHD

One of the models where the proliferation or survival of Tregs is of paramount importance is graft vs. host disease or GVHD (Koreth 2013). Earlier, when discussing Treg FAS/FASL sensitivity to apoptosis due to the lack of a source of IL-2 during allogeneic HSC transplant treatment (HSCT) for leukemia, it was also mentioned that donor Tregs expanded and ameliorated GVHD by inhibiting responding donor T cells as long as the patients did not develop CD4 lymphopenia (Matsuoka 2010). However, when studying HSCT in a mouse model it was determined that Tregs inhibited the response of GVHD-inducing donor allogeneic responding T cells by inhibiting DC-induced T cell activation by cAMP injection of the cells. Phosphodiesterases (PDEs) are enzymes that inhibit cAMP and inhibitors of PDE increase the GVHD inhibiting capabilities of Tregs in this situation (Weber 2013). Therefore, during this type of transplantation therapy, cAMP and as will be shown adenosine, play a critical role in the therapeutic outcome because of the absolute requirement of Tregs, which control GVHD-inducing T cells. Using A2A receptor (A2A-R) agonist in this same model it was shown that not only did donor Tregs inhibit GVHD-inducing T cells, but also TGF-ß dependent Treg proliferation occurred during the transplant. Treatment with several different A2A-R analogues actively mediated a diminution of GVHD symptoms and increased survival rates dramatically. It was determined that not only was there an increase in Treg numbers in the periphery, but also in the colon and skin. In addition, serum levels of pro-inflammatory cytokines such as TNF-α, INF-γ, IL-6, and GM-CSF were reduced in A2A-R agonist treated recipients, while the anti-inflammatory cytokines TGF-ß and IL-10, which both participate in Treg induction/proliferation were significantly increased. In this study it was thought the increase in Treg numbers was due to TGF-ß induction of FOXP3 expression due to the significant increase in TGF-ß in the serum. However, it was conceded that this might not be the case; rather the increased TGF-ß in the sera was an indirect effect of this type of transplant-related T cell immune response (Han 2013). This is an interesting situation because on the face of it, Tregs should not be able to proliferate under A2A-R activation given the inhibitory nature of the build-up of cAMP and the resulting T cell anergy induced by ICER/NFAT complexes.

The immunological environment during HSCT for leukemia and other cancers is one of heightened inflammation. The inflammatory site does not merely consist of the multi-millimeter space surrounding a growing tumor or infectious area. Nor does it involve multiple joint interfaces such as the case with arthritis. During these transplantation treatments using lymphoid cells the inflammatory site is the entire body and more specifically the lymphatic and peripheral circulatory systems. As previously mentioned, peripheral blood levels of pro-inflammatory cytokines increase during HSCT. In addition adenosine, (produced by Tregs during an inflammatory response of this type and multiple cell types in response to injury) levels become critically high. One of the harmful effects of continued exposure of tissues to adenosine is the development of fibrosis in the lungs and liver by the A2AR-induced elevation of collagen levels in these tissues (Chan 2010). Therefore, extended periods of systemic inflammation can be dangerous, but because of the activities of Tregs, which dampen inflammation, this period should be brief. This is one of the many reasons why Treg proliferation under these conditions is a critical factor in not only the development of GVHD, but also the development of fibrotic tissue in the lungs and liver. Yet it seems almost impossible for Tregs to enter the proliferative phase due to the anergic conditions not only already present in Treg immunobiology, but also the ones dictated by cAMP build-up, activation of the PKA pathway, and subsequent inhibition of proliferation via blocking NFAT/AP1 activation of proliferative genes such as IL-2, as well as the inhibition of the T cell proliferation inducer NFATc1's promoter by ICER or ICER/NFAT complexes. In addition to these Treg cell intrinsic anergic factors there is a negative extrinsic factor, which is the dwindling supply of IL-2 that becomes in short supply as responding T cells succumb to the effects of A2AR activation. However, this reduction in the supply of IL-2 available to Tregs is actually the beginning steps toward Treg proliferation.

Adenosine, Treg Proliferation, and the Adenosine Receptor

Clearly it is apparent that adenosine production by Tregs is an essential mechanism used by these cells to control inflammation during standard inflammatory responses as well as during tumor-induced inflammatory responses and GVHD. It was shown that a deficiency in ecto- 5' –nucleotidase or CD73 resulted in unabated T cell responses and the upregulation of proinflammatory cytokines such as INF-γ and IL-6, which causes an enhanced expansion of GVHD-inducing T cells mediated by donor T cells (Tsukamoto 2012). However, the fact is that there is very little difference between a donor's T cell that causes GVHD and the same donor's T cell that attacks the tumor. Therefore, during the process of inflammation reduction by adenosine through the A2AR, anti-tumor T cells are also inhibited. The balance between donor anti-tumor T cells and GVHD-inducing T cells is of critical importance to the survival of the transplant recipient (Thompson 2013). This is where the study of A2AR agonist revealed that there was a benefit (lessen GVHD) to increased stimulation through this receptor. Consequently, it was determined that A2AR agonist induced a massive increase in the Treg population during GVHD and in vitro. This was a direct result of Treg proliferation during an active inflammatory response. As mentioned earlier there are two types of Tregs, which are innate (derived in the thymus) and adaptive (T cells converted into Tregs) that constitute the two major types of Tregs. In this study it was found that there was both innate and adaptive Treg expansion and the expansion of adaptive Tregs was the result of conversion of CD4+ CD25- T cells into CD4+ CD25+ Tregs. However, it was pointed out that adaptive

Tregs were a small minority of the Tregs contained within the Treg expanded population and for the most part innate Tregs represented the majority of Tregs generated by the stimulation of Treg A2AR. In addition, it was shown that Tregs expanded by A2AR agonist displayed a four-fold increase in suppressive ability when compared to controls (Ohta 2012). More than likely the primary reason why adaptive Tregs are not either being created or proliferating has to do with the low levels of both IL-2 and TGF-ß produced by responding T cells under the influence of A2AR stimulation. However, recently it was determined that as a result of the activation of the PKA pathway by cAMP inhibits the ability of TGF-ß to induce FOXP3 expression in CD4 T cells. In addition, a PKA site-specific activator (6-MB-cAMP), which can substitute for cAMP-induced PKA activation demonstrated significant, but not complete reduction in the ability of TGF-ß to induce FOXP3 expression. This inhibition of the ability of TGF-ß to induce adaptive Tregs is the result of the cAMP-induced PKA blocking of ERK and JNK activation, which augments TGF-ß induction of FOXP3 (Cao 2013). As previously mentioned in Chapter 1, TGF-ß activates SMAD2 and SMAD3 in conjunction with P38 activation during the process of FOXP3 induction in naive T cells. A study that closely examined TGF-ß induction of FOXP3 expression revealed that TGF-ß does not act alone in inducing FOXP3, but that another member of the TGF-ß supergene family called bone morphogenetic proteins (BMP) synergize with TGF-ß during this process. It was found that BMP-4 augmented the ability of TGF-ß to induce FOXP3 expression through the activation (phosphorylation) of ERK1/2 and JNK (Lu 2010).

Adenosine, Treg Proliferation, and Anergy

From the evidence presented so far it is apparent that Tregs do indeed proliferate during inflammatory episodes, be it a localized/systemic, bacterial/viral infection, GVHD episode, or the site of a growing tumor. Each and every one of these situations beg the question: How in the world can these cells, which are basically anergic, gain the ability to increase their numbers in the face of fluctuating IL-2 concentrations and limiting amounts of TGF-ß. One of the things that have to be understood is the fact that Tregs display a remarkable 'plasticity' in their response in any given the situation. For instance, the example above describes how innate, but not particularly adaptive Tregs proliferate during GVHD. However, in other situations like viral/bacterial infections or at a growing tumor site, adaptive Tregs are not only created, but also proliferate. The reason why this section concerning the role of Treg-secreted adenosine has been so elongated is that it has shed some light on the intricacies of Treg immunobiology. One of the characteristics of Tregs, be they innate or adaptive is the retention and build-up of cAMP (Ohta 2012). The next section, which concerns itself with cell-to-cell contact Treg effector mechanisms will demonstrate how Tregs inject responding T cells with cAMP, thus rendering them useless as effector T cells. This is a major effector mechanism used routinely by Tregs to gain control over inflammatory situations. However, the temporary depletion of cAMP stores within the Treg during its use of this effector mechanism may be related to how Tregs manage to proliferate despite their anergic phenotype. Steady-state cAMP levels in not only Tregs, but in other cells of the body are increased or decreased for various reasons that are almost always (except for Tregs) related to cellular stress. Adenyl cyclases (ACs) are the enzymes that synthesize cAMP and are a family of enzymes that can either be transmembrane-bound or found in a soluble form. As far as cAMP regulation is concerned, phosphodiesterases (PDEs) that were mentioned previously are enzymes that hydrolyze cAMP into 5' –AMP (Gancedo 2013). PDE activity in Tregs is important because inhibition of this enzyme by PDE4 inhibitors not only increased the suppressive properties of Tregs (Bopp 2009), but also increased their ability to delay skin allograft rejection (Feng 2011). Once IL-2 activates Tregs, AC activity and cAMP production are increased, which is the opposite for responding CD4 T cells where these events are decreased (Bazhin 2010). Therefore, Tregs actively regulate AC activity by degrading cAMP with PDEs and as previously discussed, cAMP through CREB inhibition of transcription, restrain Treg proliferation as long as cAMP is present.

Earlier, when discussing T cell anergy induced by the single-signal received by T cells when the TCR, but not CD28 is ligated together on the T cell surface it was determined that this activity led to T cell anergy. Amongst the myriad of inhibitory signals received by the T cell during this process, there is also the recruitment of cAMP into lipid rafts at the inner cell membrane that activate the protein kinase A (PKA) pathway. As previously discussed, the members of the CREB protein family are phosphorylated, which results in the transcriptional inhibition of pro-T cell activation events such as activation of the NFATc1 promoter. However, once CD28 is engaged with the T cell receptor, beta-arrestin and cAMP-specific PDE4 enter the lipid rafts and deactivate cAMP (Bjorgo 2006). This process is important because it involves activation of LCK and phosphatidylinositol 3-kinase (P13K pathway) as well as the interaction of protein kinase B (PKB) with the plextrin homology (PH) domain. Here, PKB is viewed as an adaptor that brings together both P13K and cAMP signaling. This is where P13K activation and subsequent phosphatidylinositol- (3,4,5)-triphosphate (PIP3) production facilitate the formation of multi-molecular complex consisting of protein kinase B (PKB), beta-arrestin, and PDE4 linked to the lipid raft by the PKB PH domain that results in the degradation of cAMP and T cell activation (Bjorgo 2010). Related events like this one will be covered in more detail during the second half of this chapter concerned with the translational pathways associated with Treg effector mechanisms. However, at this moment it is vital to understand the sequence of events that occur at this activation intersection (P13K and cAMP) because it is undoubtedly related to the ability of Tregs to proliferate during their apparent anergic state. In order for Tregs to proliferate they must first be able to experience these early activations events because the P13K/Akt pathway leads to a plethora of activities associated with proliferation.

Adenosine, Treg Proliferation, and Their Unique Immunobiology

The ability of Tregs to proliferate is quite different from that same ability associated with responding T cells. First of all the TCR of innate Tregs, as selected in the thymus, has a specificity for the recognition of 'self.' This is a logical determination given the fact that Tregs seek-out T cells that threaten self as was discussed in the second chapter concerning autoimmunity. In order for Tregs to perform their duty, which is in effect control the T cell immune system, they must be able to adapt and thrive in situations where responding (autoimmune) T cells would die. The key to this adaptation comes in the form of the high-affinity IL-2 receptor and what it does for regulatory T cells. Without delving too deeply into responding T cell proliferation, it is apparent that the normal IL-2 receptor provides a means-to-an-end. In other words, induction of proliferation, which means cell division and replication of a T cell that bears a TCR specific for its target albeit viral, tumor, or self is the main function of the IL-2 receptor. In contrast to this, there is the usage of the IL-2 receptor by the Treg. First of all, IL-2R signals support the expression of FOXP3 in Tregs (Long 2010), and secondly activation of the IL-2R in Tregs induces STAT5 activation, which not only supports FOXP3 activation, but also independently activates the P13K/Akt and MAPK signaling pathways that lead to Treg cell proliferation (Cheng 2011). Therefore Tregs, unlike responding T cells do not need the two-signal (TCR and CD28) scenario in order to multiply. In fact, Tregs only require what would be called "bye-stander" stimulation much like the situation previously described for memory T cells. Maintenance of the memory phenotype requires the contact with antigens that are similar, but not exactly the true antigen. For instance in the case of vitiligo, memory T cells exist as a result of an anti-melanoma T cell response. These memory T cells see normal melanocytes as a source of passive stimulation. Given T cell activation conditions that require a source of exogenous IL-2, these anti-melanoma T cells actually attack normal melanocytes causing melanoma-related vitiligo. However, for Tregs their ability to proliferate is tightly linked to available IL-2 and the recognition of 'self.' The signals Tregs receive though the IL-2R and their TCR are sufficient to induce a proliferative response (Zou 2012).

Adenosine and Treg Proliferation: The Why and How

Think about this for a second. There's a really nasty inflammatory response going on and responding T cells rush to the site, set-up shop, and form a barrier between it and the rest of the body. These T cells go on the attack. They slaughter billions of bacteria, microbes, or cancer cells. Yes, cancer cells. You, me, and everybody else has had cancer and because of the efficiency of the T and NK cell systems we never know it, but tumor-specific memory T cell are left behind (Cobbold 2013). The response to these threats is swift and deadly, but unfortunately some normal cells and tissue systems get damaged. It's the job of the regulatory T cell system to insure that this doesn't happen. Tregs have the ability to go into these very active T cell responses and basically reorganize the response in such a way as to lessen autoimmune responses. The previous chapter was about that very thing. This is the short version of 'why.' The 'how' is a bit more complex. At any given moment a Treg can be incredibly resistant to death, but in other situations very labile to extinction based on the rules of the T cell immune system. Tregs use cAMP as a tool to control other T cells that would ultimately do harm to the body if left unchecked. As mentioned previously, injection of cAMP into effector T cells induces T cell paralysis through the activation of the cAMP PKA pathway, which interfere with T cell proliferative pathways related to NFATc1 production and a myriad of other translational pathways that lead to T cell proliferation (Bodor 2012). Resting Tregs, unlike effector T cells are full of cAMP and to a certain extent, it contributes to the Tregs "state of anergy" for the very same reasons it leads to anergy in responding T cells when they are injected with it. However, Tregs must proliferate and have an active ability to inhibit the AC pathway through conversion of cAMP into 5 –AMP by PDE4s. Recently it was determined that Tregs upon inhibition of the AC pathway undergo robust cell division. Blocking cAMP with pharmacological agents interferes with AC pathway downstream events that result in the inhibition of NFATc1 expression and consequently Treg proliferation occurs via NFATc1 expression (Vaeth 2011). Here, under AC pathway blocking conditions, NFATc1 was activated and NFATc1/aA was expressed, which is a characteristic of proliferating T cells (Serfling 2012). It was also determined that over expression of PDE did not affect the Tregs "anergic state," which is related to the sequestration of PDE isoforms throughout the cell. In addition, it was found that antibodies that blocked IL-2 where found to also reduce inhibited AC pathway-induced Treg proliferation because IL-2 is needed for Treg proliferation (Klein 2012).

It appears obvious that in order for Tregs to proliferate cAMP must be reduced to a level that releases the control of the proliferative pathways in the cell. The fact that that IL-2 itself can inhibit the AC pathway under specific conditions (presence of membrane-bound PKC, Ca++ and ATP) that may occur (Becker 1987) as the Treg finds itself in an inflammatory environment flooded with ATP. In addition, the membrane-bound PKC and Ca++ are more than likely due to low-level stimulation of the autoantigen specific TCR of the Treg. However, one of the many the roles of IL-2 during the normal functioning of Tregs is to upregulate AC activity and produce intercellular cAMP (Bazhin 2010). The conditions above where pharmacological inhibitors were used to induce Treg proliferation gives a clue to actually what happens as Tregs proliferate during inflammatory responses such as GVHD and anti-tumor T cell responses. One of the first things that begin to occur in these situations is that as mentioned before, the supply of IL-2 becomes rapidly depleted and for the most part, by the T cell cytokine inhibitory process induced by Treg secreted adenosine. Another reason why IL-2 begins to disappear is that the high-affinity Treg IL-2R is absorbing it, which is the next non-cell-to-cell contact Treg effector mechanism to be discussed (Pandiyan 2008). Therefore, during the natural course of an inflammatory response Tregs are carrying out multiple functions related to controlling the T cell response. Most, but not all of these functions have been discussed up to this point. However, one of the most important functions as far as induction of Treg proliferation is the use of cAMP during inflammation because the simple depletion of it from Treg cellular stores sets off a series of events that lead to Treg cell division. This is a relatively simple process to imagine given the fact that responding T cells during most inflammatory responses; vastly outnumber Tregs. Each Treg has to inject multiple responding T cells with cAMP and eventually find themselves in the conditions (presence of membrane-bound PKC, Ca++ and ATP) described above where limiting amounts of IL-2 begin to reduce the amount of intercellular cAMP via inhibition of the AC pathway. Once cAMP levels fall within the cytoplasm, the CREB system begins to fail, and the inhibition of T cell proliferative signals halts because of the lack of promoter blocking ICER and ICER-NFAT complexes. Tregs begin to proliferate using bye-stander TCR signals and the utilization of the limited amount of IL-2, yet do not secrete IL-2 and retain their ability to be suppressive.

When this section on the secretion of adenosine by Tregs and it's use as a non-cell-to-cell contact effector mechanism began, it was stated that the examination of this particular effector mechanism would shed light on the unique T cell immunobiology of the Treg. One of the first and most important aspects of this system is redundancy. The term "redundancy" was used in Chapter 2 to explain the translational pathways involved during the creation and maintenance of the Treg phenotype (Fu 2012). Within the Adenosine/cAMP system it refers to dual effects of engagement of the adenosine receptor and injection of cAMP on responding T cells. In both cases, the responding T cell is rendered "anergic." The difference here is that one mechanism operates at a distance while the other is an "up close and personal" encounter between the Treg and the responding T cell. Another interesting aspect concerning these mechanisms is the concept of anergy. Throughout this discussion it has been apparent that Tregs exist in an "anergic state" and it is interesting that most powerful and inclusive of the Treg effector mechanisms (secretion of adenosine and injection of cAMP) induce that very state in their target cells. Tregs can and do kill effector T cells (Grossman 2004), but for the most part, responding T cells are paralyzed by a state of anergy that over time wanes. This was discussed earlier as a way the T cell immune system preserved itself by allowing responder T cells to survive and either respond again or differentiate into the memory T cell state. Even though the state of anergy induced by the Treg response during either a system-wide inflammatory event or induced by multiple tumor sites can render that person susceptible to secondary infections, the alternative is far worse. There are actually two major alternatives as far the effector capabilities of Tregs is concerned and both are discussed in this book. First, defects in Treg function bring about a plethora of autoimmune disorders focused on the inability of Tregs to control the autoreactive immune T cell responses. The second alternative is where Tregs exert too much control over the immune response, which can lead to tumor development via Tregs inhibiting the anti-tumor T cell response. Looking at the systemic homeostatic control of the immune system by Tregs it can be concluded that for all intents and purposes, this is a successful endeavor because most humans do not succumb to these two alternatives except during the latter stages of aging. However, despite the aging process Tregs constantly retain the ability to exert control over the T cell immune system without direct contact with those cells. The Tregs ability to control the lymphokine IL-2 is a perfect example of this.

IL-2 Deprivation Treg Effector Mechanism

Unique Relationship between IL-2 and Tregs

Of all the various types and sub-types of T cells in the T cell immune system Tregs are found to have a unique relationship with the primary lymphokine needed by all T cells, which is IL-2. In general, there are two aspects of the relationship between IL-2 and Tregs that no other T cells share and those are the fact that Tregs do not secrete IL-2 and the continual expression of a high-affinity multi-functional IL-2 receptor. The more important of these two as far as Treg development (Cheng 2013), general function (Fontenot 2005), and effector efficiency is the IL-2 alpha-receptor. The specialized functions of this high-affinity Treg IL-2R have been covered in the previous chapters as well as just recently when discussing Treg function during a inflammatory response where their use of IL-2 shuts-down anergy via the induction of low-level translation of the cAMP/PKC pathway (Becker 1987). Tregs use IL-2 in ways totally different from responding CD4 and effector CD8 T cells do and this gives them an advantage. This difference in IL-2 utilization allows Tregs to control T cell responses. The IL-2 alpha receptor is not expressed on naive or memory T cells, but is transiently expressed on activated CD4 and CD8 T cells as they respond to antigens and need IL-2 in order to multiply. However, Tregs continually express this receptor despite the fact that they only proliferate under specialized circumstances as was mentioned during the waning moments of an inflammatory response. Therefore why do Tregs, which really don't proliferate, express such a high-affinity IL-2 receptor? The answer is related to how they use it.

Throughout this entire discussion of Tregs it is apparent that these cells use the signals (receptor/ligand) from the IL-2 receptor to arm themselves, unlike naïve T cells, which simply use it to multiply when activated. Aside from the activities mediated by the Treg IL-R such as expression of FOXP3, participation in the adenosine/inflammation activities of Tregs, and the signaling of apoptosis in Tregs, the IL-2R is a sensor of responding T cell activity that can occur anywhere in the body. Once CD4 or CD8 responders become activated by peptide antigens presented by APC that results in their secretion of IL-2, the first cell type that appears on the scene is the Treg (O'Gorman 2009). Tregs get there first because of their ability to move faster based on the expression of an activated form of the LFA-1 integrin ligand that uses the ICAM-1 receptor, a ubiquitous cell surface protein that is used by LFA-1+ Tregs to move about the body (Horn 2009). Once there, Tregs begin to orchestrate control over T cell responses and the activities of DC, which has been discussed at length previously. What has not been discussed is how and why Tregs use their high-affinity IL-2R to arrest not only responding T cell IL-2 dependent proliferation, but also most importantly inhibit the initiation of naïve T cell antigen specific IL-2 dependent cell division.

IL-2 Deprivation by Tregs and Control of the T Cell Response

The control of available IL-2 during a T cell immune response can be viewed as a way to remodel the T cell immune response in such a way as to maximize its effectiveness and to minimize autoimmune T cell responsiveness. As far as CD4 T cell differentiation is concerned, IL-2 is the main ingredient in their change from naïve T cell to type 1 or 2 T helper cell, TH17 CD4 effector, or follicular helper TH(fh) cell. These differentiation pathways are controlled by the interaction of naïve/activated CD4 T cells with APCs and other lymphokines such as INF-γ. This holds true for not only the various differentiation stages of CD8 T cell, but also the development of central and effector memory CD4 and CD8 T cell populations. Each one of these various stages of differentiation in both CD4 and CD8 T cells has been mentioned thus far. All of these stages, with the possible exception of the conversion of CD4 Tregs to CD4 TH17 T cell effectors, require the cells to enter the cell cycle and initiate a proliferative burst either during or afterward the differentiation process, or both. The single element necessary for proliferation in all these cases is IL-2. Tregs have been shown to "skew" the population of CD4 responders to the TH2 phenotype by inducing DC to secrete IL-4 (Tokoyoda 2004), thereby activating antigen specific antibody production. The reason for this is that the T cells, which facilitate the induction of B-cells in the germinal centers to produce specific antibodies are TH(fh) CD4 cells require IL-4. As has been discussed previously, the interaction of IL-2 with the IL-2R induces the activation of STAT5. It was found that the differentiation signals that allow for the formation of TH(fh) CD 4 T cells is controlled by the transcription factor BCL6. However, when STAT5 is activated it in turn activates BLIMP-1 an inhibitor of BCL6. Therefore, STAT5 activation by IL-2 is inhibitory to the formation of TH(fh) CD4 T cells and without or with minimal levels of IL-2, TH(fh) can provide help to antibody producing B-cells in the germinal centers (Johnston 2012). For example, if Tregs are removed from mice during influenza viral infection not only is the formation of TH(fh) T cells inhibited, but also the formation of influenza-specific germinal centers (Leon 2014). IL-2 activation of STAT5 can inhibit TH17 differentiation and IL-17 secretion by CD4 T cells. It was discussed earlier that the differentiation of CD4 T cells or CD4 Tregs into TH17 secreting CD4 T cells was dependent IL-6 activation of STAT3 (Hirahara 2010). In addition, it was determined that the expression of STAT5 by IL-2R activation inhibited the differentiation of CD4 T cells into TH17 T cells. As previously mentioned, TH17 CD4 T cells are an essential type of effector cell when it comes to the response to pathogens (Bettelli 2008). In both of these cases, the activation of STAT5 by IL-2 is inhibiting the development of specialized T cells (TH(fh) and TH17) that play a major role in the host's T cell immunity to two significant threats, which are viral and pathogen infections. In addition, both of these threats are negatively impacted by the ability of Tregs to deprive T cells of IL-2.

Indirect Use of Treg IL-2 Deprivation Effector Mechanism

Anti-Viral

The first one of theses threats are viral infections, which require the production of viral specific antibody that allows for viral clearance and antigen processing/presentation of viral antigens by APC as well as the formation of memory T cells. As mentioned above, limiting IL-2 availability during the early stages of an immune response by Tregs insures the differentiation of CD4 T cells into TH(fh) cells and therefore, the secretion of antigen (viral) specific antibodies occurs rapidly. Another way that this limiting of IL-2 availability by Tregs aids an anti-viral T cell response is the effect that it has on CD8 responding T cells. Once CD8 responders differentiate into short-lived effector cells (SLEC) they require the continual presence of secreted IL-2 to kill their targets and proliferate. Therefore, as Tregs absorb IL-2 and make it unavailable to SLEC it diminishes the possibility that normal cells will be killed. As had been mentioned in the previous chapter, there are two types of memory T cells. The first are the effector memory (Tem) CD4 or CD8 T cells, which have the ability to home to sites of inflammation and contain high levels of perforins making them highly cytotoxic. The second type of memory T cell is the central memory (Tcm) CD4 or CD8 T cell. These cells home to the lymphatic system, have a higher response to antigen, and produce large amounts of IL-2, INF-Γ, and IL-4 upon stimulation (Sallusto 2004). It has been determined that unlike the CD8 SLEC that are dependent on high levels of IL-2, Tcm require only transient or low levels of the lymphokine to differentiate into Tcm from the antigen-activated CD8 pool (Williams 2006). Therefore, during the early stages of an anti-viral response when Tregs begin to limit the amount of IL-2, SLEC activity drops and Tcm cells are created. It is thought that this effector mechanism is used by Tregs to not only limit autoimmune damage caused by SLEC as mentioned above, but also to ensure the development of a T cell memory to guard against re-infection (Kastenmuller 2011).

Anti-Pathogen

The second of these immunological threats that are negatively affected by this Treg effector mechanism are pathogens, but this time IL-2 depravation by Tregs results in the creation of an anti-pathogen effector cell mentioned above called the TH17 CD4 T cell. A model pathogen that exposes this positive side effect of the Treg IL-2 deprivation is a fungus called *Candida albicans*. It is a common human pathogen, which is a "commensurate" or common organism that in healthy people is benign. However, immunosuppressive conditions such as found in HIV infection can turn this benign fungus into a life-threatening infection. The onset of HIV in the 1980's generated interest related to the T cell immune response to *C. albicans* because many HIV patients died from the infection. Shortly thereafter, it was determined that the T cell immune system controlled *C. albicans* pathology at the molecular level in healthy individuals through pattern recognition receptors (PRR) such as the Toll-like receptors (TLR) expressed by APC. Once APC recognized molecular patterns associated with specific glycoprotein configurations of the fungus, particular combinations of lymphokines are secreted causing differentiation of CD4 or Treg CD4 T cells into phenotypes designed to respond to that specific type of fungus. In the case with *C. albicans,* the lymphokines IL-1B, IL-23, and IL-6, but not IL-2 are secreted by APC expressing the appropriate PRR. These secreted lymphokines in combination with TGF-ß have the ability to differentiate into TH17 CD4 T cells that have the ability to secrete IL-17 (IL-17A), IL-22, and IL17F. The anti-microbial effect of IL-17 involves its ability to recruit neutrophils and the induction of anti-microbial peptides that are directly toxic to the fungus (Hernandez-Santos 2012).

During infection with *Candida albicans* Tregs actually promote IL17 secretion by CD4 T cells because not only are TH17 differentiation lymphokines secreted by APC, but also because of the stimulatory nature of the infection, large amounts of IL-2 are also secreted. Once this IL-2 is absorbed by the high-affinity IL-2R of the Tregs, differentiation of responding T cells into TH17 CD4 T cells is actually stimulated. This absorption of IL-2 by Tregs occurs in close proximity to the CD4 responders because separation of the cells by permeable membranes fails to promote Th17 differentiation. However, the IL-2 deprivation of responding T cells can lead to apoptosis. As previously mentioned, BCL-2 members BAD and BIM initiate caspase mediated mitochondrial apoptosis, which can be induced by Treg IL-2 deprivation of responding T cells. The responding T cells that don't die are sent into an anergic state and unable to secrete inflammatory lymphokines such as IL-4 and IL-2. The T cells that are not killed by Treg IL-2 depravation are called T0 because they are basically inert, but still alive. Tregs indiscriminately halt all responding T cell responses regardless of the specificity of the T cell response (Pandiyan 2007). This condition was previously discussed as a mechanism used by the T cell immune system to preserve the responding T cell pool. However, a curious phenomenon occurs during an acute TH17 response not only to *C. albicans*, but also during inflammatory bowel disease (IBD) where TH17 T cells are thought to contribute to the pathology of this disorder (Liu 2009).

In both cases, during the early phases of the response, there is a transient drop in the ability of Tregs to suppress responding T cells. This phenomenon occurs as Tregs begin to absorb IL-2 during the *C. albicans* fungal infection just prior to the augmentation of TH17 development. Within the same study it was also found that Tregs temporarily lost the ability to suppress T cell responses during the early stages of TH17 CD4 T cell-induced IBD (Pandiyan 2011). An additional study focusing on only IBD documented the very same decrease in Treg effector function. The authors came to the same conclusion that was mentioned in Chapter 1, which was that during the conversion process of naïve CD4 T cell to TH17 T cell there was also a reprogramming event involving the reprogramming of Tregs into TH17 T cell effectors. Two things happen. The first is that susceptible Tregs under Th17 conversion conditions (mentioned earlier) begin to flux. This means the cells for a moment, are in indecision about what they are becoming. This sounds like a person trying to cross the street, but calculating when to step off the curb and yes, that may be a horrid example, but for Tregs at an inflammatory site, this is most likely what that flux moment is like. This is an important concept and it has to do with Treg "plasticity" (Jijon 2013). This activity is fluid and the response to the situation faced by Tregs is critical. In fact, during disseminated *C. albicans* infection where the fungus is found in the blood stream, Tregs are not only recruited from the innate pool, but also adaptive Tregs are created in the spleen. However, the exact thing happens where Tregs are reprogrammed to secrete IL17 as if the creation of Tregs was for that very purpose (Wibley 2014). There is a battle going on between Tregs and the T cell immune system where the victor or vanquished claim the prize and that prize is the elimination of the threat. As far as the CD4/Treg conversion/reprogramming is concerned the balance between Tregs and TH17 T cells is important. In type-1 diabetes the predominance of TH17 T cells in comparison to Tregs invokes vascular angiopathy, which leads to poor vascular circulation in diabetes patients (Ryba-Stanislawowaka 2013). However, in many cancerous situations the predominance of TH17 T cells over Tregs promote on-site inflammation, which can lead to an anti-tumor T cell response (Gaur 2012). IL-2 deprivation by Tregs seems to be a subtle effect caused by these cells that come into an inflammatory site possessing a high-affinity IL-2R. However, a non-subtle effect is how Tregs use the IL-2 they absorb to become effector cells that secrete a plethora of lymphokines designed to trim and cull the T cell response. This simple act of absorbing IL-2 initiates this battle, but also demonstrates the high degree of plasticity Tregs posses (Feinerman 2010).

In order to conclude this non-cell-to-cell contact Treg effector mechanism section it is only fair to mention how Tregs influence the T cell response by their elaboration of IL-10, which is an anti-inflammatory lymphokine that has inhibitory effects on APCs (Schwarz 2010), responding T cells (Zou 2013), and also contributes to the generation of new Tregs (Adeegbe 2013). In addition, as Tregs have the ability to secrete GrB during an inflammatory event to not only damage the cell membranes of CTL during Treg: CTL immunological synapse formation (Gondek 2005), but to also remodel the extracellular matrix causing increased cellular permeability at the site (Buzza 2005). However, the most powerful way Tregs control the T cell response during inflammation and an anti-tumor T cell response at a distance is through the elaboration of adenosine and the consumption of IL-2. Without these two effector mechanisms possessed by Tregs, rampant autoimmunity and viral/pathogenic infections would occur in the body. However, again the downside is if this Treg system is working the way it was designed precancerous cells, which take a long time to develop into cancer are protected from destruction. Needless to say, this topic will be revisited in the second half of this chapter and in the next one that has to do with the clinical aspects of Treg control. However, now it's time to address those Treg effector mechanisms that involve the direct contact between the Treg and its target. Tregs are much more aggressive in situations where massive destruction of self-tissue systems is concerned. As discussed earlier in this section, Tregs are armed with the very same effector mechanisms as the most efficient killer cell of the immune system, which is the CD8 CTL. Those effector mechanisms are the granzyme/perforin system and the FAS/FASL system. Despite the fact that these effector mechanisms are cell-to-cell contact based, they will only be indirectly mentioned in the next section because there has already been an exhaustive examination of these two effector mechanisms as far as Tregs are concerned. Instead, there will be a focus on the Treg interface with their target at the membrane level and how Tregs use this cell-to-cell contact interface to control APC and effector T cells. Now it's important to understand that interface, which is called the immunological synapse.

Cell-to-Cell Contact Treg Effector Mechanisms

The Immunological Synapse

This cellular junction between cells of the immune system (T cells, APCs, and B-cells) was originally discussed in terms of the TCR, CD28, and LFA-1 making contact with peptide antigen-loaded MHC class I & II, CD80/86, and ICAM-1 proteins of APC in a supramolecular contact site at the cell surface of the two cells (Bromley 2001). However, since then the meaning of the immunological synapse (IS) has expanded to include T cell contact between a variety of cells since this phenomenon is now extended to include contact between effector T cells and their targets. In addition, and pertinent to this discussion, cell-to-cell interactions between T cells also requires the formation of this complex cell-to-cell interaction. The interactions at a membrane level, between cells of the immune system are a complex process involving multiple protein molecules of both cells. Some of theses protein-protein interactions lead not only to T cell proliferation, but also affect the APC. This is the case where LFA-1 expressing Tregs interact with DCs expressing the ICAM-1 receptor, which results in increased Treg motility (Horn 2009) and inhibition of DC-mediated T cell activation functions (Onishi 2008). This called an "inside-out" activation phenomenon and occurs during formation of stable IS complexes. However, these cell-to-cell contacts vary based on a number of conditions between the cells such as detection of specific antigenic peptide sequences on the APC, which match the configuration of the T cell receptor. These conditions almost always lead to stable IS formation and activation of both the T cell and the APC. Translational signals flow from the IS contact point, carrying instructions to the cytoplasm and nucleus of both cells. This will be covered in detail during the translational pathway section of this chapter, but right now the scope and importance of type of contact between T cells (Tregs) and other cells of the immune system must be examined from a functional point of view because of its relevance to Treg immunobiology.

One of the basic facts about this interaction is that it is the basis of a fundamental T cell and NK cell immunological process called "immunosurveillance." It was described in detail in the *Introduction* section of Chapter 1 because this is where it all begins for the T cell immune system. It was mentioned that the T cell and NK cell systems effectively sample every cell (except immune privileged sites) in the body repeatedly over a 24hr period. Fooksman and co-workers (2010) who will be cited below refer to this interaction, which is related to immunosurveillance as a *hapsis.* This is an ancient Greek word that was almost lost to obscurity and incidentally describes close planetary body alignments. Later, the word was used by psychologist to describe perception through touch and recently has been used to create the positive psychological term "haptonomy," which refers to physical and emotional contacts that foster psychological well-being (Hall 2010). This is ironic because the immunosurveillance process does that same thing for the body except that it would be called "immunological" well-being. Nevertheless, as a result of the interaction of T cells with other cells in the body there are two separate "states." The first state is an impermanent one and similar to the activity of immunosurveillance where T and NK cells briefly make contact with cells through low affinity interactions such as between CD4 molecules on the T cell and its ligand MHC on the APC. This interaction without the involvement of other receptor/ligand systems (TCR/peptide/MHC, CD28/CD80/86, and LFA-1/ICAM-1) do not result in T cell activation, but are strong enough to allow momentary contact between the two cells. This type of interaction is referred to as an immunological "kinapse" or IK (Fooksman 2010). The IK does play an important role in the formation of stable IS complexes through the initiation of the plasma membrane scaffolding protein called, transmembrane adapter linker of activation in T cells or LAT. The LAT protein has the ability to organize the TCR signaling axis, which leads to T cell activation pathways (Salek 2013). Its been shown that kinapse formation in the form of uropod (filamentous membrane extensions) contact between naïve T cells and APC induces the localization of LAT at the contact zones prior to T cell activation (Azar 2013). Kinapse formation is the initial step in the development of large supramolecular signaling complexes containing tyrosine kinase Lck (lymphocyte-specific protein kinases), which are initiated by LATs to form the formerly mentioned, lipid rafts (Ventimiglia 2013).

The formation of the IS is a complex process and is the result of a coordinated adhesion event, which involves an array of receptors and ligands is still under study. Because this interaction is the basis for every T cell immune response researchers have focused their attention to not only the basic primary interaction, which is the TCR, peptide/MHC complex, but also the necessary secondary ligand/receptor events. In order to understand how Tregs interface with other cells of the immune system such as T cells, APC, and normal tissue cells of the body, it is important to understand the basics of the IS. Once an activated, T cells interact with APCs or target cells and there is the formation of what is called a central supramolecular activation complex or SMAC. This is the primary contact involving the TCR and peptide/MHC complex that forms a central ring, which is the result of the clustering of TCR molecules on the APC (target cell) membrane and called the central SMAC or cSMAC. A secondary ring forms composed of the interactions with the T cell's LFA-1 and the APC's ICAM-1 molecules and is called the peripheral SMAC or pSMAC. A third ring is formed that is the result of the protein tyrosine phosphatase receptor type C or CD45 interactions with the APC cell surface and is called the distal or dSMAC (Monks 1998). This third ring is very important because initially there is T cell transcriptional activity during the first two stages (cSMAC and pSMAC), but after the all three interactions are complete transcriptional activity pauses.

This pause has to do with a decision made through CD45 to initiate the transcriptional events leading to T cell activation or not (Freiberg 2001). There are four major reasons why this happens. First of all, T cells interact with APCs that are neither targets nor cells presenting antigen to induce a T cell response. There are cases where an APC expresses peptide in the context of MHC, but lack secondary ligands such as the one for CD28, which are the CD80/86 ligands. This would usually be a self/self interaction between the T cell and a normal cell such as an epithelial cell. The second situation refers to Tregs where the Treg attaches itself to a self-cell while defending it from attack by responding T cells by for instance, secreting adenosine, or inducing IL-2 deprivation/cell death of the responding T cell. The third decision has to do with killing the APC by injection, via perforin of granzymes or granulysin, which will be mentioned below in the context of the IS. The fourth reason is the decision to initiate the T cell activation/proliferation cycle. The first and second situations often result in the T cell letting go of the APC unharmed, but the third results in death and the fourth usually results in differentiation changes in the APC as a result of exposure to T cell secreted lymphokines. Each of the four decision situations mentioned above are a result the involvement or non-involvement of secondary T cell receptors such as CD4/CD8, CD28, LFA-1, and LAG-3.

The three-ringed structure of the IS acts as a platform by allowing additional TCR molecules to accumulate in the dSMAC, move through the pSMAC, and finally cluster in the cSMAC (Varma 2006). This movement of TCR molecules is dependent on cytoskeletal recruitment of actin, which actively transports the molecules that are initially accompanied by adhesion molecules such as LFA-1 to the cSMAC. Once at the cSMAC, adhesion molecules are left behind as the TCR molecules gather around a central core (Kaizuka 2007). As far as CTL recognition of APC, the central core contains the centrosome, which is where the intracellular microtubule cytoskeleton is organized. The cytoskeleton acts as a conduit for secretory lytic granules containing granzymes or granulysin to travel though the centrosome for injection of their contents into the APC target cell. As mentioned above, actin and now non-muscle myosinIIA are involved in the secretory process. As the granules reach the centrosome the actin network surrounds them. The granules themselves are surrounded by myosinIIA, which physically collapses them at the CTL/APC membrane interface releasing the granules lytic cargo (Sanborn 2011). Because of the involvement of both actin and MyosinIIA in this process and its similarity to cilia formation, it is thought that since lymphocytes are unable to form cilia that this process of IS formation and vesicular (granules) trafficking is a rudimentary vestige of primary cilia formation in lymphocytes (Finetti 2013). In this situation with CTL, the IS represents a special type of membrane specialization that results not only in the organization of important T cell surface receptors at a focal point, but in addition facilitates the coordinated release lytic proteins from intracellular cytoplasmic granules (Angus 2013).

However, if the interaction between T cell and APC is destined to result in T cell activation/proliferation the serine-threonine kinase, protein kinase-C theta (PKC-theta) is involved and begins to accumulate between the cSMAC and pSMAC rings. The localization of PKC-theta is associated with CD28 engagement and in fact, PKC-theta forms a complex with the intercellular domain of the CD28 molecule and LCK. However, once PKC-theta is activated by diacylglycerol (DAG) during the previously mentioned T cell activation pathway, PKC-theta in association with adaptor proteins such as CARMA-1, begins the process of activating NF-kB, AP-1, and NFAT that initiate IL-2 production. As mentioned above, PKC-theta activates NFAT in the context of phosphatidylinositol trisphosphate or PIP3. The main function of PIP3 in the IS is to facilitate filamentous actin (F-actin) remodeling (Le Floc´h 2013), but in conjunction with PKC-theta induces Ca2+ influx during T cell activation that leads to the dephosphorylation of NFAT by calcineurin, which allows it to enter the nucleus. As mentioned in Chapter 2 under the subheading, *Transcriptional pathways associated with TCR-only interactions that induce anergy*, if AP-1 expression is unsuccessful, NFAT mediates the induction of T cell anergy (Baine 2009). PKC-theta has a wide range of effects as far as T cells are concerned. It can promote T cell survival by not only initiating IL-2 secretion, but also by being directly responsible for upregulation of the pro-survival proteins BCL-xL and BCL-2 via activation of NF-kB. In addition, PKC-theta can phosphorylate BAD inactivating its ability to participate in the previously mentioned mitochondria apoptosis process. Because of PKC-theta's role in T cell activation, it is a possible clinical target for immune-based therapies, but because of its ubiquitous role in the body any therapy that blocks PKC-theta's activity must be approached with caution (Sun 2012). The reason why PKC-theta is important is that as far as Tregs are concerned is the fact that unlike PKC-theta's role in enhancing T cell activation in responding T cells, it actually can inhibit Tregs from suppressing T cell immune responses.

Tregs and the Immunological Synapse

One would think that a Treg T cell would conform to all T cell behavioral rules, but as previously shown, one would be wrong in that assumption. Tregs have a totally different mission and that's to control the T and NK cell responses that designed to eliminate any cell that that appears different. They do this by using two separate strategies. The first and immediate one is to latch on to their protected cell using the anti-self TCR, but they also have to interface with those two cells (effector T cells and NK cells) in a way that can stop them from killing injured cells or unfortunately in many cases precancerous tumor cells. They do this by using the effector mechanisms such as direct killing (FAS/FASL and perforin/granzymes), secretion of adenosine, cAMP injection, or IL-2 deprivation. The other strategy Tregs use is to prevent the development of effector T cells from antigen specific naïve T cells by down regulating the CD80/86 molecules on DCs to prevent or lessen CD28-mediated T cell activation. As far as the immunological synapse is concerned, Tregs have an advantage because of the way they sequester away PKC-theta from their synapse formation. As mentioned above, PKC-theta controls the ability of responding T cells to become activated and proliferate. During the synapse PKC-theta enables the adapter protein CARMA-1 to form a complex with Bc110 and MALT-1, which initiates the release of NF-kB to the nucleus where it initiates IL-2 secretion and proliferation (Rawlings 2006). For the Treg, neither of these options applies to their function so during synapse formation PKC-theta is kept away from the IS and in particular the cSMAC. PKC-theta is a negative regulator of Treg suppressive function by virtue of its role during responding T cell synapse formation and subsequent T cell activation, which is the result of PKC-theta activation of the NF-kB pathway. If this pathway is activated in Tregs the cells essentially begin to loose their Treg phenotype, which is essentially an anergic T cell that does not secrete IL-2. In fact inhibitors of PKC-theta increase the Treg's ability to inhibit responding T cell activities such as proliferation and cytotoxicity mentioned above (Zanin-Zhorov 2010).

Tregs, the Immunological Synapse, and Mobility

The IS of the Treg is quite different than that of the responding T cell. First of all, the entire interaction is more stable, which is partially due to the absence of PKC-theta in the cSMAC as noted above. The increased stability of the Treg IS is a necessary function considering the amount of time it takes Tregs to modify a target cell (DC) cell surface receptors (CD80/86). As mentioned above, Tregs prevent naïve T cell activation to specific antigen by reducing CD80/86 cell surface expression levels in DC to a point where they're unable to be used as a source of a "second signal" via the T cell CD28:CD80/86 interaction. The amount of time a responding T cell or Treg spends engaged in the synaptic state with the target cell is called, "dwell-time." This is the period of time between initial contact and disengagement. It has been known for some time now that Tregs have the ability to shorten the dwell-time between autoreactive responding T cells and DC in the lymph nodes (Tadokoro 2006) and is no doubt the result of the reduction of CD80/86 expression on the DC cell surface by Tregs. However, Treg dwell-time and stability of the IS is dependent on the interactions of CD28, PD-L1 and CTLA-4 ligands with the CD80/86 receptors. In contrast to responding T cell synapse formation where CD28 engagement promotes IS formation, with Tregs engagement of CD28 inhibits synapse formation because of its activation of PKC-theta as mentioned above. As far as CTLA-4 is concerned, its engagement inhibits responding T cell IS formation and dwell-time due to CTLA-4's ability to block CD28's interaction with the CD80/86 receptor. In contrast, CTLA-4 engagement promotes stable synapse formation and increased dwell-time in Tregs because of its ability to interfere with the CD28/CD80/86 interaction. These types of opposite effects that the CD80/86 ligands have on IS formation and dwell-time are referred to as a "mirror model." In addition to these effects mediated by CD28 and CTLA-4, the Treg expressed CD80 ligand PD-L1 has the ability to reduce Treg mobility and thereby increasing the dwell-time (Dilek 2013). This gives the Treg additional time to reduce the expression of CD80/86 on DCs.

As mentioned several times, Treg mobility is a very important part of their effector capabilities. Because of the uniqueness of not only how they move (motility), but also where they must move to (migration), these activities could be considered a separate effector mechanism these cells poses. Unlike naïve responding or effector T cells, which are usually unidirectional (from peripheral blood to the lymph nodes and inflamed tissues) Tregs often have to travel in multiple directions in order to control a T cell immune response. Migration of naïve responding/effector T cells as well as Tregs is controlled by the expression of chemokine receptors, which were mentioned previously. Each type of T cell (naïve responding or effector T cell) expresses a particular combination of these receptors that allows that cell to migrate to specific sites such as the lymph nodes, intestines, mucosal tissues, or the endothelial surfaces of blood vessels. In fact, it was determined that Tregs use their anti-self TCR to move along endothelial surfaces based on INF-Γ secretion by inflammatory T cells and the consequent expression of MHC-class II proteins by endothelial cells that line blood vessels near the inflammatory site (Fu 2014). Each combination is specific for that type of cell. For instance, with responding T cells TH-1 T cells express CXCR3, CCR5, and CXCR6 where as TH-2 T cells express CCR3, CCR4, CCR8, and prostaglandin D2 receptor CRth2. However, because Tregs are developed in the thymus (innate) and developed in the periphery (adaptive) from either naïve or differentiated T cells, they have command and control of the expression of the chemokine receptors from not only responding T cells, but also differentiated effector T cells (Ding 2012). This means that Tregs can basically migrate to any location where responding T cells appear and can leave those sites at a moments notice. Treg migration and its timing is an essential component of their ability to control an immune response. It was discussed earlier how LFA-1 expressing Tregs interact with the ICAM-1 molecule on DC and how this increases Treg motility (Horn 2009). This fact, and the expression of the high-affinity IL-2R by Tregs, allows them to be the first of many cell types that appear at an active T cell immune response (O'Gorman 2009). Because of their unique use of immunochemical intracellular pathways Tregs are masters at T cell mobility.

In general, heighten T cell motility is associated with an increased ability to respond to specific antigen. In other words, the less mobile a T cell is the less sensitive it is to activation by antigen. For instance antigen-sensitive memory T cells are not only more mobile than naïve T cells, but they also express different chemokine receptors that allow them to access a wider variety of tissues (Baaten 2013). T cell motility itself is governed by the activation of Rho-family GTPases, which cause the rapid polymerization of the actin cytoskeleton into a meshwork that becomes polarized forming a contractible microtubule (Wantanabe 2004). This process is Ca++ dependent and has been shown to be the result of P13/Akt activation of PKC-theta. Moreover, this pathway is active in highly mobile T cell lines versus their non-mobile counterparts. In addition, it was found that mobile T cells were more highly sensitive to TCR stimulation and produced significantly greater amounts of IL-2 via the PKC-theta/NF-kB pathway despite the fact that there were no differences in the expression of LFA-1 or IS formation with APC (Kim 2013). The interesting aspect of studies like this one that dissect responding T cell motility is that the motility of Tregs is an order of magnitude greater than the most mobile T cell, which is the memory T cell. Since calcium influx is an essential component of T cell mobility and this influx is PKC-theta dependent, it can be assumed that PKC-theta also plays a role in Treg motility. In fact, it was found that higher amounts of PKC-theta (six times) were recruited to the Treg cell membrane versus responding T cells when CD28 was activated by CD80 in planar membranes during IS formation (Zanin-Zhorov 2010). Despite the fact that this PKC-theta is sequestered away from the cSMAC during IS formation due to its ability to activate NF-kB and reduce Treg inhibitory function, the additional amount of PKC-theta recruited to the Treg membrane no doubt is involved with the increased ability of Tregs to move rapidly from site to site during an immune response. In support of this theory it was determined that despite the fact that synapse formation in Tregs is highly stable, PKC-theta can induce the IS destabilization by inducing myosinIIA contraction. MyosinIIA contraction promotes rapid amoeboid cell mobility by the inactivation of the LFA-1/ICAM-1 bonds at the trailing edge (Fooksman 2010). This activity not only releases the cell from the pSMAC contact point, but also allows the Treg to quickly move away.

Injection of cAMP into Effector T Cells by Tregs

Now that it is established that Tregs, unlike responding T cells, form highly stable synapses with not only APC, but also other T cells and that instead of Tregs using PKC-theta to induce NF-kB expression, it is used to increase Treg mobility during an immune response, it is time to examine one of the most effective Treg effector mechanisms. The reason why injection of cAMP into responder/effector T cells is such an effective mechanism is that the effects on the target cell are not lethal. It was discussed earlier how Tregs can kill APC and responding/effector cells using either the FAS/FASL system or the perforin/granzymes system, which operates through the formation of the IS unlike the FAS/FASL system that uses a receptor ligand interaction. The injection of cAMP into responding/effector T cell uses an entirely different mechanism to deliver the cAMP into the cytoplasm of the target cell. This mechanism will be discussed at length momentarily, but now there will be a short review of the cAMP build-up caused by the injection. The reason for the review has to do with the regeneration of the Treg population during extreme T cell immune responses during viral, bacterial, and transplantation-related inflammatory reactions. Once the method of delivery is described it will be easier to understand just how dependent Tregs are on encountering these sometimes rare, but also common inflammatory T cell responses.

Ironically, the information concerning the effects of the build-up of cAMP in responding/effector T cells after injection of cAMP by Tregs comes from studying the Treg itself, which as a part of its phenotype, stores vast amounts of cAMP in its cytoplasm. In fact, the anergic characteristics of Tregs, which are not only the inability to proliferate via TCR ligation, but also their total dependence on exogenous IL-2 because they are unable to secrete it; are for the most part due to their accumulation of cytoplasmic cAMP. As far as the lack of IL-2 secretion is concerned Tregs, which constituently express high levels of cAMP, also expressed high levels of inducible cAMP early repressor (ICER) and cAMP response modulator (CREM). ICER is a transcriptional repressor protein derived from the 3' end of the CREM gene. ICER protein can form complexes with NFAT. These complexes can specifically bind to NFAT/AP-1 sites within the IL-2 promoter region. This effectively blocks the ability of NFAT/AP-1 complexes from inducing IL-2 secretion (Bodor 1998) and this is the primary reason why Tregs do not secrete IL-2. When responding T cells were examined that had been induced to become anergic by either increased cAMP build-up due to Treg-secreted adenosine or cAMP directly injected into these cells by Tregs, a very similar transcriptional pathway involving another member of the NFAT family called NFATc1 was involved. NFATc1 is one of five NFAT family members (NFAT, NFATc1, c2, c3, and c4), but unlike NFATs c2, c3, and c4 that induce T cell anergy, reduce T cell proliferation, and increase the sensitivity to activation-induced cell death (AICD) respectively, NFATc1 expression enhances T cell proliferation and resistance to AICD (Serfling 2013).

When expression of NFATc1 is inhibited T cell proliferation ceases. This is exactly what happens when ICER alone or ICER/NFAT complexes bind to the NFATc1 P1 promoter, which results in the blockage of gene transcription (Vaeth 2011). It was also later determined that ICER could form complexes with NFATc1 and c2 with the same result (Bodor 2012). NFAT/AP-1 binding sites are also present in the promoter regions of several important cytokines such as TNF-α, IL-4, IL13, and GM-CSF, which are all susceptible to transcriptional suppression by NFAT/ICER complexes (Hogan 2003). Therefore, the induction of cAMP in responding T cells can result in more than simple inhibition of IL-2 secretion; it can lead to the induction of anergy just as in the single-signal model of anergy discussed earlier. Concerning the inability of Tregs to proliferate, adenyl cyclases (ACs) are the enzymes that synthesize cAMP and are a family of enzymes that can either be transmembrane-bound or found in a soluble form. As far as cAMP regulation is concerned, phosphodiesterases (PDEs) that were mentioned previously are enzymes that hydrolyze cAMP into 5' –AMP (Gancedo 2013). PDE activity in Tregs is important because inhibition of this enzyme by PDE inhibitors not only increased the suppressive properties of Tregs (Bopp 2009), but also increased their ability to delay skin allograft rejection (Feng 2011). Once IL-2 activates Tregs with or without TCR ligation, AC activity and cAMP production are increased, which is the opposite for responding CD4 T cells where these events are decreased (Bazhin 2010). Therefore, Tregs actively regulate AC activity by degrading cAMP with PDEs and as previously discussed, cAMP through CREB inhibition of transcription can restrain Treg proliferation as long as cAMP is present. Therefore, the mere presence of increasing amounts of cAMP in not only Tregs, but also their responder/effector T cell targets renders both cell types anergic. The only difference in anergy between the two cell types is that for the Treg, the more anergic the cell is the more inhibitory it becomes as evidenced by the treatment of Tregs with inhibitors of PDE's that increase cytoplasmic cAMP and as a result, increase their inhibitory capacity.

System Used to Inject cAMP into Responding/Effector T Cells by Tregs

One of the most interesting aspects of this effector mechanism is that as mentioned previously, it is very effective and essentially temporary because once the target cells are full of cAMP they cease functioning as responding/effector cells. Only after an extended period where the cAMP is being degraded by the cells PDEs do the cells return to functionality. This interaction between the Treg and the target T cells only temporarily removes them from participating in the inflammatory response, but when they wake-up there are a lot more Tregs than there were to begin with. The reason for this was discussed earlier and will be revisited shortly, but now exactly how Tregs inject cAMP into responding/effector T cells will be described. Tregs do this through what is called "gap junctions" or "hemichannels" that form between not only immune cells, but also multiple cells of the body and are formed by a protein family called connexins that play a major role in the communication pathways between immune cells (Ernesto Oviedo-Orta 2013). Gap junctions between cells are responsible for the transfer of small (less than 1kD) molecules such as small metabolites, ions, IP3, prostaglandins, ATP, and cAMP. Once these small molecules are transferred between cells multiple signaling pathways can be affected such as those associated with cell cycle, tissue homeostasis, migration, motility, and oxidative stress. Connexins themselves (21 family members) come in multiple molecular weights and form (oligomerize) a small hexametric pore on the cell surface and when two of these pores on different cells dock there is the formation of a gap junction. Usually, but not always, the same molecular weight connexins associate to form the same channel, but the variations that occur exclude or include the import or export of molecules that may or not be modified by biochemical modifications such as phosphorylation (Burra 2011). Needless to say that this is a complex system that is just now being understood in the context of the immune system.

As far as Tregs are concerned it was recognized that Tregs could inhibit responding T cells proliferation and IL-2 production using a cell-to-cell contact effector mechanism. This was initially based on the observation that naturally occurring Tregs contained high levels of cytoplasmic cAMP. It was also determined that after co-culture with Tregs responding T cells also had an increased amount of cytoplasmic cAMP and were unable to secrete IL-2 or proliferate (Bopp 2007). Later it was determined that and inhibitor of the hydrolyzing cAMP enzyme PDE called rolipram increased the inhibitory function of Tregs in a clinical setting where there was a significant reduction in asthmatic airway inflammation due to increased inhibition of T cell responsiveness by Tregs (Bopp 2009). Eventually, the mechanism of responding T cell inhibition by cAMP was determined, which was the activation of the PKA pathway, expression of the transcriptional inhibitor ICER, and its subsequent inhibition of not only IL-2 synthesis and CTLA expression of T cells, but also the reduction of CD80/86 expression on APC (Bodor 2012). Another clinical application of the inhibition of PDEs in Tregs was the use of PDE inhibitors during allogeneic bone marrow transplantation and the subsequent inhibition of GVHD that would occur as a result. It was found that PDE inhibitors effectively suppressed GVHD caused allogeneic anti-MHC T cell responses by not only direct Treg-induced T cell inhibition, but also by the suppression of DC activation (Weber 2013). This was an important finding because it demonstrated how effective cell-to-cell transfer of cAMP by Tregs was at controlling this specialized type of inflammatory reaction. Despite the fact that Tregs are essentially anergic T cells and under normal T cell activation conditions (TCR, CD28 ligation, and IL-2) Tregs do not multiply, but they are able use this and other major inflammatory reactions to increase their numbers.

Injection of cAMP by Tregs Leads to Treg Proliferation

The mechanisms by which Tregs proliferate during an inflammatory response originate from multiple lines of evidence that seem to be contradictory, but in essence demonstrate the "plasticity" of the Treg phenotype. Experiments similar to the one below examining the inhibition of GVHD induced by PDE inhibitors reveal that in addition Tregs were induced to proliferate (Feng 2011). Since PDE inhibition increases the amount of Treg intracellular cAMP, it would seem impossible for Tregs to proliferate since increased cAMP increases Treg anergy as described above. It was also observed that adenosine receptor (A2A) analogues or agonist not only ameliorate GVHD as PDE inhibitors do, but also increase the numbers of Tregs during allogeneic transplantation (Han 2013). As described in the *Non-cell-to-cell contact Treg effector mechanisms* section activation of the adenosine receptor on responding T cells induces the generation of cAMP and activation of the protein kinase A (PKA) pathway, which results responding/effector T cell anergy. In addition, it was also mentioned that Tregs were also affected in a similar fashion due to the fact that they also express A2A. During these types of inflammatory responses (allogeneic transplantation) there is massive T cell proliferation of donor T cells responding to recipient tissue-associated MHC antigens. Inflammatory cytokines such as TNF-A, INF-γ, IL-6, and G-CSF are secreted in large amounts. Often after treatment with either PDE inhibitors or A2A agonist there is a reduction of these cytokines and an increase is anti-inflammatory cytokines such as TNF-A and IL-10. Both of these cytokines in conjunction with TCR activation can create new Tregs from the antigen specific T cell pool by the upregulation of FOX-P3 expression. This can lead to the creation of "new" Tregs and add to their numbers, but existing Treg proliferation appears to still be a problem based on the fact that they contain significant amounts of cAMP.

Recently it was demonstrated that cAMP production by Tregs was stopped by the inhibition of the AC pathway using specific AC inhibitors or by increasing the expression of Treg PDEs, which resulted in the loss of Treg-induced responding T cell inhibition mediated by cAMP and induced Treg proliferation. The cAMP depleted proliferating Tregs retained their expression of FOX-P3, did not revert to responding/effector T cells, and were still unable to secrete IL-2. Once cAMP production was stopped there was a decrease of ICER and increase in the translocation of NFATc1 to the nucleus, which induced T cell proliferation. The proliferation of Tregs in this situation was independent of TCR engagement, but was dependent on minute amounts of exogenous IL-2 (Klein 2013). As mentioned previously, the high-affinity IL-2 alpha receptor possessed by Tregs not only supports proliferation, but also has the ability to regulate cellular processes related to the functionality of Tregs. For instance, in contrast to responding T cells, the IL-2 receptor of Tregs induces the upregulation of the AC pathway, which results in the production of cAMP (Bazhin 2010). In addition, it was determined that Tregs could indeed proliferate in the absence of TCR ligation as long as there was a source of IL-2 (Zou 2012). Despite the fact that Treg proliferation was demonstrated in this system and allogeneic transplant systems described above; these systems are still somewhat artificial because specific inhibitors were used. The question is how do Tregs increase their numbers during normal inflammatory conditions? The answer to this question is related to the function of the delivery system used by Tregs to deliver responding/effector T cell inhibiting cAMP to their target cell.

As mentioned above, functional gap junctions (GJ) of oligomerized connexins proteins in a hexametric formation that connect two cells are formed between Tregs and responding/effector T cells. GJ that connect adjacent cells are more that mere size-limiting pores based on the molecular weights of their composite connexin proteins. They do function as permeability channels that allow small molecular weight substances to equilibrate between the cells in contact. This permeability is selective as mentioned above, and based on the molecular weights of the interfacing connexins, which in many cases may be different. These pairings and consequent channel formation between connexin proteins of different molecular weights are referred to as heterotypic-heterotypic GJ channels and they are thought to represent special permeable configurations for specific purposes (Burra 2011). In addition to their permeability characteristics, GJ serve as electrical conduits during conjugation. Often many of the small molecules that pass though the GJ are either charged or polar in nature. The conductance of these molecules becomes a factor as they pass between cells. Therefore, not only do GJ channels act as molecular sieves, but also as electrical filters that allow high or low electrically charged molecules to pass between cells (Ek-Vitorin 2013). This is particularly relevant as far as the passage of cAMP between cells.

The conductance of GJ channels formed by 3 separate homotypic pairings of connexin hexametric configurations (Cx43, Cx40, and Cx26) during the passage of cAMP was measured. Current was determined on a single (doublet) cell level as cAMP was transiting (diffusing) between cells and there was a steady increase over time with all three connexin configurations. However, the Cx43 configuration exhibited the widest range of conductances when compared to either Cx40 or Cx26. In addition, Cx43 channels were ten times more permeable to cAMP than the other channels, which may mean that these channels in addition to their smaller pore size are not suited to select larger negatively charged molecules such as cAMP. Conversely, it appears that the conductance and pore size of the Cx43 channels are designed to for the rapid diffusion of cAMP into a cell so fast that PDEs are unable to degrade it before inhibitory pathways such as PKA are activated (Kanaporis 2008). Given this information and the fact that during an inflammatory response cAMP containing Tregs, which are vastly outnumbered by responding T cells, must inject multiple target cells and thereby quickly become depleted of cAMP. The injection of cAMP into responding T cells is swift because it is not only based equilibrium permeability where the cytoplasmic concentration of cAMP within the Treg tries to equilibrate with the cAMP concentration of the target responder T cell, but the transfer is also aided by the increase in channel conductance mentioned above as cAMP flows into the target cell. Once this occurs the Tregs undergo proliferation as described above and just as quickly become armed with newly synthesized cAMP induced by the IL-2A receptor using IL-2 generated by responding T cell activation. This cycle continues until most responding T cells are rendered anergic and unable to secrete IL-2.

Significance and Scope of Treg Cell-to-Cell Contact Effector Mechanisms

The cell-to-cell contact Treg effector mechanisms mentioned above are the major effector mechanisms in this category. There are others that operate much like the degradation of responding T cell membranes by the short-range secretion of granzyme B by Tregs such as the expression and excretion of β-galactoside-binding protein or βGBP. Treg secreted or expressed βGBP has the ability to inhibit autoreactive CD8 T cell responses by blocking the ERK/MAPK and Akt signaling pathways, which were previously discussed as important pathways for the induction of TCR activation. In this case TCR antigen activation of the affected CD8 T cells is temporarily blocked because other aspects of TCR activation such as the phosphorylation of CD3zeta, ZAP70, and PKC-theta are unaffected (Baatar 2009). During the examination of both Treg non cell-to-cell and cell-to-cell contact effector mechanisms it is apparent that aside from Tregs inducing responding T cell apoptosis through the use the perforin/granzyme and FAS/FASL systems, the most effective and wide-ranging mechanisms are the ones that have systemic implications. The secretion of adenosine by Tregs allows them to not only control inflammation locally, but also minimize its spread. There is a systemic effect that is in operation at distant sites during Treg control of a local inflammatory event such as a bacterial infection or the site of a growing tumor. Even though at times were inflammatory events occupy the attention of many of the Tregs in the body and leave it vulnerable to autoimmune attack, the effects of adenosine secretion and particularly direct cAMP injection of responding T cells can exacerbate the situation by creating system-wide immunosuppressive conditions, which can lead to pathogenic infections.

As had been discussed throughout this section, the result of both secretion of adenosine and cAMP injection by Tregs is the induction of T cell anergy in the responding/effector target T cell. These anergic T cells are not simply T cells that as per the definition of T cell anergy, which is: a long-lasting, partial or total unresponsiveness induced by partial activation (Lechler 2001). Even though this definition applies to T cells that have experienced the "single-signal" type of anergy induction, it was made clear earlier that the anergic "state" induced by the use of the Treg adenosine secretion/cAMP injection effector mechanisms is identical. Anergic T cells can have a profound effect on the immune system in general because they still express functional receptors. Despite the fact that these anergic T cells cannot respond to antigen, functional receptors such as the TCR, CD4, CTLA-4, LFA-1, and LAG-3 can occupy their ligands thereby blocking their access by functional T cells. In fact, some CTL still have the capability to kill targets despite the fact that they have been rendered anergic (Otten 1991). In addition, one of the salient features of T cell anergy is that there are multiple levels of anergy, which means that some states are partial and others allow cells to function using mechanisms such as cytotoxicity that are not dependent on IL-2 responsiveness/secretion or cell division (Arnold 1993). Anergic T cells have been shown to have the capacity to induce suppressive DC in vitro by the down-regulation of CD80/86 and MHC-class II using a cell-to-cell contact mechanism (Vendetti 2000). Since this report was published just prior to the characterization of Tregs, it was thought that these anti-CD3 antibody generated anergic T cells were actually Tregs. However, several years later anergic T cells generated the same way with identical suppressive properties were shown to not be Tregs by virtue of the fact that CD25 expression was not an identifiable characteristic of these anergic T cells (Abraham 2008). Therefore, mechanistically anergic T cells in general are suppressive through their ability to inhibit APC function.

As far as the effects of Tregs rendering responding/effector cells anergic by adenosine secretion or cAMP injection, the results of this activity mean that massive numbers of anergic T cells are created. The anergic effector cells, if still capable of killing, do so until granzyme and granulysin granules are depleted. Being unable to regenerate because of the inability to respond or secrete IL-2, or divide the cells more than likely begin to disperse into the surrounding tissues and possibly into the circulation. Because these cells are full of cAMP they pose an immunosuppressive threat. Eventually, these cells will return to normal in terms of their ability to respond to TCR stimulation and secrete and respond to IL-2. However, in order for this to happen the cells must get rid of the cAMP. The way this occurs can be a problem. Because these anergic T cells have functioning receptors they have the ability to attach themselves to APC via the TCR, CD4, and CD28. Once attached, the exact thing that caused them to be anergic happens, but this time in reverse. When Tregs inject responding T cells with cAMP they express the exact same variety of connexin hexametric pores as not only the responding T cells, but also antigen presenting DC and both of these interactions result in the formation of homotypic-homotypic GJ channels (Mendoza-Naranio 2011). Therefore, the cAMP containing anergic responding T cells discharge their excess cAMP into DC causing the reduction of MHC-class II and CD80/86, just as adenosine does when it attaches to the A2A receptor expressed by DC (Weber 2009). Because anergic responding T cells have been rendered non-functional their migratory patterns are somewhat directionless and as mentioned above, these cells tend to diffuse away from the inflammatory site and can end-up almost anywhere. This means that at distant locations cAMP anergic responding T cells are inducing immune suppression by discharging their cAMP into DC, which may be needed for other purposes. The up side to this phenomenon is that the suppressive affects exerted upon the DC are temporary. The other good thing about this situation is that as soon as responding T cells discharge their cAMP they too return to normal and can now respond to the initial antigen that caused the inflammatory response. However, now they are far away from that site, but if any pathogens, tumor cells, or virus-infected cells escaped the inflammatory site, the newly awakened responding T cells can detect them and respond.

By examining the complexity and sheer elegance of Treg effector mechanisms it is expected that the entire cellular immune system is sensitive to the control of any immune response that is subject to these effector mechanisms. Despite the potential immunological danger associated with effects of these mechanisms, much like the one above with anergic responding T cells, these effects do have benefits. There is the concept of the "bystander" effect where immune cells not involved in the primary immunological event become affected, which could lead to additional infections. However, some infectious agents recruit Tregs to protect them from TH-1 CD4 T cell responses such as with *Helicobacter pylori* infection where the bacteria induce mucosal DC to secrete only TGF-ß, which induces Treg formation instead of TGF-ß and IL-6, which favors anti-bacterial TH-17 T cell development. As an additional consequence, *H. pylori* specific TH-1 CD4 T cell are unable to respond because of the presence of Tregs (Kao 2010). Here the bacteria usurp the "bystander" effect, but in some cases this bystander effect is purposely used by Tregs to add an additional layer of control. For instance during an immune response responding T cells often home to a regional lymph node to be primed or stimulated by DC that are presenting processed antigenic peptides. They do this by following chemokines released by the DC. During low or nominal T cell immune responses Tregs have the ability (show in this chapter) to directly attack responding T cells and suppress their response. However, if the T cell immune response is high, for instance where a high-affinity T cell receptor is used, Tregs abandon their direct attack on responding T cells and concentrate on turning off the ability of DC to attract T cells by secreting T cell homing chemokines (Morlacchi 2011).

The control of DC lymphokine secretion by Tregs has been discussed previously. One aspect of this control is the ability of Tregs to inhibit DC maturation and not allowing them to secrete proinflammatory lymphokines such as IL-12. However, in other cases there is an alteration of intracellular pathways in DC caused by the interaction of Treg ligands such as LAG-3 (Liang 2008). Here, LAG-3 cross-links the MHC-class II molecules on the DC and cause lipid rafts (Cho 2010) and Fc-receptor domains to coalesce. These contain ITAMs (Underhill 2007) that recruit ERK and SHP-1, which are phosphorylated and inhibit IL-12 production (Liang 2008). In addition, activation (phosphorylation) of ERK induces the increased secretion of IL-2 and IL-10, which are both important as far as the creation of adaptive Tregs (Slack 2007). This is called the ITAM inhibitory pathway, which when activated by this interaction between LAG-3 and MHC-class II leads to the degradation of internalized MHC-class II proteins; effectively reducing MHC-class II expression (Graham 2010). As far as increased IL-10 production by DCs is concerned, it was found that when DCs were induced to secrete IL-10 by yeast extract zymosan the cAMP response element (CRE), which is part of the cAMP PKA pathway is involved because both the CRE binding protein (CREB) was up regulated and associated with MAPK/ERK activation (Alvares 2009). This activity links ERK activation, increased IL-10 production, and decrease in MHC-class II expression to the induction of the cAMP/PKA pathway and will be discussed in detail in the next section that deals with translational pathways. This is related to the effects of cAMP injection and adenosine/A2A receptor activation on DC function. Even though at the present time it is not know what pathways are altered that arrest chemokine secretion by Tregs, but it is important to understand the intersections of the biochemical transduction pathways. This will be a part of what will be discussed in the next section, which will examine some of the intracellular pathways associated with Treg effector mechanisms. Because many of the pathways were highlighted during the descriptions of Treg effector mechanisms, the discussion will focus on the interrelationships between those that were discussed and new pathways directly responsible for effector mechanism function.

Translational Pathways Associated with Treg Effector Mechanisms

Introduction

Some of the Treg effector mechanisms that are shared by effector T cells such as the FAS/FASL and perforin/granzyme systems adhere to the signal transduction rules that are followed by effector T cells. The ability of granzyme B (GrB) to activate mitochondrial-induced apoptosis via cytochrome *c* (Bao 2007) through the ability of caspases to degrade BID (Wang 1998) and allow BAX and other death regulators (Gross 1999) to disintegrate the mitochondrial membrane and release pro-apoptotic factors (Moldoveau 2013) is an example of the activation of specific pathways that result in target cell death. Because of commonality with standard T cell effector mechanisms, these transduction pathways associated with Treg effector mechanisms will not be discussed. However, because the Treg-only effector mechanisms are unique to Tregs, there will be an effort to understand why Tregs possess them and how these mechanisms use the responder/effector T cell transduction pathways to subvert their function. For instance, the serine protease inhibitors or serpins act as serine protease substrates and take the place of naturally occurring serine expressed in the membranes of DC. These protease inhibitors (PIs) absorb the proteolytic function of GrB and protect DCs from lysis by Tregs, which secrete GrB. PI-9 is one of the most important of these inhibitors because it protects effector T cells and DC from secreted GrB (Sun 1996). PI-9 not only protects DC from Treg-secreted GrB lysis, but also from FAS/FASL induced caspase proteolytic activity (Cunningham 2007). The expression of PI-9 is tightly linked to the maturation process of DCs because it is expressed in conjunction with CD80/86, but not with the secretion of IL-12 and its expression is also dependent on the p38 MAPK pathway, which is linked to DC activation (Bots 2007). However, this is not a problem for Tregs because if GrB secretion doesn't work, Tregs attack with adenosine secretion and cAMP injection to reverse DC maturation and reduce the expression of P-9, or in extreme cases use perforin/granzyme cytotoxicity, which actually bores a hole in the DC membrane causing death. Either way in the end, the DC is suppressed.

This redundancy, which was mentioned earlier, is the hallmark of Treg control of the T cell immune system (Hagness 2012). Responding/effector T cells, macrophages, DC, and NK cells have just one mission and that is to respond, kill, and make sure the invader disappears. This process is very effective and often misdirected toward autoimmunity, but nature invented a control mechanism called the regulatory T cell system. It is a system because there are natural (innate) and created (adaptive) Tregs that have the ability to recruit other cells of the immune system such as DC to carry out their mission of controlling the T and NK cell systems. Tregs are a built-in control mechanism because Tregs can be created from the responding T cell population itself. For instance, if a viral infection occurs and there is a high–affinity TCR available to respond, the responder/effector T cells rush in and begin to kill every one of those virus-infected cells. Killing of the virus-infected target cells is based on the recognition of viral peptides in association with MHC molecules on the cell surface. As mentioned previously, there is some promiscuous killing of normal "bystander" cells. Once these cells are lysed APC (macrophages and DC) begin to present self-antigens, which is a process similar to autophagy, but involves ingestion of cellular debris from autologous (self) cells. Because Tregs are drawn to an inflammatory response via detection of IL-2 released by responding/effector T cells and the detection of chemokines, they become activated by these self-antigenic peptides presented by APC and in some cases attach themselves to the tissue under attack. At this point Tregs begin to seek out and destroy any anti-self promiscuous CTL that approaches that tissue. Tregs will actually kill these types of CTL without hesitation (Grossman 2004). However, this is unlike their ability to render foreign antigen-reactive responder/effector T cells anergic by either adenosine secretion or cAMP injection during an inflammatory response. The transduction pathways associated with these two effector mechanisms are important to understand because their activation can completely change the behavior of the target cell and thus change the direction and intensity of an inflammatory T cell response.

Translational Pathways Associated with Adenosine Secretion by Tregs

Remodeling the T Cell Response during an Inflammatory Response

The effects of adenosine attaching to just one of its receptors (A2A) on cells of the immune system is incredibly complex, but yet designed to specifically tailor the T cell response in such a way as to make it more specific and less likely to do damage to normal cells. For instance, it was discussed how A2A receptor signals activate adenyl cyclase to produce cAMP. This reaction is catalyzed by heterotrimeric G proteins and leads to the activation of the PKA pathway. It also was discussed how lymphokine (IL-2) secretion was inhibited through the binding of inducible cAMP early repressor (ICER) protein/NFAT complexes to the IL-2 promoter NFAT/AP-1 binding sites (Bodor 1998). What was not discussed was the specificity of DC-induced lymphokine profile after cAMP production. As a result of the activation of the PKA pathway, type 1 (IL-2, INF-γ, and TNF-α), but not type 2 (IL-4, IL-5, and IL-10) lymphokines secreted by TH-1 and TH-2 CD4 T cells respectively are inhibited and as mentioned previously, activation of the PKA pathway through cAMP can skew the T cell response to a TH-2 phenotype where autoantibodies are produced (Tokoyoda 2004). This again calls more Tregs by virtue of the fact that DC begin endocytosis of self cells coated with autoantibodies through a process called "opsonization" where antibody coated cells are endocytosed via the DC Fc receptor. The reorganization of the T cell phenotypes during an inflammatory response from a TH-1 to a TH-2 type response is not the only rearrangement of the T cell population. Activation of the PKA pathway by either the engagement of the adenosine receptors or the direct injection of cAMP into cells of the immune system can totally change the nature and composition of the T cell response during inflammatory responses.

Most of these changes in the cellularity of the T cell response are through the alteration of lymphokine secretion induced by this purinergic pathway. This term, "purinergic pathway" not only defines the effects related to Treg, CD73/39 produced adenosine, but also the effects of ATP binding to its receptors P2Y and P2X. However, one of the main forces involved in the changes in T cell phenotypes is the transcription factor cAMP response element binding protein or CREB. Many of the lymphokine genes associated with inflammation such as IL-1, IL-6, IL-10, and TNF-α contain cAMP responsive elements (CRE). Similar motifs have been found in the promoters and enhancers of TCR alpha and TCRV-beta genes. CREB is a phosphorylation-dependent transcription factor and a member of a family of proteins that are CRE transcription activators. Once CREB is phosphorylated at serine-133 it interacts with a co-activator protein called CREB-binding protein (CBP) or p300 in order to initiate transcription or termination of CREB-responsive genes. CREB is involved with multiple cellular processes such as cellular proliferation differentiation, glucose homeostasis, spermatogenesis, and can be considered both an activator and inhibitor of transcription (Mayr 2001). It was discussed earlier that NF-kB activation in conjunction with AP-1 and the activation of Akt leads to among other things the induction of IL-2 secretion in responding T cells. It was also mentioned that APC respond to bacteria and fungus by the use of pattern recognition receptors (PRR) such as Toll-like receptors (TLR) and the response of APC to these PRR is to secrete proinflammatory lymphokines (Hernandez-Santos 2012) such as the ones mentioned above that posses CRE. Activation of the NF-kB pathway is responsible for the activation of these lymphokine genes through direct contact with their promoters. Prior to the activation, NF-kB exists in the cytoplasm while bound to the inhibitor molecule IkB. Once TLRs are activated, the MyD88 and TRIF adaptors, which are indispensible for TLR-induced DC differentiation/maturation (Kolanowski 2013), initiate the degradation of IkB that releases NF-kB (RelA/P65 and p50 subunits) from the cytoplasm where it travels to the nucleus. In order for NF-kB to activate these genes it must bind to them using the same CBP/p300 that phosphorylated CREB (pCREB) uses to bind and inhibit gene activation (Gosh 2008). It is thought that the increased production of pCREB, as a result of activation of the PKA pathway, inhibits NF-kB binding via competition for available CBP (Parry 1997).

In this case, CREB is an inhibitor of transcription, but like mentioned above CREB can be an activator of transcription such as in the case with IL-10. IL-10 is included in the list of lymphokines that has a CRE within its promoter and is an anti-inflammatory lymphokine that has profound dampening effects on the T cell immune system including the induction of newly created Tregs (Saraiva 2010). This is related to the discussion at the end of previous section where IL-10 secretion was augmented by the treatment of DCs with zymozan and there was a corresponding up-regulation of pCREB, which was associated with activation of the MAPK/ERK pathway (Alveres 2009). TLR ligands such as LPS also induce the increased secretion of IL-10 by APC via the activation of the NF-kB and MAPK pathways ERK1/2 and p38. This leads to direct phosphorylation of CREB and AP-1 by the kinases MSK1 and MSK2 (MacKenzie 2013). Once pCREB and pAP-1 bind to the IL-10 promoter, increased IL-10 secretion commences. However, there is a negative feedback loop because MSK1/2 also induces the transcription of the dual-specificity protein phosphatase-1 (DUSP1). DUSP1 inhibits p38 thus reducing ERK1/2, p38 activation of MSK1/2. In addition, there is a positive feedback loop that involves the ability of IL-10 to induce the production of glycogen synthase-3B (GSK-3B), which increases the binding of pCREB to the IL-10 promoter and inhibits NF-kB by decreasing the interactions between it and CBP/p300 (Martin 2005). While CREB is phosphorylated it can inhibit pro-inflammatory lymphokines such as IL-2, IL-6, TNF-α, and at the same time stimulate the production of anti-inflammatory lymphokines such as IL-10 and INF-γ. Pathways that lead to or are the result of CREB include PKA, PKC (PKC-A and PKC-theta), Ras, ERK1/2, MAPKs, p38, and MSK1/2. In addition, TCR activated CREB is involved in the TGF-ß generation and maintenance of FOXP3 by binding to the previously mentioned Treg demethylation region (TSDR) after demethylation by TGF-ß. This stabilizes the FOXP3 gene and the expression of the Treg phenotype (Kim 2007). All of this points toward the importance of CREB and the role of CRE in T cell immunobiology of inflammation (Wen 2010).

DC-Induced Remodeling of the T Cell Response by Treg-Secreted Adenosine Controlled by Two cAMP Activated Transcriptional Pathways: PKA and EPAC

When considering the changes induced by Tregs in the types of T cells that develop during an inflammatory response as they secrete adenosine or inject cAMP, the one cell that must be considered is the DC. During the previous non-cell-to-cell contact section under the subheading *Adenosine and DC* there was a somewhat detailed description of the effects induced by cAMP activation of the PKA pathway. The PKA pathway, via cAMP intracellular increases, occurs not only as adenosine interacts with its receptor on the DC surface, but also as levels of cAMP are increased by TLR ligands (MacKenzie 2013) and the interaction of ATP with the purinergic receptors P2Y and P2X (Wilkin 2001). However, when examining the effect of the presence of increased intracellular cAMP on DC maturation there are conflicting reports. DC maturation or lack thereof is critical in dictating not only nature of the T cell response, but also the types of T cells that develop during an inflammatory response. It has been determined that increase in intracellular cAMP leads not only to the secretion of anti-inflammatory lymphokines, but also retards DC maturation and the ability to stimulate T cell activation/proliferation due to the reduction of MHC class II and CD 80/86 expression (Wilson 2008). In contrast, it also has been shown that the very same increase in intracellular cAMP leads to the differentiation of immature DC to fully mature DC expressing increased amounts of both MHC class II and CD80/86 (Wilkin 2001 and Schnurr 2000). In both of these cases not only is intracellular cAMP increased, but also there is activation of the PKA pathway. The difference between these two situations is how the cAMP levels within the DC were increased. In the first case, where LPS-induced DC maturation was retarded, cAMP was generated by A2B adenosine receptor activation, which initiated the PKC pathway. The reduction of inflammatory lymphokine secretion such as IL-12 was likely due to the inhibitory effects of CREB (mentioned above) since in addition, IL-10 secretion was increased (Wilson 2008). In the second case where immature DC were differentiated into fully mature DC, the cells were also induced to mature with LPS with TNF-A, but this time ATP binding to the P2Y purinergic receptor was used to activate the cAMP PKA pathway. IL-12 secretion as well as the expression of CD83 (DC maturation antigen) and CD80/86 was increased. In addition, it was determined that heightened intracellular levels of cAMP were present (Wilkin 2001 and Schnurr 2000).

Modulation of DC Function by the Purinergic System

For some time now it has been recognized the source of DC (bone marrow or peripheral blood monocytes) and the DC maturation process profoundly affected the T cell response to not only inflammatory responses (viral, bacterial, autoimmune, or cancer), but also the fate or end result, which could lead to chronic disease or death. DCs, despite the fact that they literally commanded by the T cell immune system to function in specialized ways, can actually control the fate of most T cell responses. However, it was found that there was multiple activation of transcriptional pathways such as ERK1/2, p38 (MAPK pathways), PKA, PKC, and P13/Akt and that were sequentially responsible for migration, lymphokine secretion, and maturation. The conclusion from these observations was that there was a "modular integration of function," which was the result of the formation of "functional units of molecular networks" (Luft 2006). This sounds complex and considering the pivotal role DCs play in the T cell immune system, the word 'complex' seems like an insufficient term to apply to such intricate processes as antigen processing/presentation, lymphokine secretion, migration, and chemokine detection/secretion. DCs and their involvement in the T cell response have been the topic of discussion in every chapter of this book and the previous one called, *Immune-based Cancer Treatment. The T lymphocyte Response* for one singular reason. That reason is what would be called, "multi-directional tasking" and is a term used to describe an immune cell that both takes and gives orders to and from the T cell immune system. If you exclude cells of the granulocyte/monocyte series and examine the functions of the other cells of the immune system such as T cells, B cells, and NK cells what you will discover is that over 90% of their time, they are fulfilling their function as either responder/effector T cells, antibody producing cells, or rudimentary effector cells. However, if you examine the functional commitments of the ultimate differentiated granulocyte/monocyte lineage cell, which is the DC, T cells dictate roughly half of their function, but the other half is committed to directing cellular functions to that very same T cell immune system. This is why the intracellular transcriptional pathways in DCs are so complex.

The conflicting reports concerning the build-up of intracellular cAMP and DC maturation, lymphokine secretion, and migration are not only a testament to the complex nature of the transduction pathways operating in DCs, but also the built-in redundancy related to the translational pathways of the purinergic system. This system includes the effects of ATP detection via the P2Y and P2X receptors (Schnurr 2000), adenosine/adenosine receptor activation (Hasko 2000), and the direct gap junction injection of cAMP into DCs by Tregs (Boop 2007) and discharge of cAMP into DC by cAMP-loaded responder/effector T cells (Mendoza-Naranio 2011). The one common outcome of these actions is the build-up of intracellular cAMP in DCs. The relationship between ATP and DC, which results in the increases intracellular cAMP and augmentation of DC function as far as stimulation of allogeneic T cell responses (increased DC MHC-class II expression), increased CD80/83/86 expression (Jacob 2013), and changes in DC migration are in effect, at odds with the inhibitory effects of adenosine/adenosine receptor and injected cAMP. These discrepancies associated with the increase of intracellular cAMP are in large part due to the complexity of the purinergic system and to some extent reflect the built-in redundant systems put in place to combat totally different immunological threats, which create distinct immunological conditions. For instance, when discussing how CREB, after being phosphorylated was able to inhibit NF-kB activation of inflammatory cytokines by competing for the NFkB cofactor CBP/p300 (Wen 2010). In contrast, pCREB also has the ability to promote cell survival, which is important during pathogen infection by activating anti-apoptosis genes in the BCL-2 family of survival genes (Sandoval 2009). As far as redundancy is concerned with the PKA system, both ICER and CREM modulate lymphokine secretion, but ICER acts immediately and specifically targets lymphokine genes such as IL-2 that are associated with T cell activation (Bodor 1998). The pro-survival aspects of CREB were first noticed in macrophages that were stimulated to proliferate by incubation with forskolin. Proliferation was Akt phosphorylation-dependent and was inhibited by an inhibitor of the PKA pathway. However, it was determined that this proliferation induced an increase in EPAC and Rap-1 and consequently it was determined that both PKA and EPAC pathways, which are both activated by cAMP were involved in pCREB promotion of macrophage proliferation and survival (Misra 2005).

Modulation of DC Function by the Activation of PKA and EPAC Pathways

EPAC (exchange protein directly activated by cAMP) that was briefly described earlier is a Rap-1 (anti-Ras oncogenesis GTpase) guanine-nuclear-exchange factor, which is activated by direct binding of cAMP to a specific cAMP-binding site (Rooij 1998). Since its discovery EPAC has been recognized as a second cAMP sensor pathway other than the cAMP-dependent protein kinase, PKA. It is theorized that the existence of two separate pathways, which are activated by cAMP binding, allow for the diversity associated with cAMP specifically, but also the purinergic system in general. Within immune cells many, but not all of the consequences of membrane adenyl cyclase activation and production of cAMP via G-protein coupled adenosine receptors have already been discussed. It was thought, before the discovery of the EPAC pathway, that many of these effects were the result of the PKA pathway only. The PKA pathway itself is far from simplistic and as a matter of fact quite complex because of the presence of two classes (PKA-I and PKA-II), which include multiple C and R subunit genes. As far as EPAC is concerned, and as mentioned before, there are two isoforms (EPAC-1 and EPAC-2) with EPAC-2 having limited tissue distribution while EPAC-1 is found in all tissues of the body (Cheng 2008). Since both PKA and EPAC pathways are activated in response to increased cAMP, activities such as the inhibition of apoptosis, which was mentioned above and thought to be due to activation of the PKA pathway, have been found to be the result of cAMP induced EPAC activation through the use cAMP analogues that bind to either PKA or EPAC (Grandoch 2009).

The discrepancies described above related to intracellular cAMP build-up during the maturation (P2X and P2Y/ATP/TNF-A and LPS stimulation) or inhibition of maturation (adenosine/adenosine receptor activation) in DCs can be partially explained by the activation of PKA and EPAC pathways as well as the interaction of extracellular ATP with the P2X and P2Y receptors. As far as DC maturation or its inhibition in relation to the interaction of ATP with the P2 receptors is concerned, there are two separate pathways based on the affinity for ATP of the P2 receptors and the concentration of extracellular concentration of ATP detected by the DC. The P2Y11 receptor has a high affinity for ATP and the P2X7 a lower affinity. When intercellular concentrations of ATP are increased due to cellular damage caused by massive cell death the low-affinity P2X7 receptor is activated, which leads to Ca++ influx that induces calcineurin to dephosphorylate both NFAT and NFkB. This leads to DC maturation and the secretion of proinflammatory lymphokines in order to create an inflammatory response against whatever caused cell death and the release of high quantities of ATP. However, when lower amounts of ATP are present at the end of an inflammatory response, the high-affinity P2Y11 receptor gets activated, which directly induces the production of cAMP by adenyl cyclase and thereby activates the PKA/EPAC pathways leading to arrested DC maturation, inhibition of secreted inflammatory lymphokines, and secretion of IL-10 (Gorini 2013). Immune cell proliferation and survival is undoubtedly linked to the activation of NF-kB and is as discussed above, responsible for the elaboration of inflammatory cytokines during an inflammation. It was determined that NF-kB activation was mediated by EPAC-1 during LPS stimulation of macrophages by using the EPAC-1-only cAMP analogue CPT (Moon 2007). In support of this, it was recently discovered that EPAC promoted the ubiquitin-proteasome degradation of the above mentioned co-factor p300 by inhibition of p38 MAPK activation (Jeong 2013). As mentioned earlier, the co-factor p300 is used by pCREB to bind to the IL-10 promoter and negative regulation via MSK1/2 activation, which leads to inhibition of p38 and therefore reduces phosphorylation of pCREB and limits its ability to activate the IL-10 gene (Martin 2005). In the above study where p300 was degraded, it demonstrates that EPAC itself participates in the inhibition of p38 MAPK activation. Another recent study that examined the effects of cAMP analogues specific for activation of either the PKA or EPAC pathways during LPS stimulation of human monocytes. It was shown that PKA-specific cAMP analogues globally inhibited lymphokine secretion in monocytes, but not B cells where IL-10 secretion was stimulated as it is in macrophages. EPAC-only analogues only inhibited IL-10 secretion while allowing IL-1, TNF-A, and IL-12 to be secreted (Gerlo 2010).

The main function of the EPAC proteins is to activate RAP-1 and RAP-2, which regulate some of the most fundamental cellular processes such as proliferation, differentiation, migration, apoptosis, and cell movement. EPAC-1, which is ubiquitous and involved in cAMP regulation of the immune system is unlike EPAC-2 because it contains only one cAMP-binding domain (CBD) whereas EPAC-2 possesses two and is restricted in tissue distribution. However, the binding affinity of cAMP to the CNB domain of EPAC-1 is lower than that of PKA, which means that PKA is activated first and as the intracellular cAMP concentration increases, EPAC-1 becomes active (Shirshev 2011). This difference in binding affinities for cAMP between PKA and EPAC may explain how the limited amounts of intracellular cAMP induced by activation of ATP receptors P2Y (except P2Y11) and P2X led to DC maturation and secretion of pro-inflammatory lymphokines (Jacob 2013). On the other hand, the inhibition of DC maturation caused by massive amounts of intracellular cAMP induced by adenosine receptor activation may cause cAMP to bind to both PKA and EPAC and lead to inhibitory effects of the EPAC pathway described above. However, these two cAMP activated pathways do not act independently of each other and the interactions, which are termed “crosstalk,” are just being understood. For instance, it was recently shown that PKA-induced ICER, which was thought to be the main inhibitor of not only responding T cell lymphokine secretion, but also proliferation is not essential for those functions because mice that had this gene removed developed normal responding T cell inhibitory Tregs that had an increased expression of EPAC and lower that usual levels of PDEs (phosphodiesterases), which was likely due to the need for higher levels of cAMP because of the lower affinity for the EPAC CBD (Vang 2013). Another recent study using PKA-only and EPAC-only cAMP analogues demonstrated that both pathways acted in an opposing fashion. For instance, activation of PKA only induced DC maturation and EPAC alone had no effect. However, when the two were activated together it led to the inhibition or retardation of maturation. In addition, and in support of EPAC-induced degradation of p300, it was found that EPAC reduced the level of phosphorylated CREB thereby controlling DC maturation. The same was true as far as cytokine production and proliferation in activated T cells. It was determined that the activation of adenyl cyclase and the subsequent build-up of cAMP under various conditions induced cellular changes that were not the result of PKA or EPAC acting alone, but in a coordinated fashion to control cellular activity (Garay 2010).

In conclusion, it is apparent the two major Treg-only effector mechanisms (secretion of adenosine and injection of cAMP) are linked to major transduction pathways that not only control effector/responding T cell and DC function, but also cellular differentiation, chemokine expression and the effects of inflammation on normal tissues. Aside from killing target T, NK, and DC, Tregs have the ability to divert those cell's functions in order to re-shape inflammatory responses so that they do not harm the body. As shown in the previous chapter on autoimmunity, prolonged T cell inflammatory responses can lead to not only the generation of autoimmune T cells, but also the development of cancer through chronic inflammation. Therefore, Tregs serve the purpose of reducing the inflammatory period by inducing responding T cell anergy, directing DC function away from T cell activation, and remodeling the ECM by secretion of GrB. By using these two effector mechanisms Tregs take control of responding cell intracellular transduction pathways using a system (purinergic system) that has access to basic fundamental cell processes. The translational pathways in almost every cell in the body that have to do with cell division, differentiation, apoptosis, adhesion, migration, and cellular metabolism intersect with transduction pathways activated through the purinergic system. Therefore, by carefully understanding not only the relationships between the pathways involved in the purinergic system as they relate to immune function, but also those pathways in this system that relate to the normal function of non-immune cells, it will be possible to design Treg-based clinical treatments. These treatments, which would potentially use intracellular pathway altering small-molecule componds may allow for the suspension of unwanted immune effects related to Treg function such as an array of autoimmune disorders and of course, Treg inhibition of the anti-tumor T cell response. The next chapter will examine clinical efforts to manipulate Treg immunobiology directly related to cancer treatment using immune cell-based immunotherapy or a combination of it and chemotherapy. Potential experiments or treatments that focus on altering intracellular translational pathways in Tregs, anti-tumor T cells, and tumor cells that improve the anti-tumor T cell response will be highlighted. The hope is that through the information discussed in the previous chapters, new concepts concerning development of therapeutic treatments based on immune cell function, which are dictated by translational pathways, will be revealed.

Chapter 4

Treg Immunobiology as It Relates to the Anti-Tumor T Cell Response during Immune Cell-Based Cancer Treatment

Introduction

The ability to understand and manipulate Treg immunobiology for the treatment cancer and autoimmune disease is critical to the development of future immune-based cancer therapies. However, from the viewpoint of the Treg, the response to these diseases is essentially the same, which means that development of these future immune-based therapies will be linked to autoimmunity. Future standard therapies for both of these diseases will make use of the immune system itself and may not require what is now known as chemotherapy, but the use of specific chemical agents that modify biochemical events (translational pathways) within the immunotherapeutic cell to specifically alter its behavior in a positive fashion. Immunotherapy for the treatment of cancer will use therapeutic procedures developed from the practical knowledge of autoimmunity and will be based on the alteration of specific components of the immune system such as lymphokines, immune cells (T cells, B cells, and DC), targeted antibodies, and peptides. The reason for this is the same reason that most of what has been discussed up to this point has had to do with two particular types T cell immune responses, which were autoimmune (anti-self or autoantigen) and antigen (viral, pathogen, or alloantigen) and not particularly the T cell response to tumor antigens. In reality, the anti-tumor T cell response is in essence, a hybrid response that involves the recognition of both self and non-self. This is not in reference to antigen specific T cells recognizing foreign peptide antigens in the context of self-MHC, but something much more complex and ill defined. The standard definition of a tumor antigen is a substance produced by a tumor cell that activates the immune system. However, this definition is purposely vague and tells you nothing about whether these antigens are foreign (non-self), altered self, or self. The fact that tumor antigens activate the immune system gives the impression that they are foreign, but self-antigens (autoantigens) can also activate the immune system in the form of autoimmune disease.

If the T cell immune response to a tumor were completely based on the recognition of non-self, Tregs would not be inhibiting the anti-tumor T cell response by using their complete effector mechanism arsenal. Therefore, the autoimmune aspects of the anti-tumor T cell response are as, if not more important than, the recognition of non-self. The list of tumors that have had or have been associated with Treg involvement is far too extensive to list here. What could be said is that most if not all growing tumors have at some point been associated with Tregs, which should be based on several very simple assumptions. The first of those assumptions was mentioned in the previous chapter when it was said that almost all of us have developed cancerous cells in our bodies, but these cells were eradicated by the immune system without us even knowing it. This is evidenced by the fact that anti-tumor T cells are present in individuals that have never been diagnosed with the disease (Cobbold 2013). What this means is that the T and NK cell surveillance system found the cancerous cells, mounted a response, and killed the cells immediately, but leaving memory T cells behind. Another assumption is that the first cell to appear at the site of a T cell immune response where IL-2 and chemo attractants are released is the Treg (O'Gorman 2009). The ability of Tregs to interfere with the anti-tumor T cell response can occur if there is a prolonged T cell response to pre-cancerous tumor cells, which would have to do with confusion related to whether T cells recognize self or non-self as a normal cell becomes cancerous. The way T cells approach the slow development of precancerous cells is linked to the process of inflammation, how it can cause cancer (mentioned in Chapter 2), and why Tregs protect inflamed cells. During this period, T cells respond slowly to the expression of tumor antigens that are part self and non-self. These are pre-cancerous genetically mutated altered peptides or what are called "neoantigens." The T cell immune system has problems with confronting such antigens because they are similar to self-antigens. It takes time for the T cell immune system to respond. In the meantime, Tregs have arrived at the site, begin to shut-down the attacking T cell response, and in effect set up a barrier between the developing tumor and the T cell immune system. Sometimes this barrier is composed of Tregs attached to the tumor, but as will be shown; many times it is a membrane barrier created by Tregs remodeling the extracellular matrix (EM). So this is the immunological background to the development of new immune-based cancer therapies and it's apparent from the information given that Tregs could be a problem.

In order to focus on the potential and actual problems Tregs induce during immune cell-based immunotherapy, the current therapies that make use of immune cells will be highlighted. There are many forms of immunotherapy, which are now or will be used in clinical trials and eventually as standard treatments, but the immunotherapeutic procedures that make use of T cells, DCs, and IL-2 alone or separately are susceptible to the influence of Tregs. These therapies include adoptive T cell immunotherapy (June 2007), DC-based immunotherapy (Engleman 1997), and lymphokine immunotherapy (Lotze 1987). An additional type of cancer therapy that often applies to blood-borne cancers is bone marrow transplantation and will be examined because of the important role Tregs play in GVHD (Koreth 2013). As will be shown, almost all of these therapies include additional treatments such as total body irradiation (TBI) and/or chemoablation to eliminate not only the patient's immune system, but also existing tumor cells. Some of these therapies use additional components such as the treatment of malignant lymphoma patients with autologous bone marrow stem cell transplantation (ABSCT) with or without subcutaneous injections IL-2 and INF- alpha, which is another form of lymphokine immunotherapy (Nagler 1997). By focusing on these types of immune cell-based immunotherapies it should be possible to understand just how and why Tregs have become one of the most important elements of immune-based cancer therapy. Some of the Treg-mediated effects found in immunotherapeutic clinical trials are subtle, but many are directly inhibitory. The subtle effects of Tregs on immune cell-based immunotherapies have to do with the ability of Tregs to create homeostatic conditions. Tregs have the ability to balance immune responses. This balance can be detected in the blood stream where there are lymphokines and other immune bioactive protein/peptides that reflect the current state of the immune system. During the immune response to a cancer, Tregs often induce a state of systemic anergy, which as previously mentioned, may lead to opportunistic infections. This was mentioned several times in reference to how Tregs induce anergy in T cells via the secretion of adenosine during an inflammatory reaction.

However, given the negative role of Tregs in cancer immunity, the fact is that Tregs are a positive force in the immune system, and that this activity is centered on the ability of Tregs to inhibit inflammatory T cell responses. One can imagine that in the future, Treg immunobiology will become a blueprint for the development of completely immune cell-based immunotherapeutic treatments for cancer and autoimmunity. From the information provided in previous chapter on Treg effector mechanisms, it's apparent that Tregs are by far the most efficient effector T cell possessed by the immune system. With this in mind, and knowing that tumor antigen-specific Tregs are created from the antigen-specific T cell pool, and be derived from memory Tregs (Zhang 2013), one again can imagine how these types of Tregs could be therapeutically used to fight against the tumor and not the anti-tumor T cell response. Because Tregs can shape and refocus the T cell immune system they are the perfect vehicles to use to direct the T cell immune system during immunotherapeutic procedures. In an adoptive transfer setting, genetically altered autologous Tregs generated in vitro can be transferred back to the patient for any number of immune modulating reasons. In fact, preliminary studies are being done on Tregs that have been genetically engineered to express antigen specific TCRs (Wan 2013). The value in using Tregs themselves as immune cellular therapeutic tools lies in their ability to swiftly alter a T cell response on many different levels. For instance, one of the main interactions between Tregs and other cells of the immune system is centered on the relationship between Tregs and DC. Much has been written about this interaction throughout the discussions here that have focused on the intracellular pathways, which dictate the behavior of Tregs, T cells, DC, and tumor cells as they interact during anti-tumor and autoimmune T cell responses. As will be shown in this chapter, the Treg/DC interface, much like the immunobiology this interaction, can be a good thing or a bad thing during clinical immune cell-based immunotherapy for cancer.

This chapter will at first examine the early developments of human clinical immunotherapeutic trials related to three types (adoptive T cell-based therapy, DC-based vaccines, and bone marrow transplantation) of immune cell-based immunotherapies. There will be a section devoted to each of these three immunotherapies, which will give details about the ultimate rational behind the procedures, the immune cells involved, auxiliary treatments, and the expected/actual outcome. At the end of each section there will be an examination of the role Tregs play in the successful or unsuccessful treatment of cancer with that particular type of immunotherapy. An effort will be made to confine these discussions to human clinical trials of the therapies mentioned above. However, almost all human clinical trials are preceded by similar procedures performed in animal models. Many times, but not always, immune cell-based therapies that work in these animal models fail to produce similar results in humans. There are several possible explanations for these discrepancies ranging from the inbred nature of laboratory animals to immunological evolutionary differences between animals and humans. Regardless of these explanations it may be of value to refer to some of these pre-clinical animal trials because some of the experimental discrepancies may reveal important information about the human anti-tumor T cell response.

Whenever possible during these discussions of the three immune cell-based therapies mentioned above references will be made to information that was provided in the previous chapters that had to do with Treg origin/function, responding T cell fate, autoimmune aspects of the T cell/Treg/cancer interactions, and use and consequences of Treg effector mechanisms. This approach should give a holistic view of how the immunotherapy of cancer encompasses the entire function and spectrum of the T cell immune system. The human T cell immune system is complex and full of redundant inter and intracellular systems and this must be reflected in the design of immune cell-based immunotherapy for cancer. As per the first three chapters, there will be two major sections. The first section will detail the cellular interactions involved in these therapies as their descriptions and outcomes are revealed. The second section will concern itself with the intracellular translational pathways associated with the cellular behaviors described in the preceding section. However, toward the end of the translational pathway section there will be a discussion related to altering these pathways by agents that temporarily enhance or block pathways in T cells and/or Tregs to increase efficacy of the immunotherapeutic treatment. This section will be a culmination of the information and more importantly, the rational behind the concepts contained within this book.

Cellular Interactions

Early Human Cancer Immunotherapeutic Clinical Trials

In the early 1970s there was the recognition of an immune response to cancer in animal models and the term, 'tumor-specific transplantation antigen' or TSTA was coined and described what is now know as tumor antigens (Gold 1970). After years (late 70s to early 80s) of performing immune cell-based experiments on genetically cogenic strains of mice it was apparent that not only was there an immune response to a growing tumor, but the cells that responded (T cells) were the same cell-type that responded to viral infections. During this period it was recognized that this immune response resulted in the failure of T cells to eradicate the cancer despite the fact they were present during tumor growth. This was demonstrated in mice where tumor-specific T cells could be isolated from peritoneal effusions of a growing genetically identical (syngeneic) mastocytoma tumor called P815Y. Despite the fact that these mice died from the tumor; there were functional anti-tumor cytotoxic T cells present during this process (Biddison 1977). This was a constant observation where there were responding T cells present during tumor growth, but ultimately the host animal died from the tumor. However, the model tumor system in mice that got the most attention was that of melanoma and in the mid-1970s it was recognized that immunotherapy was the vision of future cancer therapies (Rosenberg 1975). Modern tumor immunology was born in the 1970s and with the above observation being repeated in several tumor systems there was a challenge to manipulate this apparent conundrum of a constant ineffective T cell immune response to cancer by altering the immune system itself. Using a mouse model of melanoma (B16) it was determined that in order for the tumor to be eradicated there had to be a specific sequence of anti-tumor therapies. Chemotherapy to induce tumor apoptosis was first, then surgery to remove the tumor mass was next, and the final therapy was an immunotherapeutic procedure (Pendergrast 1976). This therapeutic rational will be revisited several times during this discussion because it is telling and comments on inflammation, phagocytosis, antigen presentation, and tumor immuno-selection. Studies using this particular tumor model continue to this day and are a valuable tool used to examine the basic tenants of tumor immunology, which as mentioned, may or may not relate to the human immune response to cancer.

The development and interest in this mouse model of melanoma was prompted by the prevalence of human melanoma, which during the 1960s was recognized as a relatively incurable form of cancer, yet was amongst a group of tumors that displayed spontaneous regression (Sumner 1960). One of the earliest preclinical experiments involving human melanoma was done in England in the early 1970s. These experiments involved the immunization of malignant melanoma patients with autologous tumor lysates and measuring the cytotoxicity mediated by peripheral blood lymphocytes (PBL) using recently excised adherent autologous melanoma cells as targets. Less that half (5 of 12) mounted a significant CTL response after seven days. The researchers were unable to explain the brevity of this response that only lasted two weeks after the treatment. There was no correlation between patient sera antibody binding to their melanoma cells and the lack of cytotoxicity. However, this was the first time immunologist considered the value of immunotherapy as a treatment for melanoma, but admitted that this procedure had little impact on disease progression (Currie 1971).

During this period in the US, clinician/scientists were taking another approach to actually treating melanoma by injecting cutaneous and subcutaneous melanoma lesions with Bacillus Calmette-Guerin or BCG, which is a powerful adjuvant that had been used as an anti-tuberculosis vaccine. Prior to this treatment patients were tested for immunocompetence using a skin reactivity test called delayed cutaneous hypersensitivity test (DHT) to a compound called dinitrochlorobenzene (DNCB). It was found over a 7-year period that out of 151 malignant melanoma patients treated with BCG immunotherapy, 90% of the injected lesions regressed and 17% of uninjected lesions in the same immunocompetent patients also regressed. In addition, 25% of these patients remained disease free for 1-6 years following the treatment. However, despite the fact that surgical resection of large tumor masses and removal of regional lymph nodes did improve the response to the therapy, many if not most of these patients developed recurrent disease. Another complication was that when the therapy was tried on patients who had visceral or subcutaneous metastasis the response rates were lower, temporary, and very rarely uninjected lesions regressed (Morton 1974). These were very important findings because this was the first time that immunity to a tumor could be generated within a patient as evidenced by the regression of uninjected lesions and disease-free survival. The unexplained results were that the majority of positively responding patients eventually developed recurrent disease and patients with visceral metastasis were non-responsive to treatment. These results suggest that the immune response to melanoma was complex and there was no agreement on which arm (antibodies or lymphocytes) of the immune system was responsible for the immune response because at this point there were no standardized in vitro assays to accurately measure these responses. These in vitro assays would allow clinician/scientist to identify not only the specific responder/effector cells, but also what they recognized on the tumor to allow them to respond (Mukherji 1973).

Encouraged by the positive results of studies such as these clinicians in the late 1970s took a direct approach to the treatment of melanoma by using a specific targeted approach to immunotherapy. For instance in a large clinical trial they made an addition to the BCG adjuvant therapy used above by including subcutaneous injections of irradiated (blocks cell division), neuraminidase treated (removes carbohydrates and exposes cell surface proteins) autologous or allogeneic melanoma cells. These were very complex clinical trials because in large studies such as the one discussed below there were 979 patients with various stages of melanoma in multiple locations. The stages of melanoma were classified on levels, which were associated with the thickness of melanoma lesions (level I = thinnest, level V = thickest) and based on a micro staging classification system developed by Dr. Wallace H. Clark in the late 1960s-early 1970s (Clark 1969). This classification system with another, which classified the stage (I = primary, II = cutaneous metastasis, etc) of melanoma, allowed physicians to predict the outcome of a patient's disease based on the stage and thickness of their melanoma lesion. This clinical study treated only Stage I and Stage II patients with various thickness levels. In general, and without treatment, Stage I patients survived their disease with a higher frequency than Stage II as do Clark's Level I vs. Clark's level V patients. Using this type of immunotherapy, four-year survival rates were improved for Stage I and lower Clark's Level patients (Level I-III), but there were no significant differences in survival in patients that had Stage II melanoma because of the fact that more often than not the disease had already spread to the lymph nodes. Lymph node involvement often results in the loss of immunocompetence. Despite the fact that the therapy was ineffective on melanoma patients with disseminated disease, the increase in survival rates in patients predicted by histologic staging was encouraging and supported the theory that the immune system was an important factor in the survival of melanoma (Seigler 1979).

Development of In Vitro Models Representing the Anti-tumor T Cell Response

As mentioned above, one of the difficulties in understanding the immune response to melanoma was the lack of reliable in vitro studies that would mirror the in vivo immune responses. During the late 1970s tumor immunologist began to understand the nature of the immune response to a growing tumor and as mentioned above where tumor-specific T lymphocytes had been isolated from growing tumors in mice, this response was ineffective (Biddison 1977). The most important observation was the fact that tumor immunologist began to relate standard cellular immunological concepts such as H-2 restriction (recognition of non-self in the context of self-MHC) to the immune response to cancer. In fact, during the discussion section of the large clinical trial above, it was mentioned that there were competing theories about whether two separate types of T cells were involved in the anti-tumor response, where one recognized tumor non-self antigens and the other self (Seigler 1979). It was thought that these two T cell types cooperated to form the anti-tumor T cell response, but of course that theory was misguided because there is one type of T cell that responds (CD4) and another that kills (CD8) and they recognize tumor antigens in the context of MHC-class II and MHC-class I respectively. As far as melanoma was concerned, it wasn't until the early 1980s that an in vivo/in vitro system was developed that helped explain the very nature of the cellular immune response to melanoma. In 1980 the Wistar Institute and the University of Pennsylvania School of Medicine formed what was unofficially called, "The Melanoma Research Cooperative Group." There were three major departments that collaborated on this project. The NIH funded Melanoma Program Project consisted of the Melanoma Research group at the Wistar Institute, which was headed by Dr. Meenhard Herlyn who was responsible for establishing and characterizing melanoma cell lines. These cell lines were established from patients who were seen at the University of Pennsylvania's Pigmented Lesion Clinic (PLC), which was headed by the aforementioned Dr. Wallace Clark. Diagnosis, treatment, and melanoma patient-related laboratory studies were carried out through the University of Pennsylvania School of Medicine's Department of Hematology Oncology by oncologist Dr. DuPont Guerry.

This was a coordinated effort carried out by these three groups where melanoma cell lines of patients that were established at the Wistar Institute would be grown in the Medical School laboratories, histological studies of their melanoma lesions characterized, and blood drawn from patients getting follow-up examinations at the PLC. Once the blood was drawn it was delivered to the laboratory where the peripheral blood leucocytes (PBL) were separated from the red blood cells. The PBL were further fractionated into monocytes, B-cells, and T cells. The melanoma patients, through the study of their lesions were diagnosed/classified as having either primary (Stage I) or metastatic (Stage II or greater) melanoma (Clark 1986). In the early 1980s, the Medical School laboratories developed an in vitro system that measured melanoma patient T cell responses to their own cultured melanoma cells. When comparing the T cell responses of both primary and metastatic melanoma patients to the presence or absence of a histologic lymphocytic infiltrate, which was only present in primary lesions, there was a perfect correlation. In other words, only primary, but not metastatic melanoma patients that had a brisk lymphocytic infiltrate within their resected tumor were able to mount an in vitro T cell immune response to melanoma cells cultured from those lesions. It was also determined that the T cell response was dependent on MHC-class II expression by the cultured melanoma cell line (Guerry 1984). In addition, it was observed that T cells within these primary lesions released INF-γ that was also detected during the in vitro T cell response to autologous cultured primary melanoma cell lines (Guerry 1987). In the same laboratory it was determined that unlike metastatic melanoma cell lines, which also expressed MHC-class II, primary melanoma cells had the ability to process and present not only T cell activating melanoma associated peptide antigens, but were also able to process and present exogenous antigens in the context of MHC-class II such as tetanus toxoid peptides much like normal APC (Alexander 1989). Laboratory studies such as these were the first to demonstrate a predictable in vitro T cell immune response to melanoma that was a mirror image of what was happening in the patient. This led to the latest form of cell-based immunotherapy because the technology to propagate tumor antigen specific T cells in vitro had been developed. Once it was established that T cell immunity to melanoma could be generated outside the patient's body, it ignited the vision of removing the immune cells from the patient, conditioning them to attack the tumor, and returning the now anti-tumor cells to the patient to attack their tumor.

Postmodern Human Cancer Immunotherapeutic Clinical Trials: The Treg Influence on the T Cell Response

Some of the earliest and somewhat successful cell-based immunotherapy clinical trials began in the late 1980s with metastatic melanoma patients. Tumor-infiltrating lymphocytes (TIL) were removed from resected tumor masses, expanded with IL-2, and returned to the patient during systemic IL-2 therapy. Tumor regression was observed in 60% of patients who never had IL-2-alone therapy. The percent was reduced to 40% in patients who had previously been treated with IL-2 alone (Rosenberg 1988). However, as these trials expanded using increasing numbers of metastatic melanoma patients it was apparent that only one-third of these patients responded and in some cases, suffered from the side effects of IL-2 therapy (Rosenberg 1994). Much like many of the cell-based immunotherapies that will be mentioned here, this clinical trial involved both adoptive and lymphokine therapy. However, despite the disappointing response rates to the treatment, these trials did demonstrate that there existed an immuno-competent anti-tumor response in human metastatic cancer. The next wave of cancer immune-based therapy utilized the DC as a vaccine vehicle to present immunogenic tumor peptides to metastatic melanoma patient's immune system. Initial studies focused on the immunogenicity of allogeneic tumor-lysate pulsed autologous DC. Delayed-type hypersensitivity (DTH) reactions against subcutaneous injected tumor lysates were measured after subcutaneous injection of tumor antigen pulsed DC with or without IL-2. Patient and control subject PBL were tested for INF-γ secretion after immunizations. Five patients were found to be HLA-A2+ and four of them responded in vitro to a melanoma specific peptide that had an affinity for HLA-A2. In this limited study 50% of these patients responded positively and the positive responses correlated with future disease stability and survival. In addition, there were no adverse side effects of either the DC vaccine or the dose of IL-2 used (Escobar 2005). Both of these studies (Rosenberg 1988 and Escobar 2005) were Phase I clinical trials, which as mentioned below are conducted for the sole purpose of determining if the clinical procedure is safe. Often these types of trials are conducted with written consent from patients with end-stage (Stages III-V) disease (Turkington 2005). As mentioned above, some of the melanoma patients treated with IL-2 during the adoptive transfer of IL-2 expanded TIL experienced adverse side effects associated with the IL-2 therapy. In contrast, the patients in the study using tumor lysate pulsed DC and IL-2 experienced no side effects. It was apparent the low-dose IL-2 therapy in conjunction with antigen loaded DC induced an anti-tumor response without adverse side effects. Knowing this, and the fact that DC play a pivotal role in the anti-tumor T cell response, tumor immunologist and clinicians moved forward in an attempt to augment the T cell response to cancer.

A refinement of the tumor antigen pulsed DC pre-clinical experiment was soon used in a clinical trial with renal cell carcinoma (RCC) patients. The refinement consisted of using a CTL specific peptide (MUC-1) that has a binding affinity for HLA-A2. Autologous DC generated from PBL were pulsed with the peptide and injected subcutaneously (s.c.) four times at 2-week intervals. These patients (20) were also given subcutaneous injections of low-dose IL-2. Given that this was a Phase I clinical trial to determine the safety of the procedure, none of the patients experienced adverse side effects. Out of the twenty patients, six experienced regression of metastatic lesions and four others had partial responses. Peptide-specific CTLs were detected in the PBL of the six patients with tumor regression. In addition, MUC-1 non-specific T cell responses could also be detected, which indicated the presence of lymphokine-activated killer cells. Another finding in this study was the fact that IL-2 therapy may not have been an effective addition to the treatment. In fact, it was determined that IL-2 therapy was inhibitory when observing T cell responses to the MUC-1 peptide and PADRE, a pan CD4 activating peptide (Wierecky 2006). The authors of the study gave no indication of why IL-2 therapy during the use of a DC vaccine was inhibitory, but the addition of IL-2 more than likely induced the activation of innate Tregs. As discussed in the previous chapter, Tregs have the capability to not only eliminate tumor antigen presenting DC, but also can de-differentiate mature DC into a immature form capable of inducing Treg conversion from the anti-tumor T cell pool. These were the early indications in the postmodern era of cell-based immunotherapy for cancer that there was another force resisting this form of therapy. This therapy is based on basic cellular immunological rules, which were that DC had the ability to activate an anti-tumor T cell response in naïve T cells by presenting tumor-associated peptides and secreting TH-1 lymphokines such as IL-12. However, the only way to understand what was really happening tumor immunologist again had to rely on histologic examinations of resected renal carcinoma tumors.

Postmodern Human Cancer Immunotherapeutic Clinical Trials: The Treg Influence on Solid Tumor Growth

Years after this and several other DC-based vaccine immunotherapeutic trials were performed, scientist conducted a study on histologic sections of RCC tumors and examined two parameters (DC chemokines and DC maturation) of DC immunobiology using specific antibodies to mature/immature DC and the three chemokines, MIP-3α (CCL20), MIP-3β (CCL19) and SLC or secondary lymphoid chemokine, which are involved in DC homing. This was an interesting study for several reasons. This was the first time that a detailed study of DC were made inside and outside of a tumor mass with regards to the function of DC based on their expression of antigens that characterized their maturity and homing capabilities. As has been mentioned several times; the maturity of DCs during the response to an inflammatory tumor mass is critical to the outcome of the anti-tumor T cell response by virtue of the fact that immature DCs help create Tregs and mature DCs can induce an anti-tumor T cell responses. Another reason why this study was so interesting is that through the use of specific antibodies it was possible to characterize not only the cells within the tumor mass, but also in the surrounding tissues. The authors of this study do not directly address the involvement of Tregs in the formation of these RCC tumors, but it will be shown that the influence of Tregs may have led to the structure and nature of the tumor mass and surrounding tissue. However, in order to understand the importance of these finding it will be necessary to understand the relationship between these three chemokines and DC. SLC is a chemokine expressed in secondary lymph nodes and attracts mature, but not immature DC that express the CCR7 chemokine receptor, which is strongly upregulated on DCs during inflammation (Saeki 1999). Chemokine MIP-3α (CCL20) is expressed by many cells in the body including the liver, epithelium, and can also be secreted by a wide variety of tumor cells. It is primarily a chemo attractant for immature DC, B-cells, naïve/responder T cells, and Tregs that express its receptor CCR6 (Schutyser 2003). MIP-3β (CCL19) is a chemokine produced by not only normal tissues and lymphocytes (including mature DC), but also many forms of cancer such as breast cancer (Treilleux 2004). Its receptor (CCR7) is expressed on DC as they differentiate into their mature cellular form and is thought to direct mature DCs from the periphery to the secondary lymph nodes (Foster 1999). The interesting aspect of the expression of CCR7 by DCs is how Tregs de-differentiate mature DCs by reducing expression of costimulatory proteins such as CD86. However, CCR7 expression is increased causing the DC to home to the lymph nodes and proceed to inhibit naïve T cell activation (Bayry 2007).

The study under discussion made several interesting observations concerning the location of immature/mature DC, T cells, and chemokine/receptor expression within or surrounding the solid tumor architecture. The first observation was that only immature CD1a+ DC could be detected within the tumor mass, which was devoid of both mature DC and T cells. In addition, there was the detection of "numerous" CD11c+ macrophages within the tumor. The second observation was that mature CD83+ DC with CD4 T cells clustered around them was found in the peri-tumoural area, which is near the pseudocapsule of the tumor. This area (perimeter) of the tumor is often surrounded lymphatic vessels containing these DC/T cell clusters where T cell proliferation has been detected. The cytokine MIP-3α was detected within tumor cells, tumor-associated macrophages, and cells of normal kidney origin. In contrast, MIP-3β was on expressed on CD83+ DC/ T cell clusters, but not within the tumor mass. SLC was expressed by lymphatic vessels, which were only found surrounding the tumor mass and stromal fibroblast that were associated with DC/T clusters and within the vessels themselves.

As far as the receptors for these chemokines were concerned, CD1a+ immature DC within the tumor mass expressed CCR6 (MIP-3α receptor) as well as immature DC within the DC/T cell clusters in the peri-tumoural area. However, none of the mature DC in DC/T cell clusters expressed CCR6. There was no expression of CCR7 (MIP-3β receptor) within the tumor mass, but significant expression of this receptor by both T cell and mature DC in the peri-tumoural areas. The interesting aspect of the scene of the tumor site, which was mentioned by the authors, was the fact that there was a "preferential localization" of mature DC in the peri-tumoural area that resembled the formation of DC around secondary lymphoid organs and the presence of the lymphoid chemokines SLC and MIP-3β is consistent with the formation of tertiary lymphoid tissue at the tumor pseudocapsule interface (Middel 2010).

The reason why so much time was spent on describing the "scene" or appearance of these RCC tumors undoubtedly has to do with Tregs. There are several features present that directly relate to the functional capabilities of Tregs and what maybe seen here are the aftereffects of Treg influence during the development of the tumor. The first fact that would support the conjecture that Tregs were or are still influencing the overall growth of the tumor and the immune systems relationship with it comes from the fact that the tumor cells are expressing CCL20 or MIP-3α. T cells, as well as immature DC express the CCR6 receptor, which would allow Tregs to appear even before RCC specific T cells could be generated. This has been already supported by observations that CCR6 is expressed on tumor infiltrating Tregs in RCC tumors (Oldham 2012).

Another piece of evidence is the fact that only immature DC are found within the tumor mass. Aside from the fact that immature DCs express CCR6 and would be attracted to MIP-3α, they most likely helped generate additional Tregs as the tumor grew. It was discussed earlier that when Tregs retarded or dedifferentiated DC they expressed lower levels of

CD80/86 and had augmented levels of CCR7 (Bayry 2007). However, these dedifferentiated DC would not enter the tumor mass because of the absence of MIP-3β expression. Only CCR6 expressing immature DC would be attracted to the tumor mass because of the expression of MIP-3α by RCC tumor cells. The "scene" of the tumor mass as far as the architecture of the tumor mass is concerned has the "signature" of Treg function all over it. For instance, in the peri-tumoural there are two physical structures that had to be manufactured. The first is the presence of a pseudocapsule, which is found in 66% of RCC tumors and the result of fibroblast growth due to the compression of the renal parenchyma and the subsequent re-modeling of the extracellular matrix (ECM) (Yamashita 1996). The second physical structure present that relates to the presence of Tregs is the appearance of blood and lymph vessels in the peri-tumoural area.

During the previous chapter on Treg effector mechanisms there was a protracted conversation about the secretion of granzyme B (GrB) by Tregs and its function to remodel the ECM (Buzza 2005). The induction of fibrotic tissue is a characteristic of protracted inflammation induced by GrB (Miyazaki 2004) and the presence of Tregs during the growth of these pseudocapsilated RCC tumors may point toward Treg activity during the formation of these fibrotic capsules. This activity is in line with Treg function during an inflammatory response where Tregs take command of the site and set-up conditions that isolate and dampen the inflammatory T cell response, but does not completely halt the T cell response. The main purpose of Treg function is to prevent autoimmune T cell responses, but the remodeling of the ECM does not completely cut-off the access by antigen specific T cells to their targets. As previously mentioned, Tregs can behave as inflammatory cells like mast cells that also release GrB to increase permeability of the ECM to lymphokines and cells by degradation of fibronectin, collagen, and laminin (Buzza 2005). The presence of lymphatic and blood vessels in the peri-tumoural space is the result of the secretion of vascular endothelial growth factor (VEGF) secretion by cells drawn to inflammatory responses. One of these cells that were mentioned by the authors of the histologic study of RCC DC phenotypes was the presence of numerous CD11c+ macrophages (Middel 2010). Its been shown that tumor-associated macrophages secrete VEGF in response to Treg secreted adenosine contact with all three (A1, A2A, A2B, and A3) adenosine receptors (Hasko 2012). One of the many functions of Tregs during an inflammatory response is to also secrete VEGF (Facciabene 2012), which as mentioned allows a blood supply to a tumor mass, but also facilitating tumor escape from the primary site.

In support of this concept, it been shown that the presence of Tregs in RCC tumors correlated with increased angiogenesis of the tumor mass (Ning 2012). The physical characteristics of the tumor mass and the fact that it resembles a secondary lymphoid organ points toward the involvement of Tregs during the formation of these encapsulated solid tumors. As mentioned before, the effects of Tregs in many inflammatory responses at times can be subtle such as the situation above where the tumor is carefully cordoned-off from the normal tissue, yet has access to the lymphatic system. This situation and the more direct influence of Tregs during both growth and treatment of cancer will be revised again as specific immune cell-based therapies are discussed next.

Human Cancer Immunotherapeutic Clinical Trials: Adoptive T Cell Immunotherapy

Adoptive T cell therapy (ACT) actually has a long history in animal models. However, as discussed above, the clinical trials involving the transfer of in vitro expanded TIL into metastatic melanoma patients during infusion with IL-2 where the first clinical trials approved in the 1980s by the NIH using this particular combination of therapeutic procedures (Rosenberg 1988). Again as mentioned above, the results of these trials were encouraging, but were ultimately ineffective and as time went on it was recognized that the patient's own immune system was resisting the treatment. It was shown in animal models of ACT that removal of the tumor host immune system by either chemicals (chemoablation), total body irradiation (TBI), or a combination of both improved the response rate. After almost twenty years it was determined that the main immune factor that was impeding the success of these treatments was in fact Tregs. A secondary factor was the absorption of lymphokines by not only Tregs as discussed previously, but also the intact cellular immune system, and was referred to as "cytokine sinks." This realization prompted clinician/scientists to initiate the treatment of melanoma patients with the immunosuppressive agents fludarabine and cyclophosphamide, which increased the response rate from 25 to greater that 50%. In addition, there was evidence that this procedure led to the "long-term persistence" of adoptively transferred T cells. It was determined, through the study of animal models, that an even more aggressive approach should be used that removed all of the lymphocytes of the host or lymphodepleting conditioning (Muranski 2006). During the almost twenty years after those clinical trials utilizing adoptive transfer of in vitro expanded TIL during IL-2 therapy cellular immunologist where not only able to recognize the existence of Tregs, but also had developed detailed knowledge about T cell immunobiology. This knowledge allowed them to further manipulate this process by adoptively transferring Treg-depleted CD4+ positive T cells with anti-melanoma CD8 effectors in mice, which induced tumor regression of established tumors (Antony 2005).

Human Cancer Immunotherapeutic Clinical Trials: Adoptive T Cell Immunotherapy and the TCR

Despite the recognition of the host immune system resistance to these treatments and attempts to overcome them, the strength of ACT was the effector T cell. The isolation and recognition of tumor-associated CD8 T cell recognized peptides such as the gp100 melanoma-specific epitope recognized by melanoma-specific CD8 CTL (Moreau-Aubry 1997) was the beginning of specific targeting of tumor-associated antigens that could be a source of anti-tumor T cells during ACT. The discovery and use of tumor-associated peptides that generated tumor specific CTL in vitro, using peptide-pulsed DC, became prevalent in other tumor systems (Carlisson 2004) and it seemed that soon in vitro-induced tumor peptide specific T cells could be used during ACT. However, what immunologist discovered about the nature of these peptides induced caution based on their combined use as immunogens. It was found that the melanoma-specific peptide gp100 was also expressed on normal melanocytes and as previously discussed; its recognition by CD8 effector T cells was a major cause of the melanoma-induced autoimmune disease called vitiligo (Mandelcorn-Monson

2003). In fact, it was determined that the use of several anti-tumor/anti-self peptides was detrimental to the generation of an anti-tumor T cell response (Rosenberg 2006). Obviously, this has to do with the nature of tumor-associated antigens, which was discussed previously when referring to neoantigens. The concept is that these antigens (peptides) are composed of self and non-self (Overwijk 2000). When the TCR models itself (somatic mutation) against these peptides they do respond to the cancer, but also respond to normal tissues such as melanocytes, which induces the activities of Tregs and failing in their ability to control these T cells can result in autoimmune diseases such as vitiligo. This was an added complication, which was reflected in therapies that used tumor antigens as vaccines because often auto-reactivity would be detected in conjunction with improved patient survival (Lotem 2009). However, despite this problem that pertained to several tumor systems there was an effort to collect information, correlate the findings, and try to further refine this type of therapy in order to make it much more effective (Gattinoni 2006). It became evident that the T cell used as an immunotherapeutic tool during this type of therapy had to be totally specific for the tumor, be able to function as a normal long lasting antigen specific T cells, and generate a T cell memory pool.

In order to induce the type of situation mentioned above where significant amounts of tumor antigen-specific T cells could be transferred into tumor bearing host and behave as normal antigen specific effectors that would generate an immunological memory (memory T cells), it was necessary to genetically engineer the adoptively transferred T cells. The initial focus was on the TCR because it is the central element responsible for activating the T cells to become effectors and later memory T cells. This seems like a straightforward task. However, the TCR is quite complex as is the process of delivering the genetic information for the expression of a genetically altered receptor. As previously described, the TCR is actually a complex of proteins that come together during the interaction of the cell with peptide antigens. This complex is composed of TCR-alpha, TCR-beta, and three varieties of the CD3 proteins (epsilon, delta, and gamma) as well as the CD247 accessory molecule known as CD3ς chain. These proteins not only span the cell membrane, but also protrude onto the cell surface as mentioned above. The CD3 proteins are needed to assemble the TCR alpha and beta chains on the cell surface. Two CD3ς proteins are associated with the ends of both the TCR-alpha and beta proteins on the inside of the cell membrane, protrude into the cytoplasm, and mediate the initiation of translational signals. Depending on which type of T cell (helper CD4 or cytotoxic CD8), a CD4 or CD8 protein is necessary for the contact between the APC and the T cell. If this is a CD4 T cell then there is an affinity for MHC class II (HLA-DR, DP, DQ, or DM) proteins because the CD4 protein (ligand) attaches itself to the MHC class II protein (receptor). Alternatively, a CD8 T cell has an affinity for MHC class I proteins (HLA-A, B, C) for the same reasons (Lefranc 2001). The TCR alpha and beta proteins are configured in such a way as to conform to the peptide-MHC protein complex on the surface of the APC. The TCR is now prepared to attach to the presented peptide with significant affinity to actually bind the two cells (T cell and APC) together in a semi-permanent manner. Contact is now made between the TCR-complex and the MHC-peptide complex. Included in this event is the binding of CD28 on the T cell with its ligands CD80 and CD86 expressed on the APC. Once this contact is made the T cell actually begins to spin so that all of its available receptors (TCR, CD4/CD8, and CD28) are engaged to the available ligands (MHC-antigen and CD80/86) attached APC. Once the receptors are localized on the T cell surface the intercellular domains begin to interact with cytoplasmic protein messengers.

Human Cancer Immunotherapeutic Clinical Trials: Adoptive T Cell Immunotherapy and the Genetically Engineered TCR

Aside from the complexity of the physical interaction between the TCR, stimulating peptide, and MHC molecule of the APC, there is also the activation of intracellular pathways that lead to the T cell activation/effector function. These pathways are detailed in Chapter 1 under the subheading *Intercellular signaling as a result of T cell receptor engagement* and will not be discussed here. However, there were two approaches to genetically altering the TCR. The first was to identify the genes responsible for the TCR-alpha and TCR-beta proteins that were specific for a particular antigen, clone the genes, and transfer that genetic material to a population of naïve T cells to be used as adoptively transferred therapeutic T cells (Dembic 1986). Another way cell immunologist approached re-engineering T cells utilized the fact that it is more difficult to identify tumor-specific peptide/TCR combinations on a genetic level than it is to isolate tumor-specific monoclonal antibodies. Given this disparity in tumor antigen recognition they were able to construct what are called chimeric TCRs or CARs. These receptors were composed of a single-chain construct of the variable and light-chain of a tumor-specific antibody linked to a hinge region. This is called the exodomain and it is attached to a transmembrane domain, which in turn is connected to an intracellular endodomain composed of the either the CD3ε, CD3γ, or CD3ζ (TCR ζ-chains) cytoplasmic domains of a traditional TCR or the cytoplasmic domain of high-efficiency FcRI. This is the description of the initial first generation CARs (Eshhar 1993). These intracellular domains direct specific activation events as well as the secretion of lymphokines by the use of signaling motifs of intracellular lymphokine domains. The entire chimeric gene is modular and allows researchers to not only specify which antigen the T cell responds to, but also allows them to direct the effects on the T cell after it engages its target. The modular nature of these CAR genes has resulted in the development of 2nd and 3rd generation versions able to be used to modify hematopoietic stem cells (HSC), induce specific lymphokine secretion, and insertion into developing thymocytes. These CARs are now being used in multiple clinical trials to not only treat cancer, but also to alter the progression autoimmune diseases. The development of CAR+ T cells and the introduction of these cells into patients, which have modified genetic promoters, can have safety issues, but because of their design, have the potential to revolutionize adoptive T cell therapy for cancer (Jena 2010).

Adoptive T Cell Immunotherapy: Clinical Trials Using Genetically Engineered TCRs. High-Affinity Specificity and Autoimmunity Induced by Transduced TCR Alpha and Beta-Chains

Tumor antigen specific peptides, which are identified by the response of patient T CTLs are always associated with a specific MHC class I genotype. For instance the MUC-1 RCC peptide has a binding affinity for HLA-A2 (Wierecky 2006), as well as MART-1 and gp100 melanoma/melanocyte peptide (Chang 2011). The first clinical trials using the insertion of cloned genetically engineered TCR-alpha and beta genes specific for tumor antigen peptide and MHC-class I (HLA-A2) was performed in 2006 in melanoma patients. The TCR-alpha and beta genes were isolated and cloned from the TIL of a melanoma patient that was successfully treated (near complete regression) with adoptively transferred TIL that had been expanded in vitro with IL-2. A retroviral vector was used to transfer MART-1 specific TCR-alpha and beta genes into PBL separated into CD4 or CD8 T cells. All of the melanoma patients (17) had progressive disease and had failed to show objective responses during IL-2 immunotherapy. The transfer of genetically altered T cells proceeded after lymphoablation where there was the maximum amount of lymphodepletion. Prior to infusion transduced CD4 or CD8 T cells were cultured in vitro with anti-CD3 antibodies from 8 to 11 days (cohort 1) and 6-9 days (cohort 2) for optimal cell division. Initially, all of the patients T cells were reactive to MART-1 expressing HLA-A*0201 melanoma cell lines in vitro measured by the secretion of INF-γ. The cloning efficiencies as measured by Vβ12 expression were between 17 and 67%. Flow cytometry using MART-1 peptide tetramer binding was also used to monitor levels of MART-1 specific T cell and RT-PCR was used to detect retroviral RNA. The patients were also divided into several cohorts based on T cell proliferation mentioned above. The patients in the cohorts with fastest doubling time of the transfused T cells exhibited prolong persistence of the TCR transduced T cells after ACT. Eight of these patients had a cell persistence of 17% after 50 days, with seven patients exhibiting persistence for 90 days.

One month after ACT 14 patients tested positive for viral RNA as well as increased numbers of CD8+ Vβ12 T cells. Two of the 17 patients that received this type of ACT had sustained objective regression of their melanoma where large tumor masses shrunk and they remained disease free for over 21 months. Despite the fact that for the majority of patients in this clinical trial objective responses were not as robust as the two mentioned above, this study demonstrated for the first time that TCR transduced T cells could be used during ACT because they persist in the circulation and induce the shrinkage of large tumor masses. This study, which again was a Phase I clinical trial was able to accurately expose the weakness of the procedure such as low expression of functional MART-1 TCRs due to possible mispairing of TCR-alpha and beta proteins (Morgan 2006).

Shortly after this study another clinical trial was conducted on melanoma patients with high affinity genetically engineered TCR in order to improve the anti-tumor effector function of ACT transferred T cells.

Two TCR constructs were created to the above-mentioned MART-1 and gp100 melanoma/melanocyte peptides. The TCR genes from the TILs found in the patient's resected melanoma lesions were cloned and retroviral transduced T cells recognized the MART-1 peptide. However, since it was difficult to isolate TCRs that recognized gp100 peptide in humans, HLA-A2 transgenic mice were immunized with the peptide and the TCR genes were isolated, cloned, and used as a source to produce the gp100 peptide specific TCR. Retroviral gene therapy vectors were used to transduce 48h anti-CD3 antibody stimulated patient PBL with the TCR genes. After an additional period of stimulation with anti-CD3 antibodies the cells were evaluated for surface expression and responsiveness to MART-1 and gp100 by tetramer staining and INF-γ secretion in response to HLA-A*0201 melanoma cell lines. In 36 patients the cloning efficiency for the MART-1 and gp100 TCRs was 71% and 82% respectively.

The majority of these patients, who were lymphodepleted before transfer of genetically engineered T cells, exhibited tumor specific T cell responses after 1 month. Of 20 patients who received the MART-1 peptide TCR, 30% had objective cancer regression compared to 19% of 16 patients that received the transduced mouse anti-gp100 peptide TCR. A side effect of the treatment was the initial appearance of an erythematous rash in most patients, which was the result of melanocyte destruction as evidenced by the appearance of a CD8+ T cell infiltrate that resulted in "patchy" vitiligo. In addition, 55% of the MART-1 TCR patients and 25% of the gp100 TCR patients developed anterior uveitis, which is typical of a lymphocytic response to pigment producing cells of the eye. Even the melanocytic cells of the inner ear were affected where a significant number of patients experienced hearing loss (Johnson 2009).

This apparent increase in autoimmunity induced by these high-affinity anti-melanoma/melanocyte TCRs, as the authors pointed out, was due to the increased specificity for those antigens and my not reflect the true nature of an effective anti-tumor T cell response. Such a response includes the polyclonal recognition of tumor antigen variants by T cells as well as proper lymphocyte homing.

Adoptive T Cell Immunotherapy: Clinical Trials Using Genetically Engineered TCRs. TCR-Chain Mispairing and ACT T Cell Effector Homing

As far as traditional genetically engineered TCR is concerned, one of the problems or potential problems has to do with the formation of the alpha and beta chain pairing. The problem is that the peptide specificity of the TCR is determined by the combination of peptide-MHC binding sites that span both chains. Therefore, if there is a pairing between a transduced TCR chain and an endogenous TCR chain, new peptide specificities may be created. In a mouse model it was shown that transduced TCR alpha or beta chains and endogenous TCR chains could combine and form what is called a neo-TCR. It was found that these neo-TCR could recognize self-antigens and lead to a lethal autoimmune GVHD-like syndrome. These mixed dimer TCR were a direct result of the pairing of transduced TCR-alpha or beta chains associating with endogenous TCR alpha or beta chains. It was found that during the pairing process there was an abundance of endogenous TCR chains, but if their numbers were limited by using polyclonal T cell populations or by equalizing pairing using modified retroviral vectors, it would reduce the incidence of the syndrome (Bendle 2010). This syndrome closely resembles transfusion-associated GVHD in immunocompromised patients where haploidentical donor T cells attack the recipient's immune system and organs and is always fatal (Orlin 1997). Even though this phenomenon has not been observed in human ACT clinical trials, the potential exist because the theory/evidence of TCR-chain mispairing is a reality.

Despite these potential problems with the induction of a GVHD-like syndrome due to TCR-chain mispairing, clinician/scientist continued to conduct clinical trials using genetically engineered TCR. However, this time the target was melanoma brain metastasis as this trial addressed the homing properties of genetically engineered and TIL effector cells. This clinical trial utilized not only engineered T cells, but also isolated CD8+ TILs in separate treatment protocols.

This was a comparative study involving two separate populations of patients who were older that 18, had a life expectancy of 3 months, that had stable hepatic, renal, and hematopoietic reserves. In addition, all (26) of these patients had brain lesions of less than 10 mm without edema. In the TIL/ACT group the autologous TIL were isolated from resected metastatic melanoma lesions that were grown in vitro for 14 days with anti-CD3 antibody and IL-2 before patient infusion. Some of the patients within this group received TIL that were highly purified for CD8+ T cells. In the genetically engineered TCR/ACT group PBL were stimulated with anti-CD3 antibodies and IL-2 prior to being transduced with recombinant retrovirus encoding the α and β chains of and HLA-A2 restricted TCR for melanoma/melanocyte peptides MART-1 (Morgan 2006) and gp100 (Johnson 2009). These were the same two genetically engineered TCRs used in the previous two clinical trials mentioned above. Prior to infusion with TIL or engineered T cells, the patients were lymphodepleted with non-myeloablative (depletes lymphocytes, but not monocyte/macrophages) agents cyclophosphamide and fludarabine and some received TBI at various levels. At the time of lymphocyte infusion the patients received IL-2 every eight hours as tolerated with a maximum of 15 doses.

Because these were Phase I clinical trials and a diagnosis metastatic melanoma brain metastasis results in a 3-month life expectancy, the purpose of the trial was to determine if TIL or engineered T cells could induce tumor regression and extended life expectancy. In the patient group that received the TILs plus IL-2 41% showed complete remission of their brain disease with the majority sustaining that condition from 4 to 44 months. However, several of these patients experienced brain tumor relapses within 6 months. All of the patients (17) experienced median survival rates of 8.5 months and 40% of them had an actuarial 2-year survival rate. In the patient group (9) that received the genetically engineered T cell plus IL-2, two experienced complete remissions of 8 and 25 months and the median survival rate for all 9 patients were 15 months. Considering the severity of their disease both groups in this clinical trial experienced exceptionally long median survival rates when compared to the 2-month survival rates of identical patients without treatment. There were several special aspects to this trial that were very informative. First of all, there is the issue of effector T cells crossing the blood-brain barrier to attack brain metastasis. Initially, it was thought that for a variety of reasons, and as mentioned previously, that the brain being part of the central nervous system (CNS) was an immune privileged site, which is not part of the immunological surveillance system described earlier in this text. Even though that is the case, conditions that arise that cause inflammation such as experimental autoimmune encephalomyelitis (EAE) and in this case tumor metastasis, allow T cells to enter the CNS (Wekerle 2002). However, this clinical trial was the first of its kind to demonstrate that indeed T cells may enter the brain to effectively kill tumor cells. The second aspect of this study was the possible elimination of standard procedures for these types of brain metastasis and their replacement with ACT. Normally, there is brain surgery of radiosurgery to remove the tumor mass and then whole-brain radiation therapy. This and other more radical procedures result in a 5 to 8 month survival rate, which is a 3-5 month improvement, compared untreated brain metastasis patients. Whereas the median survival rate for patients treated with TIL or engineered T cells was 24 and 15 months respectively. This clinical trial (Hong 2010) serves as an improvement over the previous two mentioned in this section because it was safe and effective in this setting.

Adoptive T Cell Immunotherapy: Clinical Trials Using Genetically Engineered TCRs. The Continual Persistence of Tregs Inhibits ACT Despite Lymphodepletion

Cancer immunotherapy as stated previously, encompasses a broad variety of therapies intended to elicit a cellular (T cell) immune response against the tumor. Some of the therapies rely on the existing immune system of the patient to mount a response through administration of defined tumor antigens/peptides with or without antigen presenting DCs or exogenous IL-2. However, ACT is a more direct approach to cancer immunotherapy because it specifically targets the tumor with specialized anti-tumor T cells that have either been specifically isolated and expanded or genetically altered to respond to or kill the tumor upon infusion into the patient. Using antigen (tumor peptides) alone or in concert with DC/IL-2 is a passive method of cancer therapy and clinically has resulted in only a 5% overall response (OR) rate in melanoma patients. Using ACT prior to lymphodepletion and with IL-2 therapy the OR rates for the same category of patients is from 40 to 76% with complete response rates of 40%. The crucial part of these ACT clinical trials has been shown to be the lymphodepletion phase. This phase of the protocol is thought to be important because it removes two important factors that impede the success of the therapy. Those are endogenous Tregs and resident IL-2 absorbing lymphocytes (Giao 2013). Despite the effectiveness of lymphodepletion (non-myeloablative agents and TBI) to increase the OR during ACT, there are serious concerns about the continued involvement of Tregs in the inhibition of this type of cancer immunotherapy. The first concern is the fact that lymphodepletion is not 100% and there is still a very small population of endogenous lymphocytes that survive the treatment. The second concern is that despite the fact that either TIL or TCR-engineered PBL are used as a source infused T cells, they are still T cells nonetheless and can be converted into tumor-specific Tregs once they enter the patient's body. This is a particular concern considering high-dose IL-2 therapy is used to augment the effectiveness of the transferred T cells. In fact it has been shown that high-dose IL-2 therapy, which has been a segment of the ACT protocol, induces ICOS+ Tregs. This type of Treg is highly suppressive because there is augmented expression of CD39 and CD73 (adenosine secretion), IL-2R (IL-2 depletion), and increased secretion of IL-10 and TGF-β (Sim 2014). Since adoptively transferred T cells are activated in vitro prior to transfer, they express the high-affinity IL-2R and transiently express FOXP3, which makes them basically indistinguishable from Tregs. Once these immunotherapeutic T cells enter the body they are exposed to conditions (therapeutic IL-2 and inflammation-induced lymphokine secretion) that foster the formation of adaptive Tregs. Studies are now underway to examine the possibility that Tregs are still an inhibitory factor during ACT despite the fact that a procedure (lymphodepletion) is in place to remove them.

Until recently there were no studies concerning the role Tregs played in the T cell immune response during ACT clinical trials similar to the one's outlined above. More than likely due to the apparent effectiveness of lymphodepletion during the therapy, researchers assumed that Tregs were no longer an important ACT resistive factor. However, in the years following these clinical trials it was discovered in an animal model of ACT, that there were chemical (non-myeloablative agents) and radiation (TBI) resistant Tregs, which induced specific inhibition of the anti-tumor T cell response during the therapy. In this study lymphodepletion was induced by either TBI or treatment with the non-myeloablative agent cyclophosphamide. The mice were given an immunogenic tumor and reconstituted with naïve

T cells. Tumor growth was diminished, but when Tregs were removed after lymphodepletion there was a significantly greater diminution of tumor growth. However, the effect of TBI on Treg numbers was studied as mice recovered from the treatment without reconstitution with naïve T cells. It was found that the percentage of Tregs (18%) in recovered mice was significantly higher than control mice (5%) not exposed to radiation. Even though the transfer of naïve T cells after TBI decreased the percentage of Tregs, there was still 2 to 3 times more than in control mice. In addition, it was determined that more Tregs infiltrated growing tumors in irradiated mice when compared to control mice. Specific removal of Tregs after TBI not only increased anti-tumor effector generation and tumor reduction, but also resulted in a reduction of Treg tumor infiltration. It was also determined that the Tregs responsible for inhibiting the anti-tumor T cell response were from the recipient and not the donor T cell pool. This study demonstrated that lymphodepletion by both non-myeloablative agents and TBI actually increased the numbers of recipient Tregs and these cells were actively involved in the inhibition of the anti-tumor effects of ACT (Baba 2012). It is apparent from these studies in mice that there are not only Tregs that survive lymphodepletion, but also actively participate in the inhibition of ACT. These radioresistant Tregs are active in terms of tumor invasion and responder cell inhibition, but seem to develop over time as either the endogenous lymphocytic milieu increased during recovery or as naïve T cells are infused alone or during ACT. The late development and growth of these Tregs is actually controlled by the presence of lymphokines produced by endogenous or ACT T cells either during steady-state conditions or during the response (inflammatory) to the tumor respectively.

A recent study of Tregs during ACT in human clinical trials revealed the detectable presence of Tregs after lymphodepletion. Samples were analyzed from over 100 Stage IV melanoma patients who participated in 5 NIH clinical trials. These ACT trials used TIL or gp100 engineered TCR T cells from PBL. After infusion all patients received 15 doses of IL-2 as tolerated. They also received chemical lymphodepletion (non-myeloablative) alone or with one of two (2 Gy or 12 Gy) doses of TBI. The patient's cells were analyzed for CD4+ FOXP3+CD3+ T cells and CD4+FOXP3+ T cells by flow cytometry. The phenotype of Tregs found in ACT patients was evaluated using antibodies detecting CD127 (IL-7 alpha receptor) CD45RO (effector cells) and Ki-67 (proliferation). In addition, the methylation status of CpGs within intron 1 of the FOXP3 gene was determined in order to identify stable CD4+Tregs (Wieczorek 2009). These measurements (except for methylation) were done 7 days prior to the initiation of ACT, 1 week, and 4 weeks after. As far as the persistence of Tregs was concerned, CD4+FOXP3+ T cells within CD3+FOXP3+Treg population were detected by flow cytometry 1 week and 4 weeks after ACT and there was a reduction in the percentage of Tregs, which continued into week 4. However, when absolute cell counts of CD4+FOXP3+ T cells were done, the number of Tregs had almost doubled between week 1 and 4. This difference was probably due to the presence of activated TIL transiently expressing FOXP3. Phenotypic analysis of patient Tregs after ACT revealed that a significant amount of them were proliferating (Ki-67+) effector (CD45RO+) Tregs. Functional assays performed on isolated Tregs indicated that they had the classic "anergic" phenotype and also had the ability to inhibit CD4+CD25- proliferation. In addition, analysis of the TIL used for infusion revealed that there were CD4+ and CD8+ Tregs, which secreted INF-γ upon stimulation. Demethylation studies of the FOXP3 revealed that PBL Tregs after ACT treatment were demethylated (32%) when compared to in vitro cultivated infusion TILs were the methylation was over 90%. Therefore, the Tregs found in PBL in ACT treated melanoma patients were innate or natural thymus-derived Tregs in contrast to TIL Tregs, which were characteristic of the adaptive Treg phenotype.

Another interesting aspect concerning the presence of Tregs during ACT has to do with the number of IL-2 doses. In patients that received just chemical lymphodepletion the percentage of Tregs in PBL was closely related to the number of IL-2 doses received. This association was diminished when TBI was added to the protocol. There also was a strong association of the presence and frequency of Tregs and the patient's response to ACT treatment. In other words, patients that had a recurrence of their disease or were refractory to ACT had higher percentages of Tregs. The absolute CD4 T cell numbers between responding and non-responding patients were the same, but the percentage of CD8 T cells was higher in responders. Furthermore, statistical analysis of this data using multiple clinical trials showed that Treg levels in melanoma patients correlated with negative clinical responses (Yao 2014).

It has been known for some time that Tregs can inhibit anti-tumor T cell responses. However, this study, using advanced statistical analysis of patient outcomes in a clinical setting, clearly demonstrates the negative influence Tregs have not only on the natural T cell response to cancer, but also the clinical treatment of the disease. This study does support the contention put forth in the murine model of ACT discussed above where Tregs survived lymphodepletion and were able to have a negative impact on this type of cancer immunotherapy. Another aspect of this study supported the intended goal of ACT, that being a reduction of Tregs through lymphodepletion prior to infusion of the adoptively transferred cells. In addition, it has been shown that not only does the procedure of ACT reduce Treg percentages, but also fosters the induction of a TH-1 CD4 T cell response (Ishikawa 2011). This is also an important finding because of the fact that CD4 T cell responses to the tumor support the activation of anti-tumor CD8 CTL precursors and generation of mature CTL (Pardoll 1998). However, despite the fact that ACT has the essential elements necessary to achieve the immunological eradication of the tumor, Tregs are still present and continue to interfere with the positive outcomes of clinical trials utilizing this type of cancer immunotherapy. Here, the discussion of genetically altered TCR alpha and beta chains has been restricted to Phase I clinical trials of late-stage melanoma due to the technological development of distinct T cell receptors against melanoma/melanocyte antigens that have been isolated, cloned, and inserted into naïve T cells. However, chimeric TCRs or CARs have also been successfully used during ACT in both solid and hematopoietic tumor systems.

Adoptive T Cell Immunotherapy: Clinical Trials Using Genetically Engineered TCRs. The In Vivo Persistence of Chimeric TCRs (CARs) during ACT

As previously described, CARs are genetically constructed TCRs that utilize the antigen-specific variable regions of the light chains derived from tumor-specific monoclonal antibodies. These TCRs function in a similar way to traditional TCR in that they activate the T cell they are inserted into and have the ability to mediate antigen-specific T cell cytotoxicity. In addition, CAR+ T cells, because of their genetic modular design, have the ability to circumvent problems associated with traditional TCRs. There are several disadvantages that traditional TCRs have when it comes to interacting with tumor cells. The first problem is that traditional TCRs must interact with both the tumor-specific peptide and

MHC of the tumor in order to either become activated to proliferate or kill. As discussed in the second chapter *Autoimmunity, Tregs, and the anti-tumor T cell immune system,* cancer cells because of their proclivity towards DNA mutations often do not express MHC proteins or do at a reduced level. The recognition of the tumor cell by CAR+ T cells does not depend on interactions with MHC proteins expressed by the tumor since the interaction is based on the binding of the variable light-chain region of a monoclonal antibody. A second problem is that many times the tumor does not express the CD80/86. These ligands interact with CD28 and provide the essential "second signal" discussed previously, which leads to T cell activation and with out it leads to T cell anergy. In addition, signaling through CD28 induces IL-2 secretion, cell cycle entrance, and cell survival (Harding 1992). As previously mentioned in the *Human cancer immunotherapeutic clinical trials: Adoptive T cell immunotherapy and the genetically engineered TCR* section above, the first-generation CARs included the TCR ς-chain in order to facilitate TCR signaling, but because of either the absence or low-level expression of CD80/86 these receptors were inefficient. To compensate for the absence of CD28 signals and to guarantee proper "second signal" activation of the CAR T cell, the intracellular domain of the CD28 receptor was added as a "cassette" in the modular genetic construct of the CAR gene. In addition, another intracellular domain was added called 4-1BB or CD137 that is a member of the TNF family and is activated by CD28 during TCR/CD28 engagement. CD137 signals enhance T cell proliferation; inhibit activation-induced cell death (Hurtado 1997), lead to CD8 T cell proliferation, and the amplify CD8 CTL responses (Shuford 1997). It was found that once both co-stimulatory cytoplasmic domain "cassettes" was added in combination with the TCR ς-chain to the CAR construct, transduced T cells had the ability to secrete and enhanced level of IL-2, INF-γ, TNF-α, and GM-CSF. This allowed CAR transduced naïve T cells to respond, proliferate, and survive after antigen activation in the absence of exogenous stimuli (Finney 2004). Soon, these CAR+ T cells would be ready for human cancer immunotherapeutic clinical trails.

The initial human clinical trials using CAR+ T cells was a Phase I trial that examined the efficacy of these T cells during ACT in patients with late-stage ovarian cancer. The target tumor antigen is called folate-binding protein (FBP), which is a 27kD protein over expressed in human ovarian carcinoma and identified by monoclonal antibodies MOv18 and MOv19 (Coney 1991). The first-generation CAR construct used the FBP-specific light chain of the MOv18 antibody and TCR ς-chain intracellular domains (Hwu 1995). Since this was an early Phase I clinical study, the safety assessment of adoptive therapy using gene-modified T cells was the main goal. All of the patients (14) had recurrent ovarian cancer that had failed standard therapy, but demonstrated intact immune systems as measured by DTH to multiple antigens such as *Candida albicans*. None of the patients were treated lymphodepleting procedures prior to the infusion of the chimeric MOv-γ genetic construct transduced anti-CD3, IL-2 stimulated autologous PBL. The MOv-γ genetic construct also contained the neomycin resistance gene (neomycin phosphotransferase), which was used to positively select transduced PBL. Selected patients were treated with escalating doses of IL-2 during ACT. Patients were monitored for INF-γ secretion in response to FBP expressing tumor cells, FBP-specific antibodies (ELISA), T cell migration (111In-oxide labeled transduced T cells), and T cell persistence (PCR of neomycin gene). The results demonstrated that the phenotype of transduced cells prior to infusion significantly varied as far as expression of CD4+ and CD8+ T cells as well as low expression of the transduced MOv-γ protein by flow cytometry. After infusion patient PBL responded to a FBP+ ovarian tumor cell line above a control FBF- melanoma cell line. Tracking studies using radio-labeled (111In) transduced PBL revealed that transduced cells were in the circulation (1%), but most had homed to the lungs and not to the tumor sites. It was also determined by PCR detection of the neomycin resistance gene that transduced PBL rapidly disappeared from circulation after two days and did not persist beyond 3 weeks. In addition, many of the patients developed anti-mouse antibody titers that inhibited transduced T cell responses to FRB+ ovarian tumor cells. This early study (Kershaw 2000) was the first to use CAR+ T cells in a human clinical trial. None of the patients responded to therapy and went on to progressive disease. Some of the patients receiving IL-2 therapy experienced adverse side effects that were manageable and the treatment itself was relatively safe. However, the transduced cells lacked the ability to home to the tumor sites and did not persist in the patient's circulation. The study pointed out several problems associated with these early ACT clinical trials. The first thing was the fact that there was no lymphodepletion. More than likely transduced cells were immediately attacked by the patient's Tregs, which could not only explain their inability to persist in the circulation, but also cellular damage in the form of Treg-secreted GrB could retard the homing properties of these transduced cells. More importantly, the lack of CD28 and or CD137 intercellular domains in these CAR genetic constructs could lead to the lack of survival due to the inability of the transduced cells to counteract apoptotic signals generated by antigen stimulation. The results of this study led directly to the development of the second and third generation of CAR+ T cells.

Adoptive T Cell Immunotherapy: Clinical Trials Using Genetically Engineered TCRs. Using Second-Generation Chimeric TCRs (CARs) for the Treatment of B-Cell Lymphomas and Leukemias during ACT

After a period of time scientist and clinicians understood the limitations of ACT using first-generation CAR+ T cells without lymphodepletion. As mentioned above, second-generation CAR+ T cells were constructed with CD28 intercellular domains as well as CD3 ς-chains. One of the earliest successful clinical trials utilizing these CAR+ T cells was performed with a single patient with a Stage IV B follicular lymphoma. The patient had a progressive form of lymphoma, which was characterized by enlarged lymph nodes containing monoclonal B-cells that expressed CD19, CD20, CD22, CD10, and IgM-kappa. This monoclonal B-cell phenotype was detected in 14.5% and 55% (CD19+ cells) of PBL and bone marrow respectively. Prior to CAR+ T cells the patient received the non-myeloablative agents cyclphosphamide and flurodarabine to facilitate lymphodepletion. The target antigen was CD19, which is expressed on normal, activated, B-cell precursors, plasma cell, and malignant B-cells. CAR retroviral vectors used to transduce anti-CD3 stimulated PBL were composed of the antigen-recognition variable regions (H and L chains) of an anti-CD19 monoclonal antibody (FMC63) connected to CD28 and CD3 ς-chain intracellular domains. After transduction 64% of T cells expressed CAR-related mouse IgG. T cells comprised 98% of the population, which was composed of 66% CD8+ and 34% CD4+ T cells. One day after lymphodepletion the patient receive two IV doses of CAR+ T cells and then received 8 doses of IL-2, eight hours apart. After treatment a there was detectable regression of the lymphoma, but at 9 months lymphoma growth continued in cervical and retroperitoneal lymph nodes. In addition, within 2 months of treatment peripheral blood and bone marrow B-cells were absent and lasted an additional 7 months, as did the absence of detectable serum levels of IgA and IgM. Five months after the treatment the patient was diagnosed with unknown type of pneumonia, but was treated and recovered. However, after 10 months immature (CD79a+, CD19-) B-cells were detected, which was an indicator that B-cell precursor development had began as normal B-cell development recovered after the treatment. Normal levels of all lymphocyte (except B cells) types and RBC returned to normal after 2 months. PCR detection of the CAR genetic construct revealed that CAR+ T cells were present in the circulation for at least 9 months (Kochenderfer 2010). These studies demonstrated that CAR+ T cells could facilitate an effective anti-lymphoma T cell response and persist for periods much longer that first-generation CAR constructs. In addition, the levels of normal lymphocytes, RBC, but also precursor B cells were recovering while the monoclonal B-cell tumor was reducing indicated a positive prognosis. However, the loss of antibody-producing B-cells from the periphery as well as the bone marrow was disturbing. Considering the fact that the patient was diagnosed with pneumonia, this procedure renders the patient seriously immunocompromized. Related to the inability of such patient to mount an antibody response was the fact that there was not an inhibition of CAR+ T cell activity due to the generation of anti-mouse IgG antibodies due to the mouse IgG used to construct the CAR+ T cells because the patient lacked antibody-producing B-cells during treatment.

The use of CD19 specific CAR+ T cells to treat B-cell malignancies basically skirts around a serious problem with these genetic constructs. The problem tends to be two-fold as far as the human T cell immune system is concerned. As mentioned during the discussion of one of the initial clinical trials using first-generation CAR+ T cells, there was the generation of anti-mouse IgG T cell response during ACT. This response activated a B-cells, which generated antibodies against mouse anti-FBP H & L-chain variable regions of the MOv18 antibody. These antibodies inhibited the ability of CAR+ T cells to effectively respond to the FBP antigen expressed by ovarian carcinoma cells (Kershaw 2000). In addition to the response of host T cells to mouse IgG, the presence of selective CAR T cell DNA genes such as neomycin (neomycin transferase) become targets of the host T cell immune system and contribute not only to the limited lifespan of these cells, but also inhibit their ability to attack their targets (Ramos 2011). These observations were made based on the use of first-generation CAR constructs. However, second and third-generation constructs present additional problems due to their expression of CD28 and CD137 intracellular domains that increase the efficiency of T cell activation. An adverse effect of such constructs was documented using a second-generation CAR construct that made the use of an anti-ERBB2 antibody variable region. The ERBB2 (Her-2/neu proto-oncogene) antigen is over expressed in many cancers that metastasize such as breast and ovarian cancer (Slamon 1989). This CAR, which contained a single-chain variable region of an anti-ERBB2 monoclonal antibody (4D5), the intracellular domain of CD28 and CD137, as well as CD3ς was used in a γ-retroviral vector to transduce the anti-CD3 + IL-2 expanded PBL of a colon cancer patient that had lung and liver metastasis. The gene was transferred into 79% of CD3+ T cells (17% CD4, 63% CD8). Prior to ACT the patient was lymphodepleted with the non-myeloablative agents cyclphosphamide and flurodarabine. However, immediately after the transfer of the transduced PBL ($1x10^{10}$) the patient experienced acute respiratory distress due to a massive pulmonary infiltrate of PBL. The patient was intubated in intensive care, but passed away 5 days later. Serum levels of INF-γ, GM-CSF, TNF-α, IL-10, and IL-6 indicated that the patient suffered from a "cytokine storm," which was mentioned during the *Introduction* section of Chapter 3. The authors of this report attributed the death to the accumulation of transduced cell responding to low levels of the ERBB2 antigen in the lungs and their subsequent release of these cytokines (Morgan 2010). Despite the fact that this a separate issue, not related to the immune response of the patient to mouse immunoglobulin or selective DNA used to isolate transduced cells, it nonetheless represents a potential danger associated with using a high-affinity antigen-specific antibody variable region in a genetically engineered chimeric T cell receptor. The cytokine storm induced in this patient, though not an autoimmune response similar to the use of high-affinity genetically engineered TCRs during the ACT clinical trials that involved gp100 and MART-1 (Johnson 2009), it was an adverse immune response generated because the use of CAR+ T cells.

Despite this unfortunate case above and the recurrence of the B-cell lymphoma discussed earlier that occurred during ACT using second-generation CAR constructs, a successful clinical trial with a chemotherapy non-responsive chronic lymphocytic leukemia (CLL) patient was performed. After several rounds of chemotherapy and a 2-year disease free period the patient developed recurrent disease characterized by rapid progressive leukocytosis (elevated WBC counts) and adenopathy (enlarged lymph nodes). T cells were collected by leukapheresis and cryopreserved. Thawed T cells were transduced with the CD19-specific chimeric receptor, which was in a self-inactivating lentiviral vector. The CAR construct contained the variable heavy and light chains of CD19 specific antibody FMC63 as well as intracellular domains of CD137 (4-1BB) and CD3ς. Prior to infusion of CAR+ T cells the patient was with the non-myeloablative lymphodepleting agents cyclphosphamide and pentostatin. After treatment 40% of bone marrow cells had the CLL monoclonal phenotype expressing kappa light chain, CD5, CD19, CD20, and CD23. There were two separated clones, which had various chromosomal deletions and lost chromosome 17p. The patient received a total of $1.42x10^7$ transduced cells during three days of escalating doses. The infusions induced very few adverse effects aside from lymphopenia and what is called tumor lysis syndrome characterized by elevated blood levels of uric acid, phosphorous, lactate dehydrogenase and acute kidney injury. After 28 days there were no detectable CD19+ B-cells and adenopathy had disappeared. Six months after ACT there was a sustained remission of the disease or normal B-cells. This clinical trial was successful and the study complete as of October 2013, which was four years after its initiation (Porter 2011). The success of this clinical trial was based on several factors associated with the design and delivery of the CAR+ T cells. Instead of using both CD28 and CD137 intracellular domains in the construction of the receptor with CD3ς domains, only CD137 was used allowing it to inhibit activation-induced cell death of the transduced T cells. As a consequence the transduced CAR+ T cells rapidly expanded over a 21-day period and comprised 20% of circulating lymphocytes and persisted for over 6 months. Another advantage was the amount and way the transduced cells were administered. The total dose ($1.4x10^7$) was much lower than the $1x10^{10}$ dose used in the ERBB2 clinical trial described above. Even though this patient experienced elevated levels of inflammatory lymphokines (INF-γ and IL-10) roughly 20 days after infusion, this was the result of a clinical response brought on by immune response to the CLL cells and not a cytokine storm. The transduced cells were also given over a 3-day period, which more than likely allowed them to freely circulate through the lungs. As far as an immune response to either the vector or the mouse Ig chains; again this treatment removes the involvement of an antibody response because it removed mature CD19-expressing B-cells.

Adoptive T Cell immunotherapy: Clinical Trials Using Genetically Engineered TCRs. Important Factors for the Future Success of ACT Used to Treat Cancer

The use of adoptively transferred autologous T cells for the treatment of cancer has the potential to be one of the most effective therapies used to treat this disease. The ultimate goal of these therapies would be to completely eliminate the harmful and most of the time, painful adverse effects associated with cancer treatment. However, despite the fact that ACT can and continues to demonstrate effectiveness in removing cancer cells from the body, harmful treatments such as non-myeloablative chemotherapy and/or radiation are still necessary. These procedures, as discussed previously are essential to aid in the engraftment and function of the adoptively transferred T cells. Lymphodepletion of a patient by either or both of these methods is an unpleasant experience for the patient an also leaves them vulnerable to a host systemic problems due to the lack of a functioning immune system. In addition, many of these ACT clinical trials using genetically engineered T cells or TIL (especially TCR-alpha/beta) require the use of high-dose IL-2 therapy, which by itself induces unpleasant side effects. Other adverse effects associated with ACT, which were mentioned previously are autoimmune responses induced by anti-tumor high-affinity TCRs and immune responses to mouse Ig variable regions used in the construction of CAR+ T cells. The immune responses to Mouse Ig don't particularly directly harm the patient, but they do interfere with the function of the CAR receptors, which result in the inhibition of their anti-tumor function. Autoimmune-like responses on the other hand can lead to multiple problems such as the cases of eye damage, vitiligo, and hearing loss in patients receiving ACT using high-affinity TCRs against the melanocyte/melanoma antigens gp100 and MART-1. Certainly the most extreme case was that of the patient who died after receiving CAR+ T cells specific for ERBB2 antigen that is over expressed in many malignant tumors, but also can be expressed at low levels in normal epithelial cells (Zajchowski 1988). It was determined that lung epithelial cells were the targets of these CAR+ T cells, which induced a fatal cytokine storm. These problems with ACT that use genetically engineered T cells can be addressed and possibly solved using new approaches to this type of cancer therapy.

One of the most serious, but essential protocols (chemotherapy and TBI) associated with ACT is lymphodepletion. As mentioned previously, they are mainly directed at reducing the interference caused by Tregs during the response of adoptively transferred T cells to the tumor. An additional reason to use these protocols is to remove the ability of autologous lymphocytes to absorb lymphokines released by the transferred T cells as they respond to the tumor. This is important because responding T cells require these lymphokines such as IL-2 to not only induce effector function, but also to survive in the circulation and at the tumor site. Regardless of this fact, the mere presence of the patient's normal complement of Tregs can render ACT ineffective at removing the tumor. This was evidenced by the fact that during the reports of early cancer therapy in the *Early Human Cancer Immunotherapeutic Clinical Trials* section above, which documented cancer clinical trials during the 1970s, very few clinical responses were seen. Aside from the disappearance of local melanoma lesions that were not injected with BCG in the one study, there was no effect on visceral metastasis (Morton 1974). These results and others, which demonstrated the loss of tumor-specific CTL activity of PBL from patients that received autologous tumor lysates (Currie 1971), pointed toward an active inhibition of cancer therapy by the immune system. Obviously, during the 1970s Tregs were unknown, but their ability to inhibit cell-based cancer treatment continued as clinical trials using IL-2 therapy and TILs isolated from growing melanoma lesions were used in the first ACT studies in the mid to late 1980s. As these clinical trials continued into the 1990s it was apparent that again there was resistance by the immune system to these ACT by virtue of the fact that less that one-third of the patients responded to the treatment (Rosenberg 1994). In addition, some cell-based immunotherapies made use of DC vaccines by virtue of their ability to induce an immune response by presenting tumor-specific peptides to patient T cells. As mentioned previously, a clinical trial such as this was conducted with RCC patients (Wierecky 2006). Many of the patients demonstrated partial clinical regressions of their tumors, but no complete regression. Furthermore, IL-2 therapy was inhibitory to the response; no doubt due to the generation of Tregs, which inhibited the ability of DCs to stimulate a naïve T cell anti-tumor response. Upon inspection of the nature and cellular composition of RCC tumor masses (Middel 2010) it was apparent that their formation, architecture, and immune cellular composition had been controlled by Tregs that were present possibly during the development of the tumor.

From the information given above and ACT studies carried out in mice it was apparent that removal of the host cellular immune system by lymphodepletion increased the effectiveness of the therapy. Eventually all clinical trials concerning the adoptive transfer of not only T cells, but also DC (see below) included lymphodepletion as a treatment protocol during the therapy. The addition of these protocols markedly the increase effectiveness of ACT used human clinical trials (Muranski 2006). However, it was clearly demonstrated that there were lymphodepletion regimen-resistant Tregs in mice (Baba 2012) and humans (Yao 2014) that actively participated in the inhibition of ACT. Despite the greatly reduced numbers of Tregs after lymphodepletion, high-dose IL-2 therapy used as a protocol in ACT can rapidly expand their numbers. As mentioned previously, high-dose IL-2 therapy can induce ICOS+ Tregs that are immunologically more suppressive due to their heightened expression of CD39, CD73, and CD25 (IL-2R) and increased secretion of IL-10 and TGF-β (Sim 2014). This is supported by the fact that memory T cells responsible for tissue rejection in mice are specifically inhibited by Tregs after TBI in mice (McFarland 2012). In addition, it was determined that Nrp-1+ (neuropilin-1, growth factor enhancer) CD4+ CD25+ Tregs increased after TBI and these cells had increased expression of cAMP and PKA protein in addition to increased secretion of TGF-β (Dong 2014). As far as radio-sensitivity of Tregs is concerned it was found that CD4+FOXP3+ Tregs were less prone to radiation-induced apoptosis than CD4+FOXP3- T cells. In addition, Tregs specifically expanded at twice the rate as they did in non-irradiated mice and secreted more IL-10. However, Tregs from irradiated mice were 2.5% less effective at suppressing T cell immune responses (Balogh 2013). Therefore, it is clear that not only does TBI not remove most resident Tregs, but may enhance their proliferative potential during the natural lymphocyte reconstitution process. Even though radio-resistant Tregs may be functionally deficient, given their dependence on IL-2 for functional development; IL-2 therapy after TBI and adoptive transfer would allow for the rapid recovery of Treg function. Heightened Treg function after ACT may very well be the case because of the apparent selective process involved with lymphodepletion and the subsequent reconstitution of the lymphocyte population after the procedure. Therefore, the very few Tregs that survive ACT lymphocyte-conditioning regiments may be uniquely armed to inhibit the anti-tumor effects of adoptively transferred T cells. Tregs that develop under these conditions may have developed specialized abilities to inhibit T cell responses due to the nature and plasticity of the Treg phenotype. As described previously, the ability of Tregs to control DC function is much more extensive when compared to responding T cells because Tregs can alter the expression of important DC cell-surface proteins.

DC-Based Immunotherapy for the Treatment of Cancer: The DC Vaccine

DC-based cancer immunotherapy began simultaneously with the development of ACT. The recognition of the increased antigen presentation functions of DC when compared to monocytes or macrophages prompted researchers to choose these cells as therapeutic vehicles for the delivery of immunogenic tumor peptides to immune T cells. Early on, the methods for producing active DC from PBL monocytes had been developed and will not be discussed here, but the ease of production and availability made them the perfect cell to use for cellular immune-based cancer treatment. In vitro experiments clearly demonstrated how DC could generate tumor-specific T cell proliferation and CTL generation. The use of DCs as therapeutic vehicles is specifically targeted to the adaptive immune system. This system, versus the genetically based innate immune system that relies on inherited receptor-based genetic elements, responds swiftly to the recognition of antigen. The adaptive system does not because it relies on the development of antigen-specific receptors that are derived through somatic mutations of receptor genes. The advantage of the adaptive system is that immunity can be generated to previously unknown (to the host immune system) antigens associated with pathogens or cancer. However, because of the time it takes to generate such responses these developing antigen-specific T cells become vulnerable to the influence of Tregs. As described numerous times, Tregs can control many very important aspects of DC function such as maturation, antigen presentation, and lymphokine secretion, but at the same time DCs can influence Tregs such as how immature DC induce the conversion of antigen-specific T cells into Tregs or the induction of IL-10 secretion in Tregs. These vulnerabilities and strengths of the DC population are based on two important features, which are numerous subsets/maturity levels and general cellular plasticity (Steinman 2007). This combined with the above-mentioned functionality of DCs enable them to be used as pliable immune cellular vaccines used to generate tumor-specific T cell responses.

DC-Based Immunotherapy for the Treatment of Cancer: Clinical Trials Using DC Vaccines and the Involvement of Tregs

Several clinical trials involving the use of DC vaccines for the treatment of cancer were discussed earlier. The first clinical trial (Phase I) was performed to examine the immune response to melanoma antigens. This study utilized the DC as a vaccine vehicle to present immunogenic tumor peptides to metastatic melanoma patient's immune system and focused on the immunogenicity of allogeneic tumor-lysate pulsed autologous DC. Delayed-type hypersensitivity (DTH) reactions against tumor lysates were measured after subcutaneous injection of tumor antigen-pulsed DC with or without IL-2. There were no real-time clinical responses in melanoma patients (Stage III-IV) who received the vaccine with or without subcutaneous injections of IL-2. Half of the patients (20) PBL responded (INF-γ secretion) in vitro to the same allogeneic melanoma cell lines, but the contribution of melanoma allogeneic MHC class II antigens was not measured. However, the patients that survived their disease longer demonstrated in vitro T cell responses to the melanoma cell lines used as a source of tumor lysates (Escobar 2005). This study added to the information indicating that DC vaccines were safe, induced measurable anti-tumor T cell responses, and caused no side effects. The next clinical trial was more specific as far as the T cell response was concerned in that it utilized a specific renal cell carcinoma (RCC) peptide shown to be recognized by RCC immune T cells. This peptide (MUC-1) is also expressed on metastatic breast cancers and ovarian tumors. This was a Phase I trial with metastatic RCC patients used this CTL specific peptide that has a binding affinity for HLA-A2. Autologous DC generated from patient PBL were pulsed with the peptide and injected subcutaneously (s.c.) four times at 2-week intervals. These patients (20) were also given injections of low-dose IL-2. Of the twenty patients, 6 demonstrated clinical responses with various stages of remission of lung and visceral tumors. One of the interesting aspects of this trial had to do with the administration of IL-2. In some patients IL-2 administration inhibited the effectiveness of the DC vaccine (Wierecky 2006). It was thought that the IL-2 therapy activated DC-controlling Tregs. This data and the results of multiple clinical trials related to the administration of DC-based vaccines in not only RCC, but also prostate cancer revealed that the use of DC vaccines had a positive and statistically significant effect on the progression of both types of cancer. This study was based on the meta-analysis of 200 clinical trials and stressed that the maturation and dose of therapeutic DCs used to present tumor antigens was a critical factor in the refinement of this type of cancer immunotherapy (Draube 2013).

Despite the fact that DCs can orchestrate the stimulation, proliferation, and induction of a cytotoxic T cell response to cancer, they still have the ability to arrest that response though the activation of Tregs. During the development of any given tumor there is the activation of CD4 T cells. The activation of these T cells does not necessarily have to do with their response to the tumor, but may have to do with the inflammation caused by the growth of cells (pre-cancerous tumor cells) that the T cell immune system has deemed as normal damaged tissue. This initial response is based on the influx of macrophages that are drawn in by stress indicators such as ATP. During the initial activation phase macrophages release chemokines that attract CD4 T cells and Tregs. In turn, these inflammatory CD4 T cells begin to elaborate a plethora of lymphokines that include GM-CSF and IL-3/IL-4. Resident macrophages and monocytes that become stationary at the site are immediately converted into DC. The interesting part follows. These converted DCs are not fully mature because they have not been exposed to a high enough concentration of lymphokines. This is an inflammatory response and immature DCs formed at the site have only one job, which is to control the T cell response and the cells responsible for this control are the Tregs. However, the development of the immature DC occurs with a minimum signal from these lymphokines (GM-CSF and IL-3/4). Immature DCs frequently induce (convert) T cells to become Tregs by the secretion of TGF-β and IL-10. One major factor in this process is the self-antigen specificity of the Treg. During an inflammatory response such as a viral, bacterial infection, or the growth of malignant cells normal cells of the tissue systems involved die. As they die (apoptosis) these cells release DNA (ATP) and their proteins are endocytosed and processed by immature DC. Since innate Tregs are selected in the thymus based on their self-specific TCR, they are immediately attracted to DCs that present self. However, if this lymphokine signal is constant DCs begin to mature and have increased expression of MHC-class I and II antigens as well as CD80 (B7.1) and CD86 (B7.2) receptors. CD4+ and CD8+ Tregs can become activated and proliferate with IL-2 provided by responding T cells, DC presented self-antigen, and B7 costimulation (Zou 2010). Therefore, if the inflammatory agent is a growing tumor this series of events can occur and more than likely do as evidenced by the physical characteristics of some solid tumor masses. Earlier in this chapter under the heading, *Postmodern Human Cancer Immunotherapeutic Clinical Trials: The Treg Influence on Solid Tumor Growth* it was evident that Tregs had actively been involved in shaping the physical "layout" of the tumor mass. This is based on the formation of the tumor mass's pseudocapsule, which is found in 66% of RCC tumors and the result of fibroblast growth due to the compression of the renal parenchyma and the subsequent re-modeling of the extracellular matrix (ECM) (Yamashita 1996). This re-modeling of the ECM was more than likely due to the secretion of GrB by Tregs while the tumor grew through the induction of fibrotic tissue, which is a result of GrB cellular damage (Miyazaki 2004). In addition, vascularization of the tissue surrounding the tumor pseudocapsule can be generated by either tumor-associated macrophages (TAM) that secrete vascular endothelial growth factor or VEGF in response to Tregs secreted adenosine (Hasko 2012) or secreted by Tregs themselves (Facciabene 2012).

Given the involvement of Tregs in not only the protection of growing tumors, but also the development of the tumor mass itself a clinical trial was specifically designed to eliminate Tregs during the administration of a tumor peptide DC vaccine to patients with melanoma. In a non-randomized study half (15) of HLA-A2.1+ melanoma patients (30) were treated with a humanized anti-CD25 antibody (daclizumab) 4 to eight days (two cohorts) prior to immunization of individual autologous DC aliquots pulsed with gp100 and tyrosinase peptides as well as KLH. Patients were all metastatic melanoma patients with normal renal and hepatic function and had previously been treated for their disease with various methods (surgery, radiofrequency ablation, radiation therapy, and chemotherapy) alone or in combination. DTH to pulsed DC were performed as well as serum levels of anti-KLH antibodies to determine the effect of removal of CD25+ T cells. Tetramer binding with gp100 and tyrosine peptides was performed to detect anti-tumor T cells. Proliferative responses of patient PBL and cytokine production after DC vaccine administration were done to measure an anti-KLH T cell response daclizumab or control treated patients. Soluble IL-2 alpha levels were measured in the urine in order to determine the effects of daclizumab treatment as wells as flow cytometry measurements of cell-bound CD25.

The results of the vaccine immunizations indicated that most patients experienced mild vaccine-related side effects such as fatigue, anorexia, fever, and erythema at the injection site. Adverse effects of the daclizumab were not detected and there was no detection of anti-nuclear antibodies, which would indicate an autoimmune response. However, one patient did develop vitiligo upon follow-up. Immediately after treatment with daclizumab soluble IL-2 alpha levels became undetectable and there was a complete removal of high-expressing IL-2R FOXP3+ CD4+ T cells. The levels returned to normal within 4 weeks. Anti-KLH antibodies were detected in control, but not daclizumab treated patients despite the fact that PBL from all patients that received KLH-pulsed DC responded in vitro through T cell proliferation and the secretion of TNF-α and INF-γ, but not IL-4. In addition, patient sera containing daclizumab that was injected after 48hrs prior was inhibitory to this anti-KLH T cell response. Two of 10 control patients not receiving daclizumab had detectable anti-tumor T cells measured by tetramer binding. In addition, 5 of 13 patients in the treatment group had anti-tumor circulating T cells, but in 3 of these five the tetramer+ T cells were non-functional in assays measuring cytokine secretion during stimulation with gp100. The clinical results indicate that there was no clinical benefit by the use of Treg depleting daclizumab because there was no effect on progression-free survival (PFS) when compared to the untreated control group. This clinical trial study (Jacobs 2010), which was to determine the effect of the transient removal of CD25+ CD4 T cells during tumor-peptide pulsed DC vaccination demonstrated how difficult it is to address the problems associated with the anti-tumor T cell inhibitory activities of Tregs. The authors admitted that the drug (daclizumab), which was designed to remove effector T cells in order to prevent graft rejection during organ transplantation, could interfere with the anti-tumor T cell response by interrupting IL-2 signaling pathways. The drug completely depleted CD4+ FOXP3+ CD25+ Tregs within 4 days, but normal levels of Tregs reappeared after 4 weeks. During that period functional proliferative T cell responses to KLH, but not tumor peptides was detected, which may indicate that IL-2-dependent CD4 helper T cell requirements for the generation of an anti-tumor T cell response are different when compared to those required for an anti-KLH T cell proliferative response. This is evidenced by the lack of an anti-KLH antibody response in patients treated with daclizumab when compared to untreated controls. Since CD25 is transiently expressed on activated CD4 and CD8 T cells as previously mentioned, "innate" anti-tumor helper T cells may have a more of a requirement for secreted IL-2, which is not secreted in an autocrine fashion by CD25+ CD4+ T cells because they have been removed by the treatment. Despite these problems associated with Tregs during the treatment of cancer using DC vaccines, clinical trails now in combination with ACT continue to be performed and many have produced positive objective clinical responses as well as complete regressions of the disease (Kandalaft 2013).

Transplantation Therapy for the Treatment of Hematological Cancers: The Role of Tregs and Their Use to Prevent Graft-Versus-Host Disease (GVHD)

In the previous chapter called, *Treg Effector Mechanisms* the treatment of hematological malignancies such as leukemia and lymphoma using the transplantation of hematopoietic cells was discussed in the context of not only how Tregs control graft-versus-host disease (GVHD), which can be viewed as a massive inflammatory response, but also how Tregs increase their numbers in the face of an almost out of control donor T cell response to the recipient's tissues. The process involved with the transplant of donor cells into lymphodepleted cancer patients is complex not only due to the process (haplotyping) of choosing the source and type of donated cells, but also the exact diagnosis of the type hematologic cancer, which often times dictates the design of the transplant procedure that includes the methods of lymphodepletion as discussed in the previous section on ACT. Because there are multiple types of lymphomas and leukemias the focus on these treatments and the involvement of Tregs will be made to narrowly focus on specific examples where the transplantation procedure clearly exposes the important aspects of this topic. Many of these observations began as preclinical studies in mice that used various models of hematological cancers and their related treatment using donor cells isolated from the bone marrow. These types of transplants are called hematopoietic stem-cell transplants (HSCT) and were often derived from allogeneic mice. These studies were prompted by the fact that leukemia patients, who could benefit from HLA-matched donor cell transplants could not because of the lack of suitable donors, had to resort to receiving HSCT from relatives that were only partially HLA-matched. There were two aspects of these treatments that were major opposing factors. The first aspect was beneficial because the partial HLA matched donor T cells would recognized the leukemia cells as foreign based not only on detectable tumor antigens, but also HLA-mismatched antigens. This response to the tumor (leukemia or lymphoma) is called graft vs. tumor leukemia or GVL. However, the opposing factor is that these mis-matched HLA antigens, which were first described in a mouse transplant system, are referred to as minor histocompatability antigens or Mls and are expressed on not only by the recipient's lymphocytes, but also by the cells of organ tissue systems. As a consequence these Mls antigens become targets of donor alloresponsive T cells (Korngold 1978).

In humans, Mls recognition by donor T cells and the subsequent powerful T cell response is the can be the basis of induction of GVHD in cancer patients receiving bone marrow transplants from HLA-identical siblings (Marijt 1993). GVHD has been the caused of a significant amount of death amongst patients undergoing HSCT because of the destruction of normal cells of the skin, digestive tract, liver and lungs. Acute GVHD can occur immediately (2-3 weeks post-HSCT) or later (4-6 months post-HSCT), which is referred to as chronic GVHD. Both of these forms of GVHD can be treated successfully in 50% of patients with immunosuppressive corticosteroids, but a significant number of patients not in this responsive group have corticosteroid-refractory disease. Because they don't respond to corticosteroids they must be treated immunosuppressive drugs such as methotrexate, sirolimus, anti-CD20 (B-cell) antibodies (rituximab), or alternative therapies such as extracorporeal photophoresis (Garnette 2013). Given the gravity of the GVHD problem that occurs during human HSCT, immunologist turned to the disease models in mice mentioned above and conducted preclinical trials that manipulated donor T cell populations in order to understand the cellular basis of the disease. It was found that GVHD was exacerbated by the removal of Tregs from the donor population (Cohen 2002). In addition, it was found that Tregs from the donor that were generated to be specific for Mls alloantigens (antigen-specific Tregs) of the recipient were significantly more effective than polyclonal antigen-non-specific Tregs in ameliorating GVHD (Trenado 2006). This was a significant finding in light of the fact that there was a reduction in the frequency of Tregs in patients who had allogeneic HSCT and had developed chronic GVHD based on the detection FOXP3+ T cells when compared to either HSCT patients without GVHD or normal controls. The same study revealed that the thymus of both GVHD positive and negative patients showed evidence of damage, but the most significant findings were that Tregs from both patient groups were equally suppressive to responding T cells. In addition, there was an inverse relationship between the Treg/CTL ratios between the two patient groups. In other words, chronic GVHD patients had less Tregs and more CTL than non-GVHD patients (Zorn 2005). Despite the complexity of the induction of GVHD during HSCT, it was time to make use of Tregs as immunotherapeutic agents to prevent the onset of the disease.

Transplantation Therapy for the Treatment of Hematological Cancers: Treg Therapy for the Treatment of GVHD during HSCT

One of the main aspects of using Tregs for immunotherapy has to do with generating a sufficient quantity of the cells to be used to effectively suppress GVHD. Normally Tregs compose less than 5% of the total T cell compartment. Studies in mice determined that the ideal ratio of Treg to responding T cell approached 1:1 for effective inhibition of GVHD. Traditional expansion methods use purified Tregs that are expanded using immobilized anti-CD3 and anti-CD28 antibodies in the presence of IL-2 (Trenado 2006). Other expansion protocols make use of Rapamycin and TGF-β (Hippen 2011), alloantigen-presenting APC, Rapamycin, IL-2, and IL15 (Veerapathran 2011) or Tregs generated from GM-CFS treated donor stem cells (Ukena 2012). Despite the fact that the human clinical trial mentioned below that utilize Tregs as immunotherapeutic cells for the treatment of GVHD is only one of a very few, preclinical trials in mice have advanced using recipient-specific Tregs (rsTregs) to prevent the disease during HSCT. One of the ultimate goals for the use of Tregs to prevent GVHD would be to used fewer (less that 1:1 ratio of Treg to responding T cell) because of the fear of systemic immunosuppression brought about by Tregs inhibiting non-GVHD immune responses. This type of situation might occur by the use of polyclonal Tregs isolated and expanded from the PB pool of the donor. One of the reasons why this is an important consideration for the donor Tregs has to do with engraftment of donor HSC and the immunosuppressive nature of the HSCT procedure. Often the recipients of these transplants develop bone marrow chimerism where a significant number of the bone marrow cells belong to the donor. Therefore, if the T cells of the donor respond to viruses and bacteria along with those of the recipient, they too would be susceptible to Treg inhibition by massive numbers of Tregs added during HSCT. In addition, cancer patients that participate in HSCT treatment are already immunosuppressed because they are subject to lymphodepletion prior to the procedure and the introduction of 20-100 times more Tregs would contribute to this immunosuppressed state.

By the use of Tregs that have TCR specific for the targets (recipient MHC antigens) of GVHD-inducing donor T cells, the need to have such high ratios of Treg: responder T cell would seem to unnecessary, but in the mouse study of GVHD and Tregs below this was not an issue due to the transient nature of the immunotherapeutic Tregs or recipient-specific Tregs (rsTregs). However, in a study of HSCT that mimicked human HSCT where thymic convolution takes place after lymphodepletion, it was found that therapeutic Tregs initially expanded, then contracted as natural Tregs of the donor increased. The convolution of the thymus that occurs during human HSCT treatments results in a non-functional thymus and the reconstitution process relies solely on the engraftment of the donor lymphocytes. Natural Tregs originate from T cell-depleted bone marrow (BM) progenitor cells as a product of the successful engraftment. Therefore, mice in this study were lethally radiated and reconstituted with T cell progenitor negative allogeneic BM cells. GVHD was induced by the addition of allogeneic T cells and the effects of rsTregs on this process was determined using a 1:1 ratio of rsTregs to T cells. Tregs immune to the recipient MHC (rsTregs) were generated from purified Tregs from the donor that had been cultured with inactivated (20-Gy-irradiated) recipient spleen cells for 3 to 5 weeks with IL-2. Mice receiving only T-depleted BM did not experience GVHD, but when allogeneic donor T cells were added all of the mice developed lethal GVHD within 30 days. However, when an equal amount of rsTregs was added with the donor T cells no GVHD occurred. Engraftment of the T cell compartment was studied using untreated T-depleted BM recipients, allogeneic T cell only, and allogeneic T cells + rsTreg treated mice. In both treatment groups there was a marked reduction (lymphopenia) in CD4, CD8, and B-cells compared to untreated T-depleted BM recipients despite the fact that the allogeneic T cell treatment group developed GVHD and the rsTreg + allogeneic T cell group did not. However, B cell percentages in the rsTreg treated mice partially recovered. In addition, analysis of the remaining T cells after treatment revealed that there were fewer effector memory (EM) T cells in the rsTreg treated mice when compared to non-rsTreg treated T cells demonstrating that rsTregs had silenced the GVHD T cell response by inhibiting host effector cell differentiation. In support of this fact, T cells from rsTreg treated mice secreted lower amounts of the inflammatory lymphokines IL-2 and TNF upon challenge. The most interesting result was the fact that initially rsTregs expanded ~5-fold within the first 15 days, but contracted back to initial levels by 30 days and subsequently disappeared after 60 days. However, donor natural Tregs that developed from the BM transplant rapidly divided in both GVHD+ and rsTreg GVHD- mice, but in rsTreg GVHD-mice the percentage of donor Tregs rose in relation to percentage of CD4 T cells as if they had a survival advantage (Gaidot 2011).

The fact that rsTregs induced a selective survival advantage to donor Tregs is in line with the effects of Treg secreted adenosine and its interaction with the adenosine receptor of the Treg. During the last chapter in the section called, *Adenosine and Treg survival* it was made clear that activation of the Treg A2A adenosine receptor induced the inhibition of not only the activation of NFAT and NF-kB, but also ERG-1 and ERG-3, which participate in FASL promoter activation of the FASL gene making Tregs resistant to this form of cell death (Himer 2010). Survival of Tregs is an important factor in their ability to control GVHD because if these cells fail to survive, donor T cells begin the process of GVHD. However, Treg proliferation during the beginning stages of the transplant is critical to the initiation of the GVHD process. The ability of Tregs to proliferate under the conditions of transplantation, which can be viewed as a massive inflammatory response, has been discussed in two separate sections of the previous chapter. Those discussions centered on how Tregs, which are normally unable to proliferate because of the build-up of cAMP due to the activation of the PKA pathway, were not only able to survive, but also increase their numbers. The activation of the PKA pathway specifically inhibits T cell proliferation by blocking the activation of T cell activators such as NFAT1c. During the donor T cell response to the recipient's minor and major tissue-specific MHC antigens, which occurs during every HSCT situation, Tregs immediately begin to attack not only responding T cells, but also antigen-presenting DC. Because the Treg can secrete massive amounts of adenosine through the conversion of intercellular ATP (released from dead cells), it has the ability to activate its own PKA pathway in an autocrine fashion, which allows them to produce more intracellular cAMP. This Treg cAMP is used to paralyze responding T cells and DC, but it gets depleted because normally Tregs compose 1% of the T cell compartment and must inject cAMP into multiple responding T cells. Once cAMP is depleted the PKA pathway ceases to function and the inhibitors of T cell proliferation (ICER, CREB) are no longer produced, which induces Treg proliferation through the NFkB/AP-1/NFAT pathway. Treg proliferation and cell cycle transit continues as long as there is a source of IL-2. Functioning responding T cells continue to supply Tregs with IL-2, but if the source of IL-2 disappears such as when HSCT patients become severely lymphopenic, Tregs become sensitive to FASL-mediated death and their numbers dwindle and as a consequence GVHD begins (Matsuoka 2010). During normal massive inflammatory responses such as viral infections this process of cAMP depletion/Treg proliferation is cyclic because as Tregs continue to proliferate their A2A receptors become activated by adenosine, the build-up of Treg intracellular cAMP begins, and Treg cell proliferation ceases. However, the conditions of HSCT dictate that the patients undergo lymphodepletion prior to the transplant and as a result sometimes the transplanted hematopoietic cells find it difficult to survive. Therefore, if there is a delay as far as engraftment is concerned and the patient develops leucopenia, GVHD preventing Tregs may not survive.

Recently, this problem was addressed in pediatric leukemia patients that were undergoing HSCT. In an effort to prevent the development of GVHD in patients that were receiving allogeneic HSCT researchers took advantage of the nature of the high-affinity IL-2 alpha receptor expressed by Tregs. This receptor is many magnitudes more sensitive to IL-2 when compared to not only naïve T cells, but also responding T cells as well. Despite the fact that responding T cells transiently express the receptor during activation and proliferation, they need high concentrations of IL-2 in order to support cell division and differentiation. However, Tregs use most of the IL-2 they absorb to arm themselves by the induction of A2A receptors that initiates the PKA pathway and subsequent build-up of cAMP, which as discussed at length in the previous chapter is used as an effector mechanism. In addition it has been show that Tregs, unlike responding T cells, do not depend absolutely on either TCR or MHC contact to proliferate in the presence of IL-2 (Zou 2012). The clinical trial in question used ultra-low dose (ULD) IL-2 to treat 2 groups of pediatric leukemia patients receiving HSCT and compared the Treg recovery after transplant to HSCT patients not receiving IL-2. One group (12) received allogeneic HSC from a relative (partial HLA match) and the other (4) received the transplant from unrelated donors (no HLA match). Injection of ULD IL-2 (3 times/week) began 30 days prior and continued 6-weeks beyond HSCT. Percent of CD4+ CD25+ FOXP3+ Tregs, IL-2 toxicity, onset of GVHD, and evidence of viral infections were monitored within 30 days. None of the patients receiving ULD IL-2 experienced toxicity. Tregs increased from a mean of 4.8% to 11.1% in ULD patients and the largest differenced were detected in the patients receiving related allogeneic HSC. No patients receiving IL-2 experienced GVHD compared to 12% of the control group. Patients receiving IL-2 also demonstrated T cell immunocompetence since only 15% developed viral infections compared to 63% of the control patients that had HSCT, but no IL-2. This clinical trial/study (Kennedy-Nasser 2014) demonstrated for the first time in humans the powerful role Treg proliferation/survival plays in the successful engraftment of therapeutic immune cells for the treatment of hematopoietic cancers. The low dose of IL-2 was well tolerated by the patients and effectively not only supported the survival and function of Tregs, but also immunocompetent responding T cells. Most importantly was the absence of GVHD in both HLA partial and non-matched allogeneic HSC donors.

The first and to date, the only clinical trial using therapeutic Tregs to prevent GVHD in patients with hematological cancers receiving HSCT was a Phase I trial in 28 patients. This was a complex study, which was focused on the ability of donor Tregs to prevent GVHD, not to create pathogen sensitivity, and not contribute to disease relapse. Adding to this trial's complexity was the inclusion requirements for eligible patients. Inclusion criteria included acute myeloid leukemia (AML) or acute lymphoid leukemia (ALL) in remission at high risk of relapse, acute leukemia with primary induction failure in chemo-resistant relapse, or in relapse after autologous transplantation, high-grade Hodgkin's or non-Hodgkin's lymphoma in relapse after 3 lines of chemotherapy and autologous transplantation. The age range was 18-65 years of age with no major lung, liver, renal, or cardiac dysfunction, no major psychiatric disturbances and lack of an HLA-identical sibling or a matched unrelated registry donor. In addition to this, donor eligibility also had to do with having a family member with one haplotype (HLA type) identical to the patient's and the ability to donate hematopoietic stem cells after treatment with granulocyte colony stimulating factor (GM-CSF) as well as undergo leukapheresis sessions for collecting hematopoietic stem cells, Tregs, and Tcons (conventional T cells). Of the 26 patients twenty-two had acute myeloid leukemia (AML), 5 had acute lymphoid leukemia (ALL), and one with high-grade non-Hodgkin's lymphoma. The complex transplantation scheme included TBI (8 Gy) with lung shielding and cyclophosphomide/fludarabine days prior to receiving freshly isolated donor Tregs (-day 4). During this time donors were treated with GM-CSF to increase bone marrow progenitor cells, which after BM aspiration were purified into CD34+ cells that were infused into the patients as HSC on day 0. On that same day the patients were also infused with purified T cells from the same donors that were collected prior to their treatment with GM-CSF. The T cell to Treg ratio in 5 patients was initially 1:4, but was increased to 1:2 in the remaining patients, which were maintained in sterile rooms. After treatment multiple parameters were monitored such as chimerism, pathogen responses, and Treg/conventional T cell phenotypes. Twenty-six of the 28 patients in the study had full engraftment of donor HSC. Only two of these 26 developed GVHD and were amongst the lower T cell to Treg ratio group. Again and as mentioned in the previous study of pediatric leukemia patients, the presence of additional donor Tregs improved the engraftment process where chimeric CD4 T cells that developed after the transplant were immunocompetent when compared to similar patients that did not receive therapeutic donor Tregs. Treg treated patients had a significant later onset of HSCT-associated infections. The patient outcomes, which in a Phase I study are not particularly improved by the experimental treatment, were morbid. Half of the 28 patients in this study died from viral/bacteria/fungal infections as well as the two who developed GVHD. However, the lack of GVHD in 26 of 28 patients, who without Treg therapy would have developed the disease within 15 days, demonstrated the positive impact of using donor Tregs in conjunction with the infusion of HSC and normal donor PB T cells as therapy for these types of hematopoietic cancers.

The Importance of Treg Immunobiology As It Relates to the Anti-Tumor T Cell Response during Immune Cell-Based Cancer Treatment

From the information provided above it is apparent that Tregs are a powerful controlling force of the T cell immune system. The ability of these cells not only mute T cell responses to cancer, but also to equilibrate (homeostasis) inflammatory responses, puts Tregs into a unique class of T cells. These T cells have frustrated the efforts of immunologist for years as they began to understand the fine intricacies of the T cell immune system. It was difficult to understand why the T cell immune system, which was so efficient at removing bacterial and viral infections, had such a hard time with cancer. Once it was understood that Tregs prevented autoimmunity, it was clear that the T cell immune response to cancer was vulnerable to regulation. Because a cancer cell was previously a normal functioning cell of the body, the T and NK cell system of surveillance pauses to evaluate a situation where the antigens it sees are not quite non-self. The pause is more than likely due to the presence of Tregs, which arrive at the site of questionable inflammatory events as soon as the first CD4 T cell secretes IL-2 and other cytokines that attract Tregs. All of this happens within the time it took to read the last few sentences. T cells do what they are genetically programmed to do and that is to kill and have the dead cell assimilated. The assimilation part has to do with antigen processing and presentation and is the purview of the granulocyte/macrophage series of cells such as macrophages and DCs or otherwise called, APC. With that being said, the job of Tregs is to prevent the destruction of normal cells, which means preventing autoimmune T cell responses caused by APC presentation of self-antigens. Tregs, which are T cells, react to the situation and respond as they do to minor inflammatory situations where a cell is damaged and eventually will return to its normal state. Tregs protect these cells from destruction through a series of elaborate effector mechanisms.

Immune-based cancer treatments (immunotherapy) hold the promise of not only being outpatient treatments for the disease, but also the end of chemical-based treatments (chemotherapy) that have serious side effects for the patient. However, it turns out that all of the immune cell-based treatments detailed above (adoptive T cell therapy, dendritic vaccines, and hematopoietic transplantation) are susceptible to the influence of Tregs. This is no surprise considering what has been described here, but what's really important is how to regulate Treg control in a positive fashion. That information exists and it has to be implemented in order for these immune-based therapies to live up to their expectations. One of the many problems associated with controlling Tregs cells as far as cancer treatment is concerned is how they can appear at a moment's notice due to the advanced mobility of native Tregs and the conversion/reprogramming process. These functions are genetically programmed responses and invariably are susceptible to manipulation. This is the goal of tumor immunologists, who now realize that immunity to cancer cannot occur without the consideration of Tregs during treatment. This does not mean that cancer is not recognized by the T cell immune system, destroyed, and leaving a memory behind of the encounter. The reality is that this happens more often than not. Most humans have developed malignant cells, but they were destroyed as a natural process of immune surveillance system. However, this system fails to end the unabated growth of many cancers because of the cancer's initial slow rate of growth. This slow transition from normal cell to precancerous cell and then to full-blown cancer presents a unique problem for the T cell immune system. This problem has to do with the recognition of self and the induction of autoimmunity when a response to self occurs. As normal cells become damaged by a myriad of insults such as burns, burses, and bacterial/viral infections two immune responses occur. As mentioned previously, the first response of the T cell immune system is to destroy these cells because they appear different from the surrounding normal cells and are considered a threat. The second immune response is directed against the first one. Because of their nature, Tregs usually arrive first at the site of these events and detect cells that need to be protected until they heal. In the case of cancer, which is viewed by Tregs as injured or inflamed cells, there usually is no healing and these cells continue to not only grow, but also undergo DNA mutation as growth accelerates. As had been discussed at length, the second immune response mediated by Tregs is at times both specific and non-specific. Unlike normal effector T cells, Tregs can not only specifically kill responding T cells by the use of the perforin/granzyme or FAS/FASL systems, but can also non-specifically paralyze them by either elaboration of adenosine or injection with cAMP. Therefore, and as discussed previously, it is apparent that even if very small percentages of the patients Tregs are present after lymphodepletion, which is required for successful outcome of the three immune cell-based therapies mentioned above, they eventually negatively affect the ability of the therapeutic cells to attack the cancer. Understanding how to manipulate Tregs in such a way as to lessen these problems has been the goal of tumor immunologists since the beginning of these clinical trials using immune cell-based therapies and in fact, prompted the use of lymphodepletion for that very purpose. However, not only was that not enough, but the procedure of lymphodepletion removes one of the most important properties of Tregs and that is their ability to induce immune homeostasis. This is why it is important to directly address the ability to selectively alter the intracellular pathways within the Treg just enough to impair its inhibitory properties while allowing these cells to create homeostasis during immune cell-based cancer therapy.

Translational Pathways Associated with Immune Cell-based Immunotherapy

Many of the translational pathways and their consequences related to anti-tumor T cells, Tregs, and cancer cells that have already been mentioned apply to the cellular interactions that occur during the treatment of cancer using immunotherapeutic approaches. For instance, the pathways in Tregs (PKA and NFAT1c) that controls adenosine/cAMP production and T cell anergy are directly related to the ability of Tregs to interfere with immune cell-based therapies. In addition, the pathways associated with tumor escape via tumor-secreted VEGF (P13K/Akt pathways) and chemotherapy/FASL-resistance (MAPK/ERK pathways) directly negatively impact the immunotherapy of solid tumors such as melanoma. Some pathways discussed previously related to Treg function such as the above mentioned PKA pathway may play a major role in one particular type of immunotherapy such as HSCT where Tregs affect the massive expansion of donor BM progenitors and the recovery of recipient lymphocytes after lymphodepletion at the same time. Despite the use of cell-to-cell contact effector mechanisms by Tregs, the number of T cells they must to control vastly outnumber the their small percentage of the T cell compartment. Therefore, Tregs resort to using the non-cell-to-cell contact effector mechanisms, production of adenosine (PKA pathway) and IL-10 secretion, which can affect numerous responding T cells at a distance. This is why Treg survival and proliferation is so important during transplant therapies. Of course DC-based immunotherapies and particularly in combination with ACT are extremely vulnerable to Treg contact because of the previously mentioned affinity these two cells have for each other. As mentioned above, Tregs exert their influence on the T cell immune system through the establishment homeostatic conditions. Many of mediators of this normalization do not have to do with contact between Tregs, DCs, or T cells, but are the result of the secretion of lymphokines such as TNF-α and IL-10. However, despite this control exerted over the T cell immune system by Tregs, Tregs themselves maybe controlled by the conditions established by the protocols and environments created by immune cell-based therapies.

From the information provided concerning the ability of Tregs to not only resist (Baba 2012 and Yao 2014) these protocols (lymphodepletion), but also phenotypically transform (Tregs to ICOS+ Tregs) into highly potent (Sim 2014) regulatory T cells, it would seem as though Tregs are responding and adapting to these therapies rather that being controlled. Nonetheless, Tregs still exert control over these therapies by virtue of their ability to create homeostatic conditions. The interesting aspect of the need to completely control or remove Tregs from the immunotherapeutic treatment of cancer equation is the fact that it cannot be done because of homeostasis. This is a reminder of what happens when Tregs malfunction or there is a gene defect in FOXP3 genes; the result of which is the development of rampant deadly autoimmune disease (IPEX) in the latter case and specific autoimmunity in the former. Therefore, if Tregs were not present after lymphodepletion patients would be thrust into this type of situation, but they are not and that is because even though there is a barely measurable, minute population of Tregs after lymphodepletion, there must be enough of them present to prevent occurrence of autoimmunity during the reconstitution process. If under these conditions Tregs can control the T cell immune response enough to prevent autoimmunity, there are more than likely enough of these cells to have a negative controlling influence on the ability of therapeutic anti-tumor T cells to remove a tumor. This is why it is important to consider other methods to control Tregs in these situations because simply removing them is not really an option. Therefore, the idea of controlling Tregs through the manipulation of intracellular pathways is an attractive alternative.

Translational Pathways Associated with Immune Cell-Based Immunotherapy: Inhibition of Treg Function and Increased Anti-Tumor T Cell Activity in the BM during HSCT

Multiple myeloma (MM), which is a B-cell malignancy is characterized by the accumulation of mature plasma B-cells in the bone marrow and its subsequent destruction was one of the hematological cancers not discussed in this section. This type of cancer is considered uniformly fatal and considered incurable. Despite the fact that survival rates have increased from 3 to 4 years to 8-9 years through the use of new FDA approved drugs, this type of cancer has been the subject of HSCT procedures similar to those described above for leukemias and lymphomas (Krishnan 2011). Recently, it was determined that HSCT with autologous stem cells increased the complete remission rate from 25.9% to 70.4% in patients that received autologous HSCT and chemotherapy (Fu 2013). One of the issues not addressed when discussing the use of Tregs to prevent GVHD during HSCT was the effect Tregs had on the anti-tumor T cell response or graft-versus-tumor (GVT) response. A characteristic of the bone marrow (BM) microenvironment is the secretion of IL-1B and IL-6 by BM stromal cells. It was discussed earlier that both IL-1B and IL-6 participate in the reprogramming of Tregs into TH17 effector T cells, as well as the ability to induce IL-17 secretion by CD4 cells. Both of these functions depend on the presence of TGF-β, which can be secreted by Tregs. It has been shown that in MM models when HSCT is used in conjunction with the addition of donor T cells, not only is GVHD inhibited, but also in addition, the GVT response is augmented (Guichelaar 2013). This is in contrast to other models that focus on Treg-secreted adenosine, which have the capability to inhibit donor anti-tumor effector T cells (Thompson 2013). This undoubtedly has to do with the magnitude of the response (both GVHD and

GVT) and the location of the tumor. The location of the hematopoietic tumor is important as far as the ability of Tregs to inhibit the GVT effect. MM and many leukemic tumors not only originate in the BM, but also initially grow there as in the case with MM. However, if the tumor cells travel out of that location (BM) similar to how the CD19+ B-cell lymphoma mentioned above, traveled to the patient's lymph nodes (Kochenderfer 2010), the anti-tumor effector T cells are more susceptible to inhibition by Tregs. This is mainly because of the secretion of IL-6 and IL-1B in the BM, but also the Treg encounters with anti-tumor T cells outside of the BM and in the lymphatic system where they can essentially mute anti-tumor T cell creation by inducing DC immaturity.

It turns out that IL-6 has a very complex relationship with T cells. IL-6, upon interaction with its receptor can initiate intracellular signaling through the dimerization of gp130. The presence IL-6, TGF-β, and minute amounts of IL-2 can create adaptive Tregs from naïve CD4 T cells (Josefowicz 2009). As mentioned previously, one of the basic cellular characteristics of Tregs is the fact that they are anergic. IL-6 initiates this process by inhibiting cyclin-dependent kinases (CDK), which are responsible for cell cycle entrance during T cell proliferation. It does this by activating JAK-1 pathway, which phosphorylates the IL6 receptor that in turn activates STAT3. Phosphorylated STAT3, which form dimers, enters the nucleus and can induce the cell cycle CDK inhibitor P27kip1. This effectively arrest cell proliferation in tumor cells as well as T cells (Mori 1999, Schmees 2005 respectively). However, this is a lymphokine-balancing act, which depends on the type and intensity of the T cell response during inflammation. If the responding T cells continually secrete IL-2, Tregs are activated through their TCR and begin to proliferate and subsequently inhibit these T cells as well as the DCs they use to respond to antigens. As the supply of IL-2 runs out because of responding cell death or anergy induced by Tregs, the stability of the expressed FOXP3 gene weakens slightly. This is a branch-point in the fate of Tregs as discussed earlier when Treg proliferation was activated by low-levels of IL-2, self-antigen activation of its TCR, and depletion of cAMP during the cyclic nature of a normal massive inflammatory event. However, if Tregs find them selves in a situation where the predominant lymphokine secreted is IL-6 another thing happens and that is they're reprogramming into TH17 T cells, which secrete IL-17 and are for all intents and purposes are inflammatory T cells that have the ability to not only induce inflammation, break immunological tolerance, but also remove pathogens and extracellular parasites as previously described in this section. In addition, it was found that TH17 CD4 T cells that were specific for a melanocyte/melanoma peptide had the ability to eradicate large melanoma tumors in mice (Muranski 2008).

As just mentioned, IL-6 mediates this reprogramming event that has serious consequences in the areas of not only the T cell response to tumor cells, but also the initiation of arthritis. Aside from the ability of BM stromal cells to secrete significant amounts of IL-6, fibroblasts, endothelial cells, macrophages and lymphocytes can also secrete this lymphokine (Camporeale 2012). The major immune modulating capabilities come from the IL-6 receptor's ability to activate STAT3 through the activation JAK-1. STAT3 enters the nucleus and activates the survival genes BCL-2, c-MYC, and JUN (Durant 2010), which are necessary for the reprogramming event to occur. STAT3 is directly involved in the reprogramming of Tregs into TH17 effector CD4 T cells because it binds to TH17 lymphokine receptor genes. During the process histone H3 elements within the promoters of these genes are demethylated. This allows STAT3 to bind to the TH17 promoters and this initiates gene transcription and the secretion of IL-17 (Thomas 2012). In addition to the ability of IL-6 to inhibit cell cycle progression by the activation of p27kip1, the MAPK/P38 pathway (Huber 2008) must also be activated by TGF-β and this is controlled by the expression of the RORgammat gene, which is the signature gene of TH17 T cells just as FOXP3 is for Tregs. It turns out that proteins produced by the FOXP3 gene directly bind to the RORgammt gene and inhibit its expression (Zhou 2008), but if IL-1B, IL-6, and IL21 are present, FOXP3 gene expression is inhibited, which allows the development of TH17 T cells from Tregs (Ichiyama 2008).

Translational Pathways Associated with Immune Cell-Based Immunotherapy: The Use of Transcriptional Pathway Inhibitors to Augment the Anti-Tumor T Cell Response

The reason why TH17 T cell development is relevant to the ability of Tregs to inhibit GVHD, but at the same time not interfere with the GVT effect has to do with the IL-1β and IL-6 secreted by BM stromal cells, which can convert Tregs into effector TH17 T cells. Unfortunately, as the tumor cells leave the BM the T cell response is susceptible to Treg control because in the periphery where IL-2 is secreted and STAT5 is activated, STAT3 is inhibited and subsequently the formation of TH17 T cells is inhibited (Lee 2011). However, the fact is that continual exposure to IL-6 can inhibit Treg function (Goodman 2009). In fact, it was shown IL-6 synergizes with TGF-β to induce FOXP3 protein degradation through the activation of ubiquitin-proteasome enzymes that release FOXP3 protein control of RORgammat (Gao 2012). This is due to what was previously mentioned concerning the "transition phase" between the Treg phenotype and the TH17 phenotype. During this transition phase FOXP3 expression is reduced, Treg inhibitory function ceases, and the RORgammat gene expression begins to take over. However, the activation (phosphorylation) of STAT3 in both effector T cell and Tregs results in the ability of effector T cells to resist the inhibitory effects of Tregs. Studies indicate that inhibition of STAT3 phosphorylation (pSTAT3) restores the ability of Tregs to inhibit effector T cells (Goodman 2011). The use of pharmaceutical inhibitors may be the answer to the regulation of not only Tregs, but also the regulation of autoreactive T cells. However, pSTAT3 has wide-ranging effects on not only T cells, but also tumor cells as far as T cell immunity is concerned. Glioblastoma multiform (GBM) is a brain tumor that is resistant to both chemotherapy and immunotherapy. Like melanoma (another neural crest tumor), it is immunogenic to host T cells, but because it is located in the brain it is subject to the rules of the blood-brain lymphocyte barrier and in an "immune privileged" location undetectable by the T cell immunosurveillance system. GBM tumor cells have been shown to express copious amounts pSTAT3. Activation of STAT3 allows these cells to down-regulate MHC-class II and secrete immunosuppressive lymphokines such as IL-10 (Herbeuval 2004). Inhibition of STAT3 by the use of siRNA prevented GBM cells from inhibiting DC maturation. As described previously, immature DCs induce Tregs, which is one of the hallmarks of immune evasion mediated by GBM tumors (See 2012).

Aside from the effects of STAT3 activation in tumor cells, responding T cells, and Tregs, other immune cells are positively affected by the reduction of pSTAT3. Case in point would be that of the DC. It was found that mature DC were induced to not only secrete lower amounts of IL-12, but also had a reduced ability to stimulate antigen specific T cell responses through the reduction of CD80/86 expression after their exposure to tumor-secreted IL-6 and subsequent induction of pSTAT3 (Alshamsan 2012). In addition, it was found that the blockade of both P38 MAPK and STAT3 pathways enabled human DCs to resist this de-maturation process induced by tumors and resulted in increased DC functions such as secretion of IL-12 and stimulation of allogeneic T cell responses (Oosterhoff 2012). As far as DC's are concerned it was found that either inhibiting STAT3 in human DCs or removing the STAT3 gene in transgenic mice results in an increased DC function compared to control DC. In mice that were transgenic for the deletion of the STAT3 gene, DC's demonstrated higher cytokine secretion in response to TLR stimulation, could activated T cells more efficiently, and were resistant to tumor induced inhibition of cytokine production when compared to normal mouse DC. In addition, the anti-tumor function of STAT3-depleted DCs was also heightened because if injected into a growing tumor of a normal littermate, tumor regression occurred at the injection site and also at distant sites of tumor growth when compared to the injection of normal DCs. In the same study, human STAT3 was inhibited by STAT3-specific short hairpin RNA and the resulting DC produced more cytokines with TLR stimulation, were resistant to human tumor-induced inhibition, and more efficiently induced tumor-peptide specific T cell responses (Iwata-Kajihara 2011). It is clear that activation of STAT3, which is more than likely due to the effects excessive exposure of DC to IL-6, causes these cells to dedifferentiate away from the TH-1 inducing phenotype. Inhibition of STAT3 in the above study did increase the secretion if IL-12 and INF-γ, which favor the induction of a TH-1, CD4/CD8 T cell response. However, it was also shown that STAT3-depleted DCs also secreted more IL-10, but the combination of IL-12 and INF-γ was still able to induce a productive anti-tumor T cell response. This secretion of IL-10 by STAT3-depleted DC relates to the intersecting nature of the STAT3 pathway with the Akt, P13K, and JAK-1 pathways.

Translational Pathways Associated with Immune Cell-Based Immunotherapy: The Use of Transcriptional Pathway Inhibitors to Alter Treg Immunobiology

The role of Tregs in the T cell response to cancer and immunotherapeutic treatment of the disease is not always detrimental. For instance increased survival in some solid tumor models have shown that TH17 T cells, which maintain an environment of inflammation and are favorable to the formation of TH-1 anti-tumor T cell responses. However, as Tregs take over as the predominant T cells as the cancer progresses (Maruyama 2010). Therefore, if Tregs within these tumors could be reprogrammed into TH17 as they are in the BM during HSCT this would favor the formation of an anti-tumor T cell response. As mentioned previously, the series of events that leads to the reprogramming of Tregs into TH17 T cells involves the synergistic activities if IL-6 and TGF-β on degrading FOXP3 proteins thus inhibits its ability to bind to the RORgammat gene and induce the TH17 phenotype. The degradation of FOXP3 in caused by the activation of ubiquitin-proteosome pathway, which controls cellular pathways that control cell growth, proliferation, DNA repair, and other transcriptional events (Chitra 2012). In fact it was show in the previous chapter that EPAC promoted the ubiquitin-proteosome degradation of the above mentioned co-factor p300 by inhibition of p38 MAPK activation (Jeong 2013). It was determined that the ubiquitin-proteosome pathway inhibitor

MG132 prevented the reprogramming of Tregs into TH17 T cells (Gao 2012). Therefore, in order to promote the reprogramming of Tregs in the tumor microenvironment into TH17 T cells, which create favorable anti-tumor T cell conditions by T cell secretion of INF-γ, it would call for the destabilization of the FOXP3 gene. It was mentioned in the previous chapter that a cofactor called p300 CPB (CREB binding protein) stabilized CREB binding to specific CREB-responsive genes such the IL-10 was indispensible for activity of not only CREB, but also NFkB (Mayr 2001). It also turns out that p300, which is a histone acetyltransferase that stabilizes the FOXP3 gene through acetylation. Increased acetylation of FOXP3 prevents degradation by the ubiquitin-proteosome pathway. In contrast, histone deacetylases (HDAC) such as SIRT-1, which exist in the same milieu, enhance FOXP3 degradation by exposing more ubiquitin-proteosome binding sites (van Loosdregt 2010). Therefore, the use of acetyltransferase inhibitors on antigen or tumor antigen-specific (genetically altered TCR or chimeric TCR) Tregs prior to their use in ACT should with the use of transient IL-6 therapy in solid tumor cancer patients, facilitate a short term Treg to TH17 T cell reprogramming event, which would stimulate an anti-tumor T cell response. These therapeutic Tregs could be used in conjunction with therapeutic anti-tumor TCR transduced or CAR T cells. The other side effect of this treatment would be the temporary paralysis of native Tregs during the procedure.

The above case is related to changing the phenotype of Tregs to one (TH17) that favors the induction of inflammatory conditions at the site of a growing tumor. However, there are situations when Tregs are needed to control immunotherapeutic situations such as HSCT where they are used to control GVHD. In some cases of autoimmunity and strong inflammatory responses such as GVHD, T effector cells become resistant to the inhibiting effects of Tregs. It was found that resistance was induced by the secretion of IL-6 and it's subsequent phosphorylation of STAT3 through the p130 (IL-6R)/JAK/STAT3 pathway in both the responding T cell and Treg. In addition, Treg control of responding T cell activity could be restored after treatment with pharmaceutical small molecule inhibitors (Stattic V and Stat3 inhibitor VII) specific for STAT3. An interesting finding was that pre-treatment of either responding T cell or Tregs with STAT3 inhibitors restored the ability of Tregs to inhibit anti-allogeneic T cell responses where large amounts of IL-6 was secreted by APC. (Goodman 2011). In another study it was determined that adaptive Treg creation in an anti-allogeneic T cell response, similar to what occurs during GVHD in HSCT, was increased using a small molecule STAT3-specific inhibitor called S31-201. Because activation of STAT3 favors the creation of TH17 T cell and inhibits Treg formation it was found that the creation of adaptive Tregs was a result of increasing the ratio of STAT5 to STAT3 caused by the inhibition of STAT3 by S31-201 (Betts 2014). The role of STAT5 in the creation of adaptive Tregs is indispensible in that when IL-2 is available, IL-2R signals support the expression of FOXP3 in Tregs (Long 2010), and the activation of the IL-2R in Tregs induces STAT5 activation, which not only supports continuous FOXP3 activation, but also independently activates the P13K/Akt and MAPK signaling pathways that lead to Treg cell proliferation (Cheng 2011). Therefore, by inhibiting STAT3 phosphorylation induced by IL-6, it not only blocks the FOXP3 destabilization and subsequent loss of Treg function, but also inhibits the formation of TH17 T cells while supporting the creation of new adaptive Tregs if there is a source of IL-2.

Another use of small molecular inhibitors on intracellular pathways that increase Treg inhibitory functions was discussed in Chapter 3 when examining the non-cell-to-cell contact effector mechanism of adenosine secretion by Tregs. In Tregs the adenyl cyclase pathway, which is activated in an autocrine fashion by secreted adenosine is responsible for the production of cAMP. The intracellular build-up of cAMP within Tregs not only maintains the "anergic" phenotype of these cells, but as previously mentioned is used as a cell-to-cell contact effector mechanism to induce anergy in responder/effector T cells during inflammatory responses. In order to control cAMP build-up Tregs as well as T cells utilize an enzyme called phosphodiesterase (PDE) to catalyze the hydrolysis cAMP into 5' –AMP (Gancedo 2013). A pharmaceutical inhibitor of this pathway called Rolipram inhibited the breakdown of cAMP by PDE and consequently increased the inhibitory capacity of the cells (Bopp 2009). As mentioned PDE inhibitors were used to prevent GVHD during HSCT by increasing the ability of Tregs to not only inhibit responding/effector cells, but also reduce the ability of DC to generate them (Webber 2013). The inhibition of Treg function and increase in Treg proliferation is focused on the AC/PKA pathway since without the production of intracellular cAMP inhibitors of T cell proliferation such as CREB, which is produced by the AC pathway are no longer able to block T cell proliferative pathways like NFAT1c. In addition, without cAMP Tregs are unable to induce anergy in responding/effector T cells by its injection. Inhibitors such as the expression of ectopic PDE or cAMP antagonist (Rp-8-Br-cAMPS) can inhibit Treg function as well as induce Treg proliferation (Klein 2012) and restore inhibited CTL function in effector T cells that were injected by Tregs with cAMP (Raskovalova 2007), respectively. The pathways associated with the synthesis and secretion of adenosine and the production of cAMP are ripe with the opportunity to use specific small molecule inhibitors, analogues, agonist, and antagonist of the transcriptional pathway regulators associated with the AC/PKA pathways (Taylor 2008). These regulators can be either enhanced or inhibited prior to their participation in activities such as inhibition of Treg proliferation, cAMP injection, and a host of other functions that control Treg interactions with responding/effector T cells.

Even though it was stated earlier that Tregs were the most advanced type of T cell in the T cell immune system; again they are nonetheless T cells and with very few exceptions, follow the same immunobiological rules followed by the rest of this class of lymphocyte. With that being said, caution has to be used when altering the intracellular pathways in Tregs because of their relation to other T cell types. As mentioned earlier, many of the transcriptional pathways that operate in lymphocytes also function in normal as well as cancerous cells. For instance, the JAK/STAT3 pathway just mentioned in DC, T cells, and Tregs that is activated by the p130 IL-6R, also operates in cancer cells. In some cases IL-6 induces tumor cell senescence (Mori 1999) or in others allows tumor cells to spread by silencing genes responsible for adhesion through the activation DNA methyltransferase-1 (DNMT1), which methylates the genes preventing adhesion protein production (Foran 2010). This type of shared function of transcriptional pathways between disparate cell types makes it very important to examine the systemic effects transcriptional pathway inhibitors have at first in animals and then humans. An interesting finding concerning a ABL/SRC-kinase inhibitor (dasatinib), which was found to be effective as a chemotherapeutic agent for patients with chronic myeloid leukemia (CML) who were refractory to previous treatments was that the drug did inhibit Treg (CD4+ CD25+) proliferation, function, lymphokine secretion, but also at the same doses inhibited CD4 CD25- proliferation as well as lymphokine secretion. However, Tregs were not only more sensitive to dasatinib treatment, but they also showed a significant reduction in FOXP3 expression. Despite this finding the drug was still inhibitory to responding T cells, which in the setting of HSCT are responsible for the graft-vs-leukemia (GVL) effect (Fei 2009). Apparently, dasatinib has more of an inhibitory effect on SRC-kinase family members in Tregs than it does in responding T cells, but the fact is that this was discovered years after the drug had been used to treat patients. These types of studies that examine standard non-immune therapy chemotherapeutic drugs have demonstrated that in hindsight many of the successful drug combinations to treat cancer also effectively inhibit Treg function. For instance, the drug sunitinib for the treatment of metastatic renal cancer, docetaxel for the treatment of metastatic prostate and breast cancer, and cisplatin plus vinorelbine for non-small cell lung cancer all significantly inhibit Treg function and increase the ratio between effector T cells and Tregs (Roselli 2013).

Importance of Treg Immunobiology As It Relates to the Anti-Tumor T Cell Response during Immune-Based Cancer Treatment

It is apparent from the clinical information concerning the immune cell-based therapies for cancer mentioned above (ACT, DC vaccines, and HSCT) that Tregs play a major role in these types of immunotherapeutic treatments for cancer. In fact, all of these therapies have a built-in protocol called lymphodepletion that directly addresses the Treg problem. However, it was shown that Tregs are not only resistant to non-myeloablative conditioning and total body irradiation (TBI), but are also capable of repopulating the host with more potent versions of themselves. More than likely this resistance is due to the lack of self-sustaining cell division by Tregs, much like that of macrophage/myeloid lineage cells that are also resistant. However, the generation of a more inhibitory Treg phenotype after regeneration is due to the unabated repopulation of either host or in the case of HSCT, donor lymphocytes. As had been discussed in the previous chapters, Tregs are not dependent on TCR signals as T cells are in order to proliferate because TCR signals are muted by the Tregs anergic state and therefore they are able to increase their numbers dramatically using minimal TCR signals and lymphokines secreted during lymphodepletion regeneration phase. The difficulties with Tregs during cell-based immunotherapies noticed as soon as clinical trials started examining the CTL response of melanoma patients that were injected with autologous melanoma cell lysates using the same melanoma cells as targets. Less than half of the patients generated measurable CTL and this response only lasted for 7 days (Currie 1971). The problems with the ineffectiveness of immune cell-based therapies continued through the 1970s and it was not until the mid-1980s when immunological techniques were developed to accurately detect and measure reproducible anti-tumor T cell responses, did improvements occur. However, despite the increased ability to measure a T cell immune response to cancer in patients receiving immune cell-based therapy, most of these clinical trials, and especially the one's involving expanded TILs/IL-2 therapy were only effective in about one-third of the patients. Through the 1990's it was finally recognized that there was something suppressing these therapies. Two things occurred in the late 1990s/early 2000s and those were a refinement of the immune cell-based therapy called adoptive T cell therapy or ACT and the characterization of regulatory T cells or Tregs. ACT was developed to be more specific in that at first, isolated and expanded tumor-specific T cells from the patient were transferred back to the patient with or without IL-2 therapy and for the first time, a new added protocol called lymphodepletion that improved the efficiency of ACT by removing the patient's cellular immune system, which included Tregs and patient IL-2 absorbing T cells.

The focus of ACT, which was the T cell, underwent a revolutionary technological change in that it was possible to create two types of genetically altered T cells that had the ability to recognize specific tumor-associated peptides or proteins. The first type of genetically altered T cell was the result of transducing or inserting TCR genes isolated from anti-tumor T cells. These new receptors were specific for defined tumor associated peptides. However, there were several problems associated with the systemic persistence of infused therapeutic T cells and autoimmunity induced by either high-affinity TCRs or TCR alpha and beta mispairing. The next type of genetically altered T cell called CAR used during ACT made use of genes encoding the antigen-specific antibody light chain of tumor-specific monoclonal antibodies. These genes were a part of a "cassette" arrangement of genes that included the intracellular signaling proteins of the CD28 and CD137 molecules, which are involved in sustaining T cell survival and proliferation. However, there were also problems associated with this type of genetically altered T cell such as the inhibition of T cell recognition by patients developing anti-mouse immunoglobulin antibodies, antigen-specificity to normal tissues, and in the early versions of CAR T cells without CD28 or CD137 cellular domains, a lack systemic persistence. Despite these shortcomings, both types of genetically engineered T cells performed well as far as positive objective responses and complete remission rates. However, as mentioned above, and at the same time as these ACT clinical trials showed promise, it was found that not only did Tregs of the patient survive the two types of lymphodepletion, but also when they regenerated, a more potent type (ICOS+) of Treg emerged. This was a significant, but exciting finding because ACT therapies had become successful and now there is the potential to increase that success by addressing the problem of resistant Tregs. ACT, despite the problems associated with the procedure itself and the resistance of Tregs to lymphodepletion, can be viewed as potentially one of the most successful immune cell-based immunotherapeutic procedures in the future. However, there are other therapies that hold promise as well and one of those is DC vaccine therapy.

DC vaccine therapy, which is termed a "passive" type of therapy because it generates an immune response, actually began before ACT because initially it could be used as a non-invasive/passive form of therapy in pre-clinical and clinical trials as a topical (subcutaneous injection) treatment. These early trials met with limited success, but demonstrated that using autologous tumor antigen pulsed DCs was safe and could generate a measurable anti-tumor T cell response. However, most of these trials had little effect on the progression of the disease. As has been described in detail, DC's are very sensitive to the influence of Tregs and this no doubt had to do with the fact that despite the fact that there were measurable T cell responses, very few of these patients benefited from these procedures. Clinical trials were performed where patients were subcutaneously injected with RCC peptide (MUC-1)-pulsed DC with or without IL-2 therapy. Only six of twenty patients showed significant clinical responses. In fact, the IL-2 turned out to mask the in vitro T cell responses, which was possibly due to the activation of Tregs since they were not removed prior to treatment (Wierecky 2006). However, despite the disappointing results of this trial a meta-analysis of over 200 clinical trials similar to this one demonstrated a statistically significant positive effect on the regression of cancer if dose and DC maturity level were taken into account (Draube 2013). Another clinical trial that was designed to remove Tregs using an anti-CD25 antibody administered or not to melanoma patients given subcutaneous injections of gp100 peptide-pulsed DC. Results indicated that despite a slightly higher percentage of patients receiving the anti-CD25 antibodies demonstrated measurable T cell responses in vitro, there were no differences in progression-free survival between the treated and non-treated groups (Jacobs 2010). In addition, many of the tumor antigen-specific T cells as measured by gp100 tetramer-binding were anergic and could not respond, which was more than likely due to the interruption of IL-2 signaling pathways. DC vaccine therapy still shows promise as an effective immune cell-based immunotherapy if used in conjunction with ACT where the influence of Tregs is lessened. With regard to the powerful influence that Tregs have over the ability of DC to induce an effective T cell response to cancer, recent preclinical studies in mice have show how DCs that have been transduced with IL-6 producing genes induce stable anti-tumor T cell responses. It was shown that Tregs were inhibited by the FOXP3-destabilizing effect induced through DC-secreted IL-6 when tumor antigen-pulsed DCs were used as a vaccine (Bhanumathy 2014).

Another type of immune cell-based immunotherapy used to treat hematological cancers such as leukemias and lymphomas is hematopoietic stem cell transplantation or HSCT. If HLA-matched twins or siblings or unrelated donors are used as BM donors it is referred to as matched or allogeneic HSCT, respectively. The concept is to remove the patient's BM cells, which is where normal and malignant cells originate and replace those cells with donor BM that matures in the recipient and recognizes the tumor as foreign, which is called graft vs. tumor or GVT effect. However, the problem is that many times the donors T cells recognize minor (matched donors) or major (allogeneic donors) histocompatability antigens on the recipient's normal tissues, which leads to an almost uniformly fatal disease called graft vs. host disease or GVHD. However, GVHD can be prevented by the use of donor Tregs, which eliminate or suppress donor T cells responding to the recipient's tissues, but not the tumor. This is the ideal situation, but the reality is that Tregs from either lymphodepleted resistant Tregs or Tregs regenerated after engraftment of the recipient or donor Tregs added during the procedure can inhibit the ability of allogeneic donor T cells to kill the hematopoietic tumor. As discussed previously, the ability of Tregs to inhibit the tumor may depend on the tumor microenvironment the Tregs find themselves in. The microenvironment of the BM is inhibitory to Tregs because of its secretion of IL-6 and the downstream translational pathways IL-6 activate that weaken the expression of FOXP3 and the subsequent reprogramming of Tregs into TH17 effector T cells. In combination with the inability of Tregs to inhibit anti-tumor donor T cells and the inflammatory conditions induced by TH17 T cells, donor responding T cells destroy the tumor cells within the BM. However, many hematological tumors escape the BM and grow in the peripheral lymphatic system. These tumors are more likely to not be killed by donor T cells because of the control Tregs have on responder T cells in the periphery where conditions allow for both inhibition of both GVHD and GVT. Understanding this aspect of HSCT is a significant finding related to the function of Tregs in different immunological environments and may indicate ways to improve this and other types of immune cell-based immunotherapy. One of the significant aspects of all three of these immunotherapies is the fact that there has been a significant improvement in positive patient responses, which in part is due to the use of new small molecule inhibitors, but also a focus on Treg function.

Chapter 5

The Functional and Translational Immunology of Regulatory T Cells (Tregs), the Anti-Tumor T Cell Response, and Cancer: Chapter Review

Chapter 1: The Immunobiology and Translational Immunology of Regulatory T Cells

From the information previously provided it is apparent that Tregs are an essential and vital component of the T cell immune system. They have the ability to control T cell responses that would otherwise do damage to normal tissues if left unchecked. In addition, Tregs provide the entire immune system with balance or homeostasis, which is essential if the immune system is to properly sense the introduction of harmful threats such as bacteria/viral infections, parasites, inflammatory situations that cause tissue damage (injury), and cancer. Tregs create homeostasis through their ability guide and control T cell immune responses, after which these responses are quickly silenced and during this process Tregs release lymphokines that temporarily prevent the generation of autoimmune T cells. This is the ideal pattern of control exerted by the regulatory T cell system and for all intents and purposes, one that should work flawlessly. As mentioned in the first chapter, Tregs originate from both a natural (innate) process of T cell selection in the thymus and are created (adaptive) in the periphery under immunological conditions that necessitate the control of T cell responses. In this chapter the importance of Tregs was discussed in terms of the consequences of their absence as far as the cause of a fatal autoimmune disease (IPEX) and the inability to achieve full-term pregnancy. However, their immediate importance as far as this discussion goes is the negative effect Tregs have on the ability of the T cell immune system to remove cancer from the body. This has been the key issue throughout and one that has exposed the complexity and elegance of the T cell immune response. The examination of Tregs shed light on both of these aspects of T cell immunobiology because Tregs poses all of the attributes of the other T cell phenotypes, but also have additional functional capabilities associated with their ability to control the entire cellular immune system.

The initial observation concerning Tregs and the anti-tumor T cell response was examined in this first chapter and relates to what is called "plasticity." This is the ability of Tregs to not only change their functional capabilities such as which effector mechanism to use and when, but also have the remarkable ability to change phenotypes in multiple directions. The later means that a naïve T cell or antigen-specific T cell (tumor-specific in this case) can be converted into a Treg, which itself can be reprogrammed into a TH17 helper/effector T cell. In addition, given completely different conditions (ie. lymphokine exposure), this process can be reversed except for the Treg-to-naïve T cell reverse conversion. Despite this, the ability to shift between totally different phenotypes and potentially back again makes the phenotype of the Treg more of a concept that concrete cell type (Sawant 2014). The plasticity of Tregs during an anti-tumor T cell response can alter that response in ways that affect other immune cells such as DC. The ability of Tregs to function in this way is rooted in the protein/biochemical pathways within each cell. Cellular receptors initiate a series of biochemical signals that when translated by the nucleus becomes the basis of cellular behavior. This topic, introduced in this first chapter, and when discussed in the context of immune cells is referred to as "translational immunology." As far as the T cell immune system and particularly Tregs is concerned, translational immunology may hold the key to the positive manipulation of the T cell immune system in order to successfully treat cancer. As a starting point in the first chapter the transcriptional pathways associated with TCR signaling and the induction of T cell activation were examined. This is the primary starting point and the beginning of the T cell response and the description of these pathways were used as a model to demonstrate the complex interrelationships as various protein/biochemical pathways intersect resulting in specific signals that are sent to the nucleus and in response nuclear factors send out signals to alter or modify the T cell's behavior. This was described because in Tregs many of these pathways that are initiated by the TCR complex become altered due to the their unique "anergic" phenotype. During this section in Chapter 1, the translational pathways that were associated with the major functional descriptions of Tregs as far as their origin in the thymus, development in the periphery, relation to autoimmunity, pregnancy, and the anti-tumor T cell response were discussed at length. This chapter ends with a detailed analysis of the translational events that occur within Tregs and DCs in relation to the anti-tumor T cell response because these events are the basis of Treg control of the entire immune system.

Chapter 2: Autoimmunity, Tregs, and the Anti-Tumor T Cell Immune System

This chapter was the most interesting from a basic cellular immunology point of view. Autoimmunity, which includes the activities of each of the immune classes of cells (T cells, B-cells, NK cells and granulocyte/monocyte series), exposes a type of complexity about the immune system that is not quite apparent at first glance. This complexity is rooted in the fact that in order for the immune system to recognize non-self it must have a thorough knowledge of self. In other words, the T cell immune system has to be completely familiar with the cells that make-up the tissue systems in the body in order to properly distinguish self from non-self. Of course this process begins in early development as the T cells are selected in the thymus and actually continues though out life with the immunosurveillance system and innate mechanisms (single-signal induction, etc.) to induce anergy in self-reactive lymphocytes (T and B-cells). This becomes apparent as this chapter unfolds. The reason why autoimmunity is an important topic as far as Tregs and the anti-tumor T cell response is concerned relates to the concept that has been mentioned numerous times and is the close relationship between a cancerous cell and a normal one. In part (a very large part) this is what makes cancer such a difficult disease to treat and eradicate. The self/non-self nature of cancer is a major problem not only in the development of the disease, but also during its growth phase because the T cell immune system develops a conflict about what to do with them. The source of the conflict comes from the fact that a developing and many times, a full-blown stem cell-like cancer, can express both normal (self) and abnormal (non-self) antigens at the same time. In addition, cancer cells can express antigens that are part self and part non-self (neoantigens) or totally non-self (tumor antigens) and this just adds to the conundrum. However, Tregs are not particularly conflicted in that they recognize that T cells are killing a cell that posses self-antigens and their function is to stop this activity. Because the Treg has a more formidable arsenal of weapons to use against its adversaries (T and NK cells) it has the ability to control the situation. This is the thought process behind what was written in Chapter 2, which is also included within the introduction of this chapter.

Part of that thought process began with a description and origin of both innate and adaptive Tregs as far as the recognition of self. The next topic introduces cancer-induced autoimmunity by describing how both the T cell immune system and the cancer changes. These changes are usually initiated by the tumor as a part of the tumorgenesis process, but the T cell immune system has to adjust to these changes. The sectional nature of this chapter begins with the section called, *Immune Cellular Interactions* and the first subsection called, *Cancer-induced Autoimmunity* begins with the classic prototypic example of a tumor causing autoimmunity and that is during the T cell response to melanoma. The induction of melanoma-induced vitiligo is introduced and what follows is an in depth description of melanoma as a tumor and as a model of the T cell immune response to a solid tumor. The most important aspect of this discussion is related to the immunogenicity of the tumor as well as how melanoma cells present tumor and traditional antigens in normal and abnormal ways. What follows is a detailed description of how the abnormal ways melanoma cells process and present antigen actually damage the T cell immune system by inducing T cell anergy. The mechanisms associated with this damage to the T cell immune system make a significant difference in the health of melanoma patients, which is not related to the induction of autoimmunity, but rather the debilitated condition of the T cell immune system and infections. All of these complex interactions between the cellular immune system and their ancillary effects begin with the formation of cancer from a normal cell and that process is important to understand in relation to the T cell response.

The next section concerns itself with the topics of carcinogenesis (induction of cancer), tumorgenesis (tumor development), and the development of cancer stem cells. These three areas can dictate the degree of malignancy depending upon how much damage is done to the DNA of the cell (carcinogenesis), whether or not this damage can be repaired (tumorgenesis), and what type of growth genes become unregulated (tumor stem cells). After an introduction, this section contains three sub-sections. The first concerns itself with how environmental carcinogens initiate the tumorgenesis process and the various types of cancer that are formed according to the type of carcinogen induction. For example UV light and melanoma, radon gas and lung cancer, as well as breast cancer/dioxin and benzene/leukemia are all examples where the molecular mechanisms of tumorgenesis are understood. Within this section tumorgenesis was explained in terms of the inability of DNA repair enzymes such as topoisomerases that either fail to repair DNA damaged by these carcinogens, or make mistakes during the repair process and inadvertently put powerful gene promoters in front of growth genes, which induces unregulated growth of the cells. The next section begins with just what the T cell immune system and Tregs are doing during the tumorgenesis process. As self-antigens, which Tregs recognize, diminish and non-self antigens recognized by the T cell immune system increase, an interesting thing happens. Instead of the T cell immune system taking advantage of this situation by mounting a full-on attack of the now almost fully formed tumor cell mass; the remaining Tregs increase the strength of their defense by unleashing multiple crippling effector mechanisms. Normally, Tregs can defend tissues by standard CTL effector mechanisms (perforin/granzymes and FAS/FASL) and by conversion of responding T cells into Tregs. These are cell-to-cell contact effector mechanisms and are effective where low numbers of responding T cells approach the protected cells. However, in the situation above where Tregs begin to loose their tether (self-antigens) to the cells they are protecting, start to become outnumbered, and some of the protected cells get killed, it triggers the activation of two additional effector mechanisms that can stop responding T cells in their tracks. During the attack on the protected cells fragmented DNA is released into the intercellular milieu, which includes ATP. As ATP concentrations increase Tregs begin to produce adenosine ectopically by activation of extracellular ecto-5' –nuclease (CD73) and ecto-NTPDase-1 (CD39). As a result, Tregs not only begin to produce extracellular adenosine, which immediately slows down the T cell response by reducing IL-2 secretion and retardation of DC maturation. In addition, through an autocrine process involving adenosine and the adenosine receptor A2, the adenyl cyclase pathway is activated and this increases the concentration of intracellular cAMP within Tregs. Under these conditions Tregs can proliferate once they deplete the cAMP from their cytoplasm by injecting responding T cells with it. This is a description of one of the adjustments caused by the tumorgenesis process.

The next major topic discussed is concerned with cancer stem cells (CSC) as far as their development, phenotypic characteristics, and effects on the T cell immune system. A cancer stem cell is defined as a cancer cell that is self-sustaining, gives rise to cancer cells that are phenotypically different from the CSC due to genetic mutation. The CSCs comprise a minority population that are generally resistant to chemotherapy and can drive the tumorgenesis process by giving rise non-stem cell tumor populations. However, what makes CSC so deadly is what they do to the T cell immune system. These cells can activate and secrete cytokines such as TGF-β and IL-10 and express CD80/86 antigens, which when detected by T cells immediately converts them into Tregs and in addition, create immunosuppressive DCs. Some CSCs have the ability to not only secrete inhibitory TGF-β and IL-10, but also inflammatory cytokines such as IL-1β, IL-6, and GMCF. This activity has the result of basically tying up the T cell immune system, which induces as state of confusion. However, many times tumors gain these capabilities the patients suffer from the previously mentioned "cytokine storm," which is a product of excessive secretion of lymphokines by both the tumor and lymphocytes. This condition can cause death as evidenced by the case report discussed in Chapter 4 where a patient received a chimeric T cell with a receptor specific for ERBB2, which is over expressed on tumor cells, but also expressed at low levels in normal cells such as epithelial cells in the lungs. This leads into the next section called *Alteration of the T cell Immune System by Cancer Stem cells that Lead to Autoimmunity* and has to do with how tumor cells secrete lymphokines or express receptors normally expressed on lymphocytes. This can have a devastating effect on the immune response. The type of immune response to a tumor is important one because the goal is to kill the tumor and leave behind memory T cells (another topic in this chapter) to prevent a recurrence. This is a TH-1 T cell response and is initiated by the activation of naïve T cells that respond to tumor antigens. This activation involves the secretion of IL-12 and mature DCs secrete this lymphokine. However, if IL-4 is secreted naïve T cells responding to tumor antigens activate follicular helper CD4 T cells in the germinal centers, which result in the secretion of antibody. It turns out that some tumor cells such as multiple myelomas (MM), chronic lymphocytic leukemia (CLL), and others can induce antibody production by IL-4 secretion. The presence of IL-4 induces a TH-2 T cell response that induces antibody production instead of cytotoxic T cells. The detrimental aspect related to this "skewing" of the T cell response to a TH-2 response is the fact that the antibodies produced are against self. These autoantibodies can induce autoimmunity in major tissue systems and as far as melanoma is concerned, that tissue system is the skin. More specifically normal melanocytes and the induction of the autoimmune disease called vitiligo. The short version of how this happens involves the phagocytosis of autoantigen-coated cells through the Fc receptor of the macrophage. The macrophages process and present self-antigens and this activates or in many cased hyper activates Tregs that as previously mentioned have self-specific TCR. Hyper activation of Tregs causes the cells to become exhausted and the loose the ability to inhibit CD4 T cells that respond to the gp100 melanocyte/melanoma antigen. These uncontrolled CD4 responders activate CD8 effector cells, which begin to destroy melanocytes that results in skin depigmentation. This is only one of several proposed mechanisms involving Tregs in both melanoma-induced and generalized vitiligo.

The next section called, *The Importance of Autoimmunity During the Anti-tumor T cell Response and Its Relationship to Treg Dysfunction and the Predisposition of Autoimmune and Cancer Patients to Contract Other Autoimmune diseases* and aside from it being a rather long title for a subsection, it describes a condition that many cancer patients, as well as autoimmune disease patients and their families face. Many of these patients and their family members are predisposed to getting additional autoimmune diseases. It is not entirely clear why this is because on face of it these patients and their families have normal immune systems; at least as far as current knowledge about immunity is concerned. Despite this, what this section is about is why during the treatment of cancer is the development of autoimmune responses a good prognostic indicator. In other words, if two patients with the same type of cancer are treated with the same anti-cancer treatment or observed over time as an immune response against the tumor develops, those patients who develop secondary autoimmune responses to tissues related to the cancer survive their disease and those without these autoimmune reactions do not. It seems that if the regulatory T cell system (Tregs) were working properly autoimmune responses caused by the T cell immune's response to the tumor would not occur. This would point toward a dysfunction of Tregs and that may very well be the case given the proven fact concerning the predisposition of autoimmunity in family members of cancer and autoimmune disease patients. However, this may or may not be the case because it was determined that once a T cell immune response is initiated by the T cell immune system, memory T cells begin to be produced as part of a total lifelong T cell immune response. As a simplification, it can be said the there are two types of memory T cells. Central memory (Tcm) T cells basically exist in an inert form for long periods of time in the body and require full activation through classical TCR requirements of a primary (TCR) and secondary (CD28) signal. Once activated, they secrete massive amounts of TH-1 lymphokines that basically alert the entire immune system. On the other hand the effector memory T cells (Tem) can exist for extended periods, but need occasional contact with antigens that are similar, but not particularly identical to their target antigen to briefly expand. However, occasionally these similar antigens can cause Tem to differentiate into effector T cells and immediately damage of kill that particular cell, which is not really the target cell, but shares antigens with it. This is what happens in melanoma-induced vitiligo and also other cancer systems where there has been a successful T cell response against the tumor. This, in combination with the exhaustive expansion of Tregs responding to the presentation of self-antigens by APC, creates conditions that allow this type of autoimmunity to occur. This hyperactivation of Tregs may be genetically controlled, which may explain why family members are predisposed to autoimmune diseases. However, if during this process there are tumor cells present they get eliminated, which can explain why cancer-related autoimmunity can be a good indicator of patient survival.

The next section, *Autoimmune Responses, Inflammation, and the Induction of Cancer* goes into detail about how chronic inflammation and cancer are related. Again using the finding that family members of autoimmune and cancer patients were predisposed to developing other autoimmune diseases, this section points toward evidence that this situation may be related to a generalized autoimmune defect within the human genome. This defect would probably be related to Tregs, but more than likely T cells as well. It was pointed out that during an inflammatory event there are substances released by inflammatory cells such as mast cells and even T cells that are harmful and even mutagenic to normal cells. Such substances would be oxygen-reactive (ROS) and nitrogen-reactive species (NOS) that are released from mast cells and macrophages and have been show to induce oxidative DNA damage similar to what was mentioned in the carcinogens section above. Lymphocytes also secrete proinflammatory lymphokines such as IL-1, IL-6, and IL-8, which can be harmful to normal cells because as previously discussed in the case of IL-6; translational pathways are activated, which alter a normal cells function such as cellular adhesion. Activation of these pathways, which are not usually activated in normal cells can cause that cell to become dysfunctional and lead to form of cellular dysplasia; a pre-cancerous state. It was also discussed how viral and bacterial infectious agents such as human papillomavirus (cervical cancer) (Bosch 2002) and *Helicobacter pylori* (stomach cancer) (Graham 2000) that induce inflammatory conditions can lead to the development of cancer. The other harmful effect of chronic inflammation is what it does to established cancers. It was shown how the inflammatory lymphokine IL-6 activated an enzyme (DNA methyltransferase-1 or DNMT1) that has the ability to inhibit the expression of genes responsible for cell adhesion. Inhibition of these genes in tumor cells allows them to travel throughout the body. Therefore, inflammation involves the commitment of Tregs, the induction of cancer, and can stimulate the tumorgenesis process of established cancers.

The Translational Events Associated with Autoimmunity, Tregs, Anti-tumor T cells, and Cancer begins with an examination of the pathways related to the expression of MHC-class II by tumor cells. As was stated in the previous *Immune Cellular Interactions* section, MHC-class II expression by tumor cells turns out to be a "double-edged" sword in that when anti-tumor CD4 T cells activate they use tumor-associated MHC-class II molecules to respond to processed tumor peptides. However, the downside to this interaction is the fact that the MHC-class II molecules on the tumor cell surface are aggregated by contact with the TCR in a concentrated region, which means lipid raft formation inside the tumor cell membrane. While in this configuration MHC-class II cytoplasmic domains initiate the c-jun NH2-terminal kinase or JNK. JNK, which is a member of the MAPK family, becomes phosphorylated which in turn up-regulates phosphoinositide-dependent kinase 1 (PDK1) expression. This leads to the activation of Akt and protein kinase C (PKC) and the activation of these two pathways leads to increased tumorgenesis. This pathway (JNK/PKC/Akt) is also involved in the carcinogenic activity of arsenic-tumor formation in human lung epithelial cells. Instead of up-regulating PDK1, JNK phosphorylates STAT3 at ser-727 that leads to Akt activation and the secretion of vascular endothelial growth factor (VEGF). This growth factor that induces angiogenesis (formation of blood vessels), allows cancerous epithelial cells to escape the primary tumor site. The next pathways under discussion have to do with the interactions of T cell (Tregs) expressed LAG-3 and its ligand on the tumor, MHC-class II. This interaction affects both cells because ligation of LAG-3 on T cells can induce anergy, but also can make tumor cells resistant to FAS/FASL and chemotherapeutic death. The inhibition of DC function by Tregs is explained next where the ITAM inhibitory pathway is activated, which results in the reduction of the surface expression of the CD28 ligands CD80/86 and subsequent reduction in the ability of DC to activate antigen specific T cell responses. The translational pathways associated with IL-6 secretion by the tumor cell and its effect on T cell pathways is detailed next by going into detail concerning the role IL-6 plays in T cell differentiation by activating the JAK/STAT3 pathway and the MAPK Ras/Erk pathway. This is the basis of inflammatory T cell formation that if not controlled, can lead to not only the autoimmune diseases such as IBD, MS, and RA, but also cancers associated with these inflammatory autoimmune diseases. As far as the role of IL-6 in tumor formation is concerned, it can activate a gene called Oct-4, which has the ability to transform non-CSC into CSC. This happens through a series of steps and the activation of JAK-1/STAT3 pathway via the phosphorylation of the IL-6 receptor (p130), which dimerizes STAT3. These dimers enter the nucleus and turn on survival genes such as BCL-xl. It also targets genes that control cell cycle regulators such as cyclin-D1and c-MYC, which in essence give the non-CSC stem cell properties. Next the translational pathways described were associated with the activation of memory T cells and the ability of p50 subunit of NF-kB to activate the secretion of INF-γ by binding directly to INF-γ gene promoter. Next, the ability of the cyclin kinase inhibitor p27kip1 to interrupt the S and G2/M phase of the cell cycle and induces cell quiescence in memory T cells and this activity can actually degrade the T cell memory pool. This is one of the many translational pathways described during the next sections that detail the function of memory CD4 and CD8 T cells. The next sections go into detail concerning pathways associated with Treg function as it relates to autoimmunity and the anti-tumor T cell response.

Chapter 3: Treg Effector Mechanisms

This chapter represents a detailed examination of the major Treg effector mechanisms that control not only the T cell immune response, but also the lymphatic infrastructure associated with sites of inflammation that include tumor masses. These Treg effector mechanisms were separated into cell-to-cell and non-cell-to-cell contact mechanisms. Treg effector mechanisms include the two major effector mechanisms used by non-Treg T cells (CD4 and CD8), which are the perforin/granzyme and FAS/FASL systems. There was an extensive analysis of both mechanisms with regard to how they cause cell death and how that cell death contributes to immune homeostasis. After an introduction that includes example of out of control T cell immune responses that result in massive deadly autoimmune responses such as the 1918 flu pandemic, the *Immune Cellular Interactions* section begins with a description of the two major effector mechanisms mentioned above that are used by both T cell and Tregs. The FAS/FASL system is composed of the FAS receptor (R) called CD95 or APO-1 and is a 36-kD cell surface protein that is a member of the tumor necrosis factor (TNF) and nerve growth factor (NGF) receptor supergene families. The FAS ligand (L) or CD178 is a type II 40-kD membrane protein and both of these proteins are expressed or can be induced on a wide variety of cells in the body. Once the FASL effector cell comes in contact with the FASR target a membrane synapse is formed and inside the target cell a complex is formed, which is called the FAS associated death domain or FADD. A precursor enzyme called procaspase binds to this complex and activates effector caspases (caspases 2, 3, 6, 7, 8, 9, and others). These caspases begin the process of dismantling the cell by cleavage of essential proteins and the activation of transcription factor proteins that bind to specific DNA promoters. These promoters activate genes that regulate pro-apoptotic factors such as the BCL-2 family of proteins that suppress survival-promoting proteins. This cascade of biochemical events leads to the fragmentation of DNA within the target cell and death. It has been determined that the immune system uses the FAS/FASL to remove immune cells after an immune response. In addition, the FAS/FASL system is also involved in the previously discussed "immune privileged" sites that are not apart of the immune surveillance circuit. It was found that in sites such as the nervous system, the eye, and testis contain cells that express FASL and any FASR expressing cells (activated T cells) are killed upon contact. This is a problem when tumors develop from these tissues because they often maintain their immune privilege status, which makes them difficult for the T cell immune system to attack them. Even though this system has a defined purpose in controlling the immune system, there is a problem with "collateral damage" inflicted on normal cells that express FASR by FASL expressing T cells. This activity can initiate autoimmunity because of the processing and presentation of self-antigens as previously described.

The next section describes the perforin/granzyme system, which involves the formation of an immunological synapse where the effector bores a hole into the target. Granzyme granules are then injected into the target cell, which kill the cell through degradation of target membrane proteins by proteolysis causing the cytoplasm to rush out of the cell. The exact physical conformation of perforin, which forms the pore in the target cells, is described in detail. After this description, the composition a characterization of the multiple (10) granzyme enzymes is described. After this there is a discussion about granzymes that are secreted by T cells and most importantly Tregs. The utilization of perforin/granzyme and FAS/FASL effector mechanisms by Tregs is the subject of the subsection called, *The Significance of Perforin/granzyme and FAS/FASL Mechanisms to Treg Immunobiology* that points out Treg use of these effector mechanisms are determined by the situation they find themselves in. In addition, the topic of secreted GrB by Tregs was introduced. This is an important use of an effector mechanism that operates at the interface between not only the Treg and its target, but also Tregs and cells of the extra cellular matrix (ECM). This activity allows Tregs to essentially "wall-off" solid tumors or abscesses from the rest of the body. Another aspect of these two effector mechanisms has to do with Treg sensitivity to their effects. Under certain circumstances Tregs become the target of effector CD4 T cells that secrete GrB under strong immunological stimulation. Tregs become susceptible to GrB induced caspase 3 activation and is dependent on the ratio of apoptosis-inducing proteins such as BAX and BIM versus anti-apoptosis proteins like BCL-xl and BCL. During these conditions of high antigenic stimulation CD4+ Tregs have this imbalance toward apoptosis-inducing proteins. In this section the mechanism of mitochondrial death induced by GrB is examined in detail. The next section looks at the function of serine proteases, which protect cells from the proteolytic effects of GrB. The immunoregulatory role of both effector mechanisms in the lifespan of Tregs is discussed and related to the differential expression of FASL and FAS on effector T cells and Tregs during periods of IL-2 secretion by effectors. During these periods effector cells express FAS and Tregs, which are absorbing IL-2 express FASL. This makes effectors susceptible to Treg attack during a T cell response where IL-2 is being secreted.

The next major section in this chapter has to do with Treg-only effector mechanisms and after and introduction starts with non-cell-to-cell contact effector mechanisms. It starts with the production of adenosine by Tregs. This is the largest single section that details a Treg effector mechanism. The reason for this is because the production of adenosine by Tregs is one of the most effective of all the multiple Treg effector mechanisms in that not only does adenosine induce effector cell anergy through its receptors, which are expressed on most cells of the body, but it can also modulate the behavior of non-immune cells in the area of inflammation. This section on adenosine is extensive because it is one of the major immunomodulatory factors associated with the Treg's ability to control almost all T cell immune responses associated with not only inflammatory responses, but also the T cell responses to cancer. After this extensive analysis of the effects of adenosine and how it is very much a unique part of the Treg's immunobiology, IL-2 deprivation by Tregs is examined. For some this activity of Tregs is not considered a true effector mechanism, but when viewed in the context of Tregs controlling the waning moments of a inflammatory response it is clear that IL-2 absorption away from effector cells is a means Tregs use to disable responding T cells. The approach to understanding this effector mechanism starts with the high-affinity IL-2 receptor expressed by Tregs. Even though this form of IL-2R is transiently expressed on T cell as they become activated, it is constitutively expressed on the surface of Tregs. Tregs use IL-2 in ways totally different from responding CD4 and effector CD8 T cells do and this gives them an advantage and this difference in IL-2 utilization allows Tregs to control T cell responses. Activities mediated by the Treg IL-R such as expression of FOXP3, participation in the adenosine/inflammation activities of Tregs, and the signaling of apoptosis in Tregs, are in addition to the use of the IL-2R as sensor of responding T cell activity that can occur anywhere in the body. The functional uses of the IL-2R by Tregs include aiding the helper activity of follicular CD4 T cells TH(fh). The formation of TH(fh) T cells is dependent on the activation of BCL6 by IL-4. However, if IL-2 is present it activates STAT5 as previously described, but STAT5 inhibits BCL6, which would inhibit antibody formation helper by TH(fh) T cells. Tregs absorb most, but not all of the IL-2 during this TH-2 response because TH(fh) need small amounts to perform this function. In addition there are circumstances where during viral infection memory T cells, which need limited amounts of IL-2 benefit from the absorption of IL-2 by Tregs. Also during infections with pathogens the formation of TH17 cells is favored by the reduction of IL-2 in these situations where IL-6 is secreted.

The next major section describes the cell-to-cell contact mechanisms. Since two of the major effector/cell-to-cell contact mechanisms (perforin/granzyme and FAS/FASL) were discussed earlier it was important to describe the immunological synapse (IS), which is the formation of the interface between effector and target cell. IS formation in Treg effectors are quite different from those formed between effector T cells and targets. The reason for this is the fact that the Treg synapse serves a totally different purpose than that of T effectors. This has to do with the ability of Tregs to alter protein expression of their target cells. This takes more time than when effectors interact with target in order to kill it, which takes a very short period of time. These differences are reflected in the arrangement of immunological proteins associated with the IS. PKC-theta is an example where in Treg synapses, unlike in responding T cells it is sequestered away from the IS because it participates in the induction of IL-2 secretion. However, the ability of Tregs to be the most mobile T cell has to do with PKC-theta because it controls calcium influx, which is essential for T cell motility. The first and only very important cell-to-cell contact effector mechanism is the injection of cAMP into responding T cells. This mechanism not only induces anergy in responding T cells, but it also can lead to Treg proliferation. Once cAMP is injected into responding T cells the PKA pathway is activated with AC activation. This leads to the inhibitory pathways described for adenosine interaction with its receptor.

The second part of this chapter that discusses translation pathways associated with Treg effector mechanisms starts off, after an introduction with the analysis of pathways activated as a result of the production of adenosine by Tregs. Since many of these pathways were previously discussed during the section on adenosine the results of the interactions with those pathways with others was discussed through the functions induced by them. The next section looks at the activation of the two pathways that regulate cAMP, ATP, and adenosine systems, which are the PKA and EPAC pathways. These are described through the function of DCs activated by either adenosine or ATP. The two pathways compliment each other in that they have different sensitivities to activation by either ATP or cAMP. EPAC, unlike the PKA pathway can activate NFkB in DC, yet it can mediate the degradation of the co-factor p300 that controls the binding of CREB to the IL-10 receptor increasing secretion. These two cAMP activated pathways do not act independently of each other and the interactions, which are termed “crosstalk,” are just being understood.

Chapter 4: Treg Immunobiology As It Relates to the Anti-Tumor T Cell Response during Immune Cell-Based Cancer Treatment

This final chapter examines some of the issues involved with the initiation and design of immune cell-based immunotherapeutic treatment of cancer and how those therapies are impacted by Treg immunobiology. The chapter takes a developmental approach to a relatively new type of cancer treatment called immunotherapy and uses a historical viewpoint to show that Tregs were not only present during early human clinical trials, but also the reason for their failure. The basic immunological concepts surrounding the development of these therapies was discussed with particular emphasis put on two immune cells used as immunotherapeutic agents. Those were T cells and DC, which are the two cells that not only initiate most immune responses of the body, but also maintain them as well. Of the many forms of immunotherapy, three were chosen because of their long history of development and also because the immunotherapeutic cell was either a T cell or DC. Adoptive therapy (ACT) and DC vaccine-based therapy were chosen mainly because of the therapeutic cell, but hematopoietic stem cell transplantation (HSCT) was used as an example where Tregs, which can prevent GVHD, are used as the immunotherapeutic cell. It was mentioned that Tregs could affect immune cell-based therapy for the treatment of cancer in two ways. The first way is a subtle interference with the therapy by the exerted effort of Tregs to control the immune response by altering the immune environment through the secretion of specific lymphokines such as IL-10 and induce a decrease in secreted IL-12. IL-10 is secreted by Tregs and negatively affects responding T cells and because Tregs inhibit DC through multiple (cell contact, Treg produced adenosine) pathways, they become unable to secrete TH-1 T cell inducing IL-12. The second way Tregs interfere with these therapies is to make direct cell contact with responder T cells and effectively inhibit their ability to respond to or kill the tumor. During HSCT Tregs of the donor inhibit allogeneic T cells from responding to recipient histocompatability antigens during allogeneic HSCT. However, it will be shown that a major concern is the ability of Tregs to inhibit the anti-tumor T cell response.

In the first section called, *Early Human Cancer Immunotherapeutic Clinical Trials* it was apparent that tumor immunologist became aware of the fact that there was something was blocking the anti-tumor T cell response based on the fact that in many cases of cancer measurable T cell responses could be detected. During the mid-1970s it was recognized the chemotherapy alone may not be effective enough to remove the tumor and a new approach to cancer treatment had to include the manipulation of the immune system itself. Early human clinical trails were performed with late-stage melanoma patients to determine if injection of these patients with autologous or allogeneic tumor cell lysates could induce a measurable CTL response in their periphery. PBL from 5 of 12 patients studied showed a measurable response to tumor lysates in the form of T cell cytotoxicity towards the immunizing melanoma cell. However, this response lasted only 7 days, which the researchers in this case could not understand. Undoubtedly, this had to do with the fact that the Tregs of the patient immediately inhibited the anti-melanoma T cells formed by the procedure. At the same time large treatment-based clinical trials using the strong adjuvant BCG, which was injected directly into metastatic melanoma lesions with or without inactivated tumor cells, were performed. The results of two studies using this method were encouraging for dermal lesions and to a lesser extent survival of a minority of patients. In the first study using the adjuvant alone 90% of the lesions regressed as well as 17% of uninjected lesions with 25% of patients surviving 1 to 6 years (normally 1 year survival) after treatment. The second study that included inactivated melanoma cells showed similar results, but with no measurable increases in the survival rate. Both procedures were unable to affect visceral metastasis. These studies did demonstrate that there was a response to melanoma in patients with the disease. The question was why did that response not remove the tumor?

During the 1980s immunological techniques had been developed that allowed tumor immunologist to not only measure the T cell response to autologous tumor cells, but also to develop in vitro models that represented the in vivo T cell response. With that knowledge it was now not only possible to study the dynamics of the T cell/tumor cell interaction, but also to identify the proteins involved in the interaction. What was most important about these techniques was the fact that now tumor immunologist were able to grow tumor-immune T cells in the form of tumor infiltrating lymphocytes or TILs in the laboratory and use them therapeutically to treat cancer. These clinical trials of cultured TIL being used in a new type of cancer therapy called immunotherapy were initiated in the late 1980s-early 1990s. The initial trials with metastatic melanoma patients demonstrated some regression of disease, but like the early trials only benefited less than one-third of the patients enrolled. These were usually Phase I trials, which for the most part were conducted to determine the safety of the procedure and they were valuable in that respect. These trials used IL-2 therapy to induce continued expansion of TIL, but there were serious side effects.

During this period DC vaccine therapy clinical trials with patients with renal cell carcinoma (RCC) were conducted using a known T cell immunogenic peptide (MUC-1) used to pulse DCs, which were injected subcutaneously with or without IL-2. Out of twenty patients 6 had detectable peptide-specific T cells and demonstrated tumor progression. It was determined that IL-2 therapy was inhibitory when observing T cell responses to the tumor specific peptide. This was an indication the innate Tregs had become activated during the immunization process by administered IL-2. Another non-clinical study was performed on RCC tumor sections stained with various antibodies in order to determine where T cell and DC were located relative to the tumor. A surprising finding revealed that the tumors had the architecture of regional lymph nodes; complete with connections to the lymphatic system. Mature DCs were found in the peripheral areas of the tumor clustered with T cells, but immature DCs were observed within the tumor. Antibody analysis revealed that immature DCs were attracted to the tumor mass because of the expression of the chemokine CCL20. This chemokine attracts immature DC, Tregs, and naïve T cells, but not mature DC. The arrangement and cellularity of the tumor mass has characteristics of the activities of Tregs in that there was tissue remodeling and an arrangement of lymphatic vessels most likely due to the secretion of VEGF by tumor-associated macrophages or Tregs themselves. Therefore, this was evidence that Tregs were intimately associated with the initial phases of tumor growth because they were able to encapsulate the tumor in a fibrous pseudocapsule due to the secretion of GrB by Tregs during tumor formation. Again, as the human clinical trials with metastatic melanoma patients using TIL and IL-2 proceeded it was determined after multiple trials that only one-third of the patients responded and despite the presence of anti-melanoma T cells many of the patients progresses. It was clear that there was resistance to the treatment and it also was apparent that the source of this resistance was the patient's own T cell immune system. Given the information about the existence of Tregs it was decided to add another protocol to this type of immunotherapy and in addition, focus on the T cell as the immunotherapeutic cell instead of TIL, which contain Tregs.

These changes in the use of immune cell-based immunotherapies that utilized T cells was called adoptive T cell therapy (ACT) and for the first time directly addressed the inhibitory effect of Tregs. The added protocol was the use of chemical-based agents (non-myeloablative) and radiation (total body irradiation or TBI) to remove the patient's lymphocytes (lymphodepletion) prior to the immunotherapeutic use of anti-tumor T cells and IL-2. The rational, which was supported by animal studies, was that not only did lymphodepletion remove Tregs, but also it removed the "lymphokine sink" caused by the utilization of IL-2 by the patient's resident T cells. In terms of the improvement of immunotherapeutic cells, instead of using whole TIL populations T cells were isolated from

TIL and expanded in the laboratory prior to patient infusion. These changes increased the response rat from 25% to over 50% in metastatic melanoma cells. Further focus on the immunotherapeutic T cell led to the concept of using tumor peptide specific T cells that were expanded using patient APC. However, there were problems associated with expanding the numbers of T cells needed for therapy. Because of this and other problems related to the persistence of therapeutic T cells in the patient's body because of the T cell's age, genetically altered T cells became more attractive. This was because it was possible to insert and express genes responsible for tumor peptide-specific TCR alpha and beta genes into naive T cells, which have a longer lifetime. There were two ways to genetically alter the ability of T cells to recognize tumor cells. The first, and as mentioned above, requires the identification of tumor peptide specific T cells. After cloning the TCR genes, they are inserted into a retroviral vector. Anti-CD3 activated T cells from the patient are transduced with the TCR retroviral vectors containing antibiotic resistant genes. These transduced T cells are selected in medium containing that antibiotic (neomycin) and expanded again with APC and anti-CD3 antibodies. The other way to control the specificity of T cells was to construct a transducible gene construct containing genes that encode antigen specific variable light chains of a monoclonal antibody specific for a tumor antigen. This construct, which contains several other genes such as the CD8 transmembrane gene and CD28 and/or CD137 intracellular domain genes were called CAR. Both types of genetically altered T cells in combination with lymphodepletion increased the efficiency of ACT therapy, but both also had problems associated with, in the case of CAR transduced T cells, inhibition of tumor-specific T cell by the development of anti-mouse Ig antibodies and cross reactivity of tumor antigens with normal tissues. TCR transduced T cells had been shown to induce cancer-induced autoimmunity and in some cases limited persistence in the patient. However, CAR T cells have been very successful in treating B-cell lymphoid tumors because lymphodepletion and the CAR treatment target the antibody producing cells of the patient not allowing them to make anti-mouse Ig antibodies. Similarly, TCR-transduced T cells are more effective against solid tumors such as brain tumors because of their homing properties.

However, during the success of the clinical trials there were several studies in mice and humans that revealed not only the existence of lymphodepletion-resistant Tregs, but also the rapid replenishment and increased functional capabilities of Tregs after the procedure. This was one of the most important findings during this period because the data demonstrated the success of new immune cell-based immunotherapies could be improved if this problem with resistant Tregs was addressed. It turns out that DC-based vaccines were even more sensitive to the control by Tregs because of the special relationship (which has been detailed throughout this book) that Tregs have with DC. Clinical trials using either tumor lysate or tumor peptide-pulsed DC with or without IL-2 therapy indicated that these therapies can induce regression of established tumors. However, some of the problems are again associated with using IL-2 therapy, which can activate Tregs and dampen the effectiveness of the procedure. It was also determined that the maturity level of the DC was important with regards to the cells being able to activate naïve T cells. Maturity of DCs is important as far as an inflammatory response (which can occur as a tumor mass develops) is concerned. Tregs are often drawn to these events by chemokines released by macrophages in response to ATP, which is a product of cell death and particularly apoptotic cell death where the DNA of the dead cell is fragmented by this process. During the initial inflammatory process GM-CSF and IL-3/IL-4 is secreted at low levels and this creates immature DC from stationary monocytes, which begin to convert T cell (antigen-specific and naïve) into Tregs. However, if those lymphokine signals increase in intensity, immature DC get converted to mature DC, which are able to induce Treg proliferation through the presentation of self-antigens, expression of CD80/86 in the presence of IL-2. These interactions are just a small part of the complex relationship between Tregs and DC that occur during an inflammatory response, which often occurs during solid tumor development.

The treatment of hematological cancers such as leukemia and lymphomas was examined next because these therapies make use of hematopoietic stem cell transplantation (HSCT) in order to remove the cancer by donor T cells, which recognize the tumor as foreign and called graft vs. tumor (GVT) effect. However, often a by-product of this type of therapy is the development of almost always-fatal graft vs. host (GVHD) disease where the donor T cells recognize the MHC antigens on normal tissues of the recipient. Using donor Tregs during or prior to the therapy has been shown to inhibit the donor T cell response to recipient's tissues. GVHD is a very serious complication of HSCT because despite finding the perfect HSC donor (an identical twin) there are still small differences in the polymorphic genes of the MHC between them. These are called "minor histocompatability antigens" and the response to them by the donors T cells can be deadly. The two forms (acute and chronic) of GVHD can be treated with a wide variety of treatments that include immunosuppressive agents that often put the recipient at risk of developing life-threatening infections. This is why immune-based treatments in the form of donor Tregs have become so important. Again, preclinical studies in mice show that if the Tregs posses TCR for the recipients MHC they have the ability to efficiently inhibit only GVHD-inducing T cell and not GVT T cells. This has yet to be included in human clinical trials during HSCT, but more than likely now as this is being read, trials such as this are already underway or have been completed. What has been done concerning human clinical trials is that Tregs have successfully been used to reduce the incidence of GVHD in patients that would otherwise have developed the disease within 15 days. The issue of Tregs inhibiting GVT T cells is an important one and similar to their effect in ACT where supposedly they have been removed. In other words, when an immune cell-based treatment seems to be successful is that success because the Treg inhibition is lessened, but not completely removed? In HSCT when the procedure is successful donor T cells attack and kill the tumor, but again the question is that attack dampened by either recovering recipient Tregs, donor engrafted Tregs, or added immunotherapeutic Tregs from the donor? The answer to that question and its solution could mean additional lives saved during the HSCT procedure. More than likely Tregs, being the powerful regulators of the T cell immune system that they are; become involved in either the success (weakened Treg control) or failure (total Treg control) of the GVT response during HSCT. There is evidence that may support variable Treg control of GVT of leukemia and lymphoma depending on the migratory patterns of the tumor.

Multiple myeloma (MM), which will be mentioned during the summary of the translational pathway section of this chapter, develops and grows in the BM and is responsible for its destruction. However because of this, MM is one of the hematopoietic tumors that respond to HSCT in contrast to some of the other tumors such as CLL and B-cell lymphoma that originate in the BM, but home to lymphatic system such as regional lymph nodes and the spleen. Because stromal cells in the BM produce IL-6, which inhibits Tregs and may reprogram them into inflammatory TH17 T cells. The reprogramming of Tregs into TH17 T cells does two things in this situation. First of all the lymphokine IL-17 exerts a powerful inflammatory influence during the immune response. Secondly, IL-17 specifically induces INF-γ secretion by CD4 T cells, which is favorable to the continuation of the anti-tumor T cell response. When donor Tregs are used therapeutically or innate Tregs from the donor enter the BM they are immediately inhibited by secreted IL-6 and are unable to prevent GVT T cells from destroying the MM. However, since other lymphomas and leukemias that originate in the BM, but leave to inhabit the lymphatic system they exists in a basically IL-6-free, DC populated environments. This makes them not only more visible and susceptible to Treg protection, but also puts donor anti-tumor T cells at a distinct disadvantage. This disadvantage has to do with how Tregs prevent T cell activation by inhibiting DC function and not allowing T cells to initiate antigen-specific proliferation. HSCT treatment for hematological cancers in theory seems rather straight forward as explained in the beginning of this section. However, this type of immune cell-based therapy for cancer is actually the most complex because it involves the active interaction of multiple immune cells (T cells, DC, macrophages, and Tregs) in order for it to have the desired effect of eliminating the tumor and the generation of memory T cells to prevent recurrence. In addition, there is the prevention of the side effects (GVHD) of the treatment, which involve using Tregs as therapeutic cells. Understanding the interactions between these multiple immune cells during successful HSCT has allowed tumor immunologist to learn a great deal about the dynamics of a controlled inflammatory response because that is exactly what HSCT is when examined through a basic immunological lens.

The next section (*Translational Pathways Associated with Immune Cell-based Immunotherapy)* of this last chapter about the clinical aspects of Tregs and the anti-tumor T cell response has to do with some of the many translational pathways associated with the immune cell-based therapy of cancer. The introduction of this section brings up several very important issues related to Tregs, their survival, and role in the immunotherapeutic treatment of cancer. The first thing was how important the presence of Tregs is to the recovery of the immune system in patients that have undergone lymphodepletion, which is a protocol necessary for all three types of immune cell-based therapies to be effective at removing the tumor. Without Tregs the patients would be at risk of developing deadly forms of autoimmune disease. The second related issue was the ability of Tregs to resist lymphodepletion procedures (non-myeloablative chemotherapy and total body irradiation) and respond by recovering as a highly potent version (ICOS+ Tregs) of itself. As far as Tregs and immunotherapy is concerned, these two issues are the most important ones because they indicate that the role of Tregs in cancer therapy is just same as it is in normal individuals; a vital and necessary element controlling the way the T cell immune system functions. The introduction also points out the fact that for the most part, many of the translational pathways discussed in the three previous chapters control the interactions that take place during all three (ACT, DC vaccines, and HSCT) immune cell-based therapies highlighted in this chapter. However, as a reminder the PKA and NFATc1 pathways were used as an example of pathways activated within Tregs that regulate Treg effector functions and proliferation, respectively and that these functions have a direct impact on the effectiveness of these immune cell-based anti-cancer therapies. In addition, other pathways in tumor cells associated with tumor escape (P13K/Akt pathways/ VEGF secretion) and (MAPK/ERK pathways/ chemotherapy/FASL-resistance) negatively impact the immunotherapy of solid tumors such as melanoma and glioblastoma. This section starts with the pathways associated with the conditions in the BM during HSCT that interfere with Treg inhibition of GVT effector T cells via the secretion of IL-6 by BM stromal epithelial cells. This has to do with the activation of the JAK/STAT3 pathway and the subsequent inhibition of Tregs caused by the weakening of FOXP3 expression due to the increase in RORgammat gene expression during the phenotypic change of Tregs to TH17 T cells. TH17 T cells create an inflammatory environment conducive to an effector T cell response. In addition, and as mentioned above, one of the TH-1 favorable things TH17 T cells do by secreting IL-17 is that it can induce the secretion of INF-γ by T cells during an inflammatory response. This no doubt is related to how TH17 T cells respond to pathogens, which was mentioned in Chapter 3 during the IL-2 deprivation by Tregs section.

However, the next section details the used of transcriptional pathway inhibitors to increase the anti-tumor T cell responses during immunotherapy for cancer. Again, STAT3 is mentioned in terms of its inhibition and the subsequent restoration of Treg function, inhibition of tumor cell (glioblastoma) down regulation of its MHC-class II expression, as well as tumor induced DC-mediated suppression of the anti-tumor T cell response. What followed were examples of the use of specific STAT3 inhibitors and their effects on DC function in both mice and humans. The next section called, *Translational Pathways Associated with Immune Cell-based Immunotherapy: The Use of Transcriptional Pathway Inhibitors to Alter Treg Immunobiology* discusses the reprogramming process of Tregs into TH17 T cells where in many tumors TH17 T cells predominate while an anti-tumor T cell immune response ensues, but at some point Tregs predominate as the tumor progresses. The ability of TH17 T cells to be de-programmed into Tregs is a possible explanation for this phenomenon. More work has to be done in this area because if this is true an entirely new approach to autoimmunity can be initiated based on the TH17 T cell's role in autoimmune disease. Despite that, it was found that the IL-6/JAK/STAT3 pathway leads to the degradation of the FOXP3 proteins by the activation of the ubiquitin-proteosome pathway leading to the release of FOXP3 protein control of the RORgammat gene. It was also pointed out that the ubiquitin-proteosome pathway is also involved in a number of other important pathways such as the ability of EPAC to activate the ubiquitin-proteosome pathway in order to degrade the cofactor p300 that plays a role in CREB binding to the IL-10 gene promoter thereby activating is secretion in DC. It was proposed that if TH17 T cells could be transiently expressed in a tumor mass that destabilization of FOXP3 might achieve this by the use of acetytransferase inhibitors (because p300 a histone acetyltransferase and stabilizes FOXP3) on antigen-specific Tregs and the use of transient IL-6 therapy during an ACT where the therapeutic cells are treated tumor-specific Tregs and TCR-induced anti-tumor T cells.

The next section of this subheading discusses the resistance of effector T cells to Treg inhibition during inflammatory responses such as the case with HSCT where donor T cells are proliferating and attacking recipient's tissues during GVHD. It was found that this too was the result of IL-6 secretion activating the JAK/STAT3 pathway in both Tregs and effector T cells. Tregs would lose their inhibitor functions as mentioned above while reprogramming into TH17 T cells begin. The Tregs in this case do not actually have to turn into TH17 T cells because the first step in the process is the destabilization of FOXP3, which is enough to inhibit Treg inhibitory functions. It was found that treatment of Tregs and responding T cells with small-molecule inhibitors (Stattic V and Stat3 inhibitor VII) specific for STAT3 restored the ability of Tregs to inhibit anti-allogeneic T cell responses where large amounts of IL-6 were secreted. Another STAT3 inhibitor called S31-201 contributed to the creation of adaptive Tregs during inflammation by increasing the ratio of STAT5 to STAT3. Since

STAT5 expression is indispensible in IL2R induction of FOXP3 expression new Tregs are created from both the naïve and antigen-specific T cell pools. Another aspect of the use of small-molecule inhibitors was the use of Rolipram to inhibit phosphodiesterases that break down cAMP produced by Tregs naturally and in abundance during autocrine stimulation of the A2A adenosine receptor. Rolipram increased the inhibitory function of Tregs on responding T cells and DC during GVHD. On the other hand inhibitors such as the expression of ectopic PDE or cAMP antagonist (Rp-8-Br-cAMPS) can inhibit Treg function/increase proliferation and restore inhibited CTL function in effector T cells that were injected by Tregs with cAMP, respectively. It was also pointed out that the adenosine/PKA/AC pathway is a good pathway to manipulate with inhibitors, agonist, and antagonist because this pathway intersects with other pathways controlling primary Treg functions such as anergy (cAMP), proliferation (NFATc1) and effector mechanisms (adenosine production and cAMP injection). However, there is mention of a cautionary approach to the used of any agent that manipulates translational pathways in immune cells because of the fact that other cells (normal and malignant) use the same pathways for different purposes. One example given is that fact that the IL-6/JAK/STAT3 pathway is not only active in T cells, but also tumor cells where its activation can lead to tumor growth arrest, escape (metastasis), as well as the creation of CSC from non-CSC tumors. This is why these transcriptional pathway inhibitors should be extensively tested in vitro and in animal models. To make a point about that fact it was mentioned that the chemotherapeutic agent dasatinib, which is an ABL/SRC-kinase family inhibitor and was used successfully to treat CML during HSCT turned out to not only be inhibitory to Tregs, but also at the same doses; it inhibited responding donor T cell function. Apparently, the drug did not completely inhibit responding donor T cells enough to block GVT, but GVHD was also lessened so there had to be either a reduction in anti-allogeneic T cell responses to the recipient's tissues or Tregs, which were also shown to be inhibited by the drug, were able to inhibit GVHD development. Of course all of this was found out many years after the drug was successfully used to treat patients. In addition, this is not the only chemotherapeutic agent that had a differential response to Tregs and T cells that was discovered well after the drug was in use. Several of these drugs and the cancers they were used against were mentioned.

As this short chapter ends so this book comes to a close and one thing is for certain, which is the direction of future cancer treatments. The treatments of the future will unleash the power of the T cell immune system to contain if not remove cancer from the body. The immunotherapeutic treatment of cancer will involve the manipulation of intracellular translational pathways to improve both the response and cure rates of the treatment until cancer is ultimately added to the list of successfully treated human diseases.

References

Abe BT, Shin DS, Mocholi E, Macian F (2012) NFAT1 supports tumor-induced anergy of CD4+ T cells. *Can Res* 72: 4642-4651.

Abe BT, Macian F (2013) Uncovering the mechanisms that regulate tumor-induced T-cell anergy. *OncoImmunol* 2: 2, e22679.

Adamopoulos IE (2010) Interleukin-17A upregulates receptor activator of NF-kappaB on osteoclast precursors. *Arth Res Ther* 12: R29.

Adeegbe DO, Nishikawa H (2013) Natural and induced T regulatory cells in cancer. *Front Immunol* 4: 1-14.

Adler HS, Steinbrink K (2008) MAP kinase P38 and its relation to T cell anergy and suppressor function of regulatory cells. *Cell Cycle* 7: 169-175.

Afford S, Randhawa S (2000) Demystified… *J Clin Pathol: Mol Pathol* 53: 55-63.

Ahmad R, Raina D, Meyer C, Kufe D (2008) Triterpenoid CDDO-methyl ester inhibits the janus-activated Kinase-1 (JAK-1)- signal transducer and activator of transcription-3 (STAT3) Pathway by direct inhibition of JAK1 and STAT3. *Cancer Res* 68: 2920-2926.

Albert ML, Pearce SF, Francisco LM, Sauter B, Roy P, Silverstein RL, Bhardwaj N (1998) Immature dendritic cells phagocytose apoptotic cells via $\alpha v\beta 5$ and CD36, and cross-present antigens to cytotoxic T cells. *J Exp Med* 188: 1359-1368.

Alexander M (2011) *Immune-based Cancer Treatment. The T Lymphocyte Response. CRC Press,* New York, NY.

Alexander MA, Bennicelli J, Guerry D (1989) Defective antigen presentation by human melanoma cell lines cultured from advanced, but not biologically early disease. *J Immunol* 142: 4070-4078.

Alexandrescu DT, Riordan NH, Ichim TE, Kauffman CL, Kabigting F, Dutton CT, Dasanu CA (2011) On the missing link between inflammation and cancer. *Dermatol Online J.* 17: 10.

Alkhateeb A, Fain PR, Thody A, Bennett DC, Spritz RA (2003) Epidemiology of vitiligo and associated autoimmune diseases in Caucasian probands and their families. *Pigment Cell Res* 16: 208-214.

Alshamsan A (2012) Induction of tolerogenic dendritic cells by IL-6-secreting CT26 colon carcinoma. *Immunopharmacol Immunotoxicol* 34: 465-469.

Alvares Y, Municio C, Alonso S, Sanchez Crespo M, Fernandez N (2009) Induction of IL-10 by zymosan in dendritic cells depends on CREB activation by the coactivators CREB-binding protein and TORC2 and PGE2. *J Immunol* 183: 1471-1479.

Ananieva O, Darragh J, Johansen C, Carr JM, McIlrath J, Park JM, Wingate A, Monk CE, Toth R, Santos SG, Iversen L, Arthur JS (2008) The kinases MSK1 and MSK2 act as negative regulators of toll-like receptor signaling. *Nat Immunol* 9: 1028-1036.

An O, Gursoy A, Gurgey A, Keskin O (2013) Structural and functional analysis of perforin mutations in association with clinical data of familial hemophagocytic lymphohistiocytosis type 2 (FHL2) patients. *Protein Sci* 22: 823-839.

Anderson MJ, Shafer-Weaver K, Greenberg NM, Hurwitz AA (2007) Tolerization of tumor-specific T cells despite efficient initial priming in a primary murine model of prostate cancer. *J Immunol* 178:1268-1276.

Angus KL, Griffiths GM (2013) Cell polarization and the immunological synapse. *Curr Opin Cell Biol* 25: 85-91.

Antony PA, Piccirillo CA, Akpinarli A, Finkelstein SE, Speiss PJ, Surman DR, Palmer DC, Chan CC, Klebanoff CA, Overwijk WW, Rosenberg SA, Restifo NP (2005) CD8+ T cell immunity against a tumor/self-antigen is augmented by CD4+ T helper and hindered by naturally occurring T regulatory cells. *J Immunol* 174: 2591-2601.

Ansari AW, Tmblay JN, Alyaha SH, Ashton-Rickardt PG (2010) Serine protease inhibitor 6 protects iNKT cells from self-inflicted damage. *J Immunol* 185: 877-883.

Apasov S, Chen JF, Smith P, Sitkovsky M (2000) A2A receptor dependent and A2A receptor independent effects of extracellular adenosine on murine thymocytes in conditions of adenosine deaminase deficiency. *Blood* 95: 3859-3867.

Arnold B, Schorich G, Hammerling GJ (1993) Multiple levels of peripheral tolerance. *Immunol Today* 14: 12-4.

Ashley CW, Baecher-Allen C (2009) Cutting edge: Responder T cells regulate human DR+ effector regulatory T cell activity via granzyme B. *J Immunol* 183: 4843-4847.

Azar GA, Lemitre F, Robey EA, Bousso P (2010) Subcellular dynamics of T cell immunological synapses and kinapses in lymph nodes. *PNAS* 107: 3675-3680.

Azzi J (2013) Serine protease inhibitor 6 plays a critical role in protecting murine granzyme B-producing regulatory T cells. *J Immunol* 191: 1-9.

Baaten BJ, Cooper AM, Swain SL, Bradley LM (2013) Location, location, location: The impact of migratory heterogeneity on T cell function. *Front Immunol* 4: 311.

Baatar D, Olkhanud PB, Wells V, Indig FE, Mallucci L, Biragyn A (2009) Tregs utilize β-galactoside-binding protein to transiently inhibit P13K/p21ras activity of human CD8+ T cells to block their TCR-mediated ERK activity and proliferation. *Brian Behav Immun* 23: 1028-1037.

Baba J, Watanabe S, Saida Y, Tanaka T, Miyabayashi T, Koshio J, Ichikawa K, Nozaki K, Koya T, Deguchi K, Tan C, Miura S, Tanaka H, Tanaka J, Kagamu H, Yoshizawa H, Nakata K, Narita I (2012) Depletion of radio-resistant regulatory T cells enhances antitumor immunity during recovery from lymphopenia. *Blood* 120: 2417-2427.

Baban B, Chandler PR, Sharma MD, Pihkala J, Koni PA, Munn DH, Mellor AL (2009) IDO activates regulatory T cells and blocks their conversion into Th17-like T cells. *J Immunol* 183: 2475-2483.

Bade B, Lohrmann J, ten Brinke A, Wolbink AM, Wolbink GJ, ten Berge IJ, Virchow JC Jr, Luttmann W, Hack CE (2005) Detection of soluble human granzyme K in vitro and in vivo. *Eur. J. Immunol* 35:2940–48.

Baecher-Allen C, Wolf E, Hafler DA (2006) MHC class II expression identifies functionally distinct human regulatory cells. *J Immunol* 176: 4622-4631.

Bahmanyar S, Montgomery SM, Hillert J, Ekbom A, Olsson T (2009) Cancer risk amoung patients with multiple sclerosis and their parents. *Neurology* 72: 1170-1177.

Baine I, Abe BT, Macian F (2009) Regulation of T-cell tolerance by calcium/NFAT signaling. *Immunol Rev* 231: 225-240.

Bailey-Bucktrout SL, Bluestone JA (2011) Regulatory T cells: stability revisited. *Trends Immunol* 32: 301-306.

Balogh A, Persa E, Bogdandi EN, Benedek A, Hegyesi H, Safrany G, Lumniczky K (2013) The effect of ionizing radiation on the homeostasis and functional integrity of murine splenic regulatory T cells. *Inflam Res* 62: 201-212.

Bao Q, Shi Y (2007) Apoptosome, a platform for the activation of initiator caspases. *Cell Death Differ* 14: 56-65.

Barbieri G, Rimini E, Costa MA (2011) Effects of human leukocyte antigen (HLA)-DR engagement on melanoma cells. *Inter Jour of Oncol* 38: 1589-1595.

Barns MJ Krebs P, Harris N, Eidenschenk C, Gonzalez-Quintial R, Arnold CN, Crozat K, Sovath S, Moresco EM, Theofilopoulos AN, Beutler B, Hoebe K (2009) Commitment to the regulatory T cell lineage requires CARMA1 in the thymus but not in the periphery. *PLoS Biol* 7: e51.

Barron L, Dooms H, Hoyer KK, Kuswanto W, Hofmann J, O'Gorman WE, Abbas AK (2010) Cutting edge: Mechanisms of IL-2-dependent maintenance of functional regulatory T cells. *J Immunol* 185: 6426-6430.

Bayry J, Triebel F, Kaveri SV, Tough DF (2007) Human dendritic cells acquire a semimature phenotype and lymph node homing potential through interaction with CD4+CD25+ regulatory T cells. *J Immunol* 178: 4184-4193.

Bazhin AV, Kahnert S, Kimpfler S, Schadendorf D, Umansky V (2010) Distinct metabolism of cyclic adenosine monophosphate in helper CD4+ T cells. *Mol Immunol* 47: 678-684.

Becker JC, Brabletz T, Czerny C, Termeer C, Brocker EB (1993) Tumor escape from immunosurveillance: induction of unresponsiveness in a specific MHC-restricted CD4+ human T cell clone by autologous MHC class II+ melanoma. *Int Immunol* 5: 1501-1508.

Bendle GM, Linnemann C, Hooijkaas AI, Bies L, de Witte MA, Jorritsma A, Kaiser AD, Pouw N, Debets R, Kieback E, Uckert W, Song JY, Haanen JB, Schumacher TN (2010) Lethal graft-versus-host disease in mouse models of T cell receptor gene therapy. *Nat Med* 16: 565-570.

Bennett MW, O'connell J, O'sullivan GC, Roche D, Brady C, Kelly J, Collins JK, Shanahan F (1999) Expression of fas ligand by human gastric adenocarcinomas: A potential mechanism of immune escape in stomach. *Gut* 44:156-162.

Bennett CL, Christie J, Ramsdell F, Brunkow ME, Ferguson PJ, Whitesell L, Kelly TE, Saulsbury FT, Chance PF, Ochs HD (2001) The immune dysregulation, polyendocrinopathy, enteropathy, X-linked syndrome (IPEX) is caused by mutations of FOXP3. *Nat Genet* 27: 20–21.

Benoit G, Cooney A, Giguere V, Ingraham H, Lazar M, Muscat G, Perlmann T, Renaud JP, Schwabe J, Sladek F, Tsai MJ, Laudet V (2006) International union of pharmacology LXVI. Orphan nuclear receptors. *Pharmacological Reviews* 58: 791-836.

Betts BC, Veerapathran A, Pidala J, Yu XZ, Anasetti C (2014) STAT5 polarization promotes iTregs and suppresses human T-cell alloresponses while preserving CTL capacity. *J Leukoc Biol* 95: doi: 10.1189/jlb.0313154.

Bettelli E, Korn T, Oukka M, Kuchroo VK (2008) Induction and effector functions of T(H)17 cells. *Nature* 453: 1051-1057.

Bharat A, Fields RC, Steward N, Trulock EP, Patterson GA, Mohanakumar T (2006) CD4+25+ regulatory T cells limit Th1-autoimmunity by inducing IL-10 producing T cells following human lung transplantation. *Amer J of Trans* 6: 1799-1808.

Bharat A, Kuo E, Saini D, Steward N, Hachem R, Trulock EP, Patterson GA, Meyers BF, Mohanakumar T (2010) Respiratory virus induced dysregulation of T regulatory cells leads to chronic rejection. *Ann Thorac Surg* 90: 1637-1644.

Biddison, W.E., J.C. Palmer, M.A. Alexander, E. P. Cowan, and L. A. Manson. 1977. Characterization and specificity of murine antitumor cytotoxic effector cells within an ascitic tumor. *J. Immunol.* 118:2243.

Billingham RE, Brent L Medawar PB (1953) Actively acquired tolerance of foreign cells. *Nature* 172:603-606.

Birmingham K (2002) What is translational research? *Nat Med* 8: 647-649.

Bjorgo E, Taskin K (2006) Role of camp phosphodiesterase 4 in regulation of T-cell function. *Crtit Rev Immunol* 26: 433-451.

Bjorgo E, Solheim SA, Abrahamsen H, Baillie GS, Brown KM, Berge T, Okkenhaug K, Houslay MD, Tasken K (2010) Crosstalk between phosphatidylinostitol 3-kinase and cyclic AMP (cAMP)-protein kinase A signaling pathways at the level of a protein kinase B/B-arrestin/cAMP phosphodiesterase 4 complex. *Mol Cell Bio* 30: 1660-1672.

Bladergroen BA, Strik MC, Wolbink AM, Wouters D, Broekhuizen R, Kummer JA, Hack CE (2005) The granzyme B inhibitor 9 (PI-9) is expressed by human mast cells. *Eur J Immunol* 35: 1175-1183.

Bluestone JA, Abbas AK (2003) Natural versus adaptive regulatory T cells. *Nat Rev Immunol* 3:253-257.

Bodor J, Habener JF (1998) Role of transcriptional repressor ICER in cyclic AMP-mediated attenuation of cytokine gene expression in human thymocytes. *J Biol Chem* 273:9544–9551.

Bodor J, Bopp T, Vaeth M, Klein M, Serfling E, Hunig T, Becker C, Schild H, Schmitt E (2012) Cyclic AMP underpins suppression by regulatory T cells. *Eur J Immunol* 42: 1375-1384.

Boissonnas A, Scholer-Dahirel A, Simon-Blancal V, Pace L, Valet F, Kissenpfennig A, Sparwasser T, Malissen B, Fetler L, Amigorena S (2009) FoxP3+ T cells induce perforin-dependent dendritic cell death in tumor-draining lymph nodes. *Immunity* 32: 266-278.

Bonnefoy F, Couturier M, Clauzon A, R√©my-Martin JP, Gaugler B, Tiberghien P, Chen W, Saas P, Perruche S (2011) TGF-B-exposed plasmacytoid dendritic cells participate in Th17 commitment. *J Immunol* 186: 6157-6164.

Bonnet D, Dick JE (1997) Human acute myeloid leukemia is organized as a hierarchy that originates from a primitive hematopoietic cell. *Nat Med* 3:730–7.

Bopp T, Becker C, Klein M, Klein-Hessling S, Palmetshofer A, Serfling E, Heib V, Becker M, Kubach J, Schmitt S, Stoll S, Schild H, Staege MS, Stassen M, Jonuleit H, Schmitt E (2007) Cyclic adenosine monophosphate is a key component of regulatory T cell-mediated suppression. *J Exp Med* 204: 1303-1310.

Bopp T, Dehzad N, Reuter S, Klein M, Ullrich N, Stassen M, Schild H, Buhl R, Schmitt E, Taube C (2009) Inhibition of cAmp degradation improves regulatory T cell-mediated suppression. *J Immunol* 182: 4017-4024.

Bosch FX (2002) The causal relationship between human papillomavirus and cervical cancer. *J Clin Path* 55: 244-265.

Bots M, de Bruin E, Rademaker-koot MT, Medema JP (2007) Proteinase inhibitor-9 expression is induced by maturation in dendritic cels via p38 MAP kinase. *Hum Immunol* 68: 959-964.

Brem R, Li F, Montaner B, Reelfs O, Karran P (2010) DNA breakage and cell cycle checkpoint abrogation induced by a therapeutic thiopurine and UVA radiation. *Oncogene* 29: 3953-3963.

Bromley SK, Burack WR, Johnson KG, Somersalo K, Sims TN, Sumen C, Davis MM, Shaw AS, Allen PM, Dustin ML (2001) The immunological synapse. *Annu Rev Immunol* 19: 375-396.

Brunkow ME Jeffery EW, Hjerrild KA, Paeper B, Clark LB, Yasayko SA, Wilkinson JE, Galas D, Ziegler SF, Ramsdell F. (2001) Disruption of a new forkhead/winged helix protein, scurfin, results in the fatal lymphoproliferative disorder of the scurfy mouse. *Nat Genet* 27: 68–73.

Buckner JH (2010) Mechanisms of impaired regulation by CD4+CD25+ regulatory T cells in human autoimmune diseases. *Nat Rev Immunol* 10: 849-859.

Burke KE, Wei H (2009) Synergistic damage by UVA radiation and pollutants. *Tox and Indus Health* 25: 219-224.

Burra S, Jiang JX (2011) Regulation of cellular function by connexin hemichannels. *Int J Biochem* 2: 119-128.

Buzza MS (2005) Extracellular matrix remodeling by human granzyme B via cleavage of vitronectin, fibronectin, and laminin. *J Biol Chem* 280: 23549–23558.

Byrne KT, Turk MJ (2011) New perspectives on the role of vitiligo in the immune responses to melanoma. *Oncotarget* 2: 684-694.

Camisaschi C, Casati C, Rini F, Perego M, De Filippo A, Triebel F, Parmiani G, Belli F, Rivoltini L, Castelli C (2010) LAG-3 expression defines a subset of CD4+ CD25 high Foxp3+ regulatory T cells that are expanded at tumor sites. *J Immunol* 184: 6545-6551.

Camporeale A, Poli V (2012) IL-6, IL-17 and STAT3: a holy trinity in auto-immunity? Front Biosci 17: 2306-2326.

Cao W, Jamieson BD, Hultin LE, Hultin PM, Detels R (2009) Regulatory T cell expansion and immune activation during untreated HIV Type 1 infection are associated with disease progression. *Aids Research and Human Retroviruses* 25: 183-191.

Carlsson B, Totterman TH, Essand M (2004) Generation of cytotoxic T lymphocytes specific for the prostate and breast tissue antigen TARP. Prostate 61: 161-170.

Castiello L (2011) 15kDa granulysin versus GM-CSF for monocytes differentiation: analogies and differences at the transcriptome level. *J Trans Med* 9: 41.

Caton AJ, Cozzo C, Larkin J 3rd, Lerman MA, Boesteanu A, Jordan MS (2004) CD4(+) CD25(+) regulatory T cell selection. *Ann NY Acad Sci* 1029: 101-114.

Chan ESL, Cronstein BN (2010) Adenosine in fibrosis. *Mod Rheumatol* 20: 114-122.

Chang GY, Kohrt HE, Stuge TB, Schwartz EJ, Weber JS, Lee PP (2011) Cytotoxic T lymphocyte responses against melanocytes and melanoma. *Jour Transl Med* 9: 122-132.

Chatterjee S, Eby JM, Al-Khami AA, Soloshchenko M, Kang HK, Kaur N, Naga OS, Murali A, Nishimura MI, Le Poole IC, Mehrotra S(2013) A quantitative increase in regulatory T cells controls development of vitiligo. *J Invest Dermatol* Dec 23 doi: 10.1038/jid.2013.540.

Chen M, Huang L, Wang J (2007) Deficiency of Bim in dendritic cells contributes to overactivation of lymphocytes and autoimmunity. *Blood* 109: 4360-4367.

Chen M, Felix K, Wang J (2011) Immune regulation through mitochondrion-dependent dendritic cell death induced by T regulatory cells. *J Immunol* 187: 5684-5692.

Chen PW, Ullrich SE, Ananthaswamy HN (1994) Presentation of endogenous tumor antigens to CD4+ T lymphocytes by murine melanoma cells transfected with histocompatability complex class II genes. *J Leukoc Biol* 56: 469-474.

Chen S, Liu Y, Sytwu H (2012) Immunological regulation of pregnancy: From mechanism to therapeutic strategy for immunomodulation. *Clin and Devel Immunol* 2012: 1-10.

Chen, W (2003) Conversion of peripheral CD4+ CD25- naive T cells to CD4+CD25+ regulatory T cells by TGF-beta induction of transcription factor Foxp3. J. Exp. Med. 198, 1875–1886.

Cheng G, Yu A, Dee MJ, Malek TR (2013) IL-2 signaling is essential for functional maturation of regulatory T cells during thymic development. *J immunol* 190: 1567-1575.

Cheng G, Aixin Y, Malek TR (2011) T cell tolerance and the multi-functional role of Il-2R signaling in T regulatory cells. *Immunol Rev* 241: 63-76.

Cheng X (2008) Epac and PKA: a tail of two intracellular camp receptors. *Acta Biochim Biophys Sin* 40: 651-662.

Chikamatsu K, Takahashi G, Sakakura K, Ferrone S, Masuyama K (2011) Immunoregulatory properties of CD44+ cancer stem-like cells in squamous cell carcinomas of the head and neck. *Head and Neck* 33: 208-215.

Chitra, S, Nalini G, Rajasekhar G (2012) The ubiquitin proteasome system and efficacy of proteasome inhibitors in disease. *Int J Rheum Dis* 15: 249-260.

Cho J.H, Kim HO, Surh CD, Sprent J (2010) T Cell Receptor-Dependent Regulation of lipid rafts controls naive CD8(+) T cell homeostasis. *Immunity* 32: 214-226.

Chougnet CA, Tripathi P, Lages CS, Raynor J, Sholl A, Fink P, Plas DR, Hildeman DA (2011) A major role for Bim in regulatory T cell homeostasis. *J Immunol* 186: 156-163.

Christopoulos P, Pfeifer D, Bartholome K, Follo M, Timmer J, Fisch P, Veelken H. (2011) Definition and characterization of systemic T cell dysregulation in untreated indolent B-cell lymphoma and very early CLL. *Blood* 117: 3836-3846.

Cifuentes M, Albala C, Rojas, CV (2008) Differences in lipogenesis and lipolysis in obese and non-obese adult human adipocytes. *Biol Res* 41: 197-204.

Clark WH Jr., From L, Bernadino EA, Mihm MC (1969) The histogenesis and biologic behavior of primary human malignant melanoma. *Cancer Res* 29: 705-727.

Clark WH, Elder DE, Guerry D (1984) A study of tumor progression: the precursor lesions of superficial spreading and nodular melanoma. *Hum. Pathol.* 15: 1147-1165.

Clark WH, Elder DE, Van Horn M (1986) The biologic forms of malignant melanoma. *Hum Path* 17: 443-450.

Clayberger C, Finn MW, Wang T, Saini R, Wilson C, Barr VA, Sabatino M, Castiello L, Stroncek D, Krensky AM (2012) 15kDa granulysin causes differentiation of monocytes to dendritic cells but lacks cytotoxic activity. *J Immunol* 188: 6119-6126.

Cobbold M (2013) MHC Class II associated phosphopeptides are the targets of memory-like immunity in leukemia. *Sci Trans Med* 5: 203ra125.

Cohen S (1990) Lymphokines and the immune response. *CRC Press, Inc., Boca Raton,* FL.

Coney LR, Tomassetti A, Carayannopoulos L, Frasca V, Kamen BA, Colnaghi MI, Zurawski VR Jr (1991) Cloning of a tumor-associated antigen: MOv18 and MOv19 antibodies recognize a folate-binding protein. *Cancer Res* 51: 6125-6132.

Crellin NK, Garcia RV, Levings MK (2007) Altered activation of AKT is required for the suppressive function of human CD4+CD25+ T regulatory cells. *Blood* 109: 2014-2022.

Cresswell AC, Sisley K, Laws D, Parsons MA, Rennie IG, Murray AK (2001) Reduced expression of TAP-1 and TAP-2 in posterior uveal melanoma is associated with progression to metastatic disease. *Melanoma Res* 11: 275-281.

Cunningham TD, Jiang X, Shapiro DJ (2007) Expression of high levels of human proteinase inhibitor 9 blocks both perforin/granzyme and fas/fas ligand-mediated cytotoxicity. *Cell Immunol* 245: 32-41.

Curiel TJ (2007) Tregs and rethinking cancer immunotherapy. *J Clin Invest* 117: 1167-1174.

Currie GA, Lejeune F, Fairley GH (1971) Lymphocyte cytotoxicity in malignant melanoma. *Brit Med J* 2: 305-310.

Czystowska M, Strauss L, Bergmann C, Szajnik M, Rabinowich H, Whiteside TL (2010) Reciprocal granzyme/perforin-mediated death of human regulatory and responder T cells is regulated by interleukin-2 (IL-2). *J Mol Med* (Berl) 88: 577-588.

Danbolt, N. C. (2001) Glutamate uptake. *Prog. Neurobiol.* 65: 1–105.

Deaglio S (2007) Adenosine generation catalyzed by CD39 and CD73 expressed on regulatory T cells mediates immune suppression. *J Exp Med* 204: 1257-1265.

Di Ianni M, Falzetti F, Carotti A, Terenzi A, Castellino F, Bonifacio E, Del Papa B, Zei T, Ostini RI, Cecchini D, Aloisi T, Perruccio K, Ruggeri L, Balucani C, Pierini A, Sportoletti P, Aristei C, Falini B, Reisner Y, Velardi A, Aversa F, Martelli MF (2011) Tregs prevent GVHD and promote immune reconstitution in HLA-haploidentical transplantation. *Blood* 117: 3921-3928.

Dilek N (2013) Targeting CD28, CTLA-4, and PD-L1 costimulation differentially controls immune synapses and function of human regulatory and conventional T-cells. *PLOS ONE* 8: e83139.

Dimitriou ID, Clemenza L, Scotter AJ, Chen G, Guerra FM, Rottapel R (2008) Putting out the fire: coordinated expression of innate and adaptive immune systems by SOCS1 and SOCS3 proteins. *Immunol Rev* 224: 265-283.

Ding Y, Xu J, Bromberg JS (2012) T regulatory cell migration during an immune response. *Trends Immunol* 33: 174-180.

Dissemond J, Gotte P, Mors J, Lindeke A, Goos M, Ferrone S, Wagner SN (2003) Association of TAP-1 downregulation in primary melanoma lesions with lack of spontaneous regression. *Melanoma Res* 13:253-258.

Doherty PC, Kelso A (2008) Toward a broadly protective influenza vaccine. *J Clin Invest* 118: 3273-3275.

Dong JC (2014) Role of PLC-PIP2 and cAMP-PKA signal pathways in radiation-induced immune-suppressing effect. *Biomed Environ Sci* 27: 27-34.

Draube A, Klein-Gonzalez N, Mattheus S, Brillant C, Hellmich M, Engert A, von Bergwelt-Baildon M (2013) Dendritic cell based tumor vaccination in prostate and renal cell cancer: A systematic review and meta-analysis. *PLoS ONE* 6: e18801.

Drake CG, Jaffe E, Pardoll DM (2006) Mechanisms of immune evasion by tumors. *Adv Immunol* 90: 51-81.

Drenou B, Blancheteau V, Burgess DH, Fauchet R, Charron DJ, Mooney NA (1999) A caspase-independent pathway of MHC class II antigen-mediated apoptosis of human B lymphocytes. *J Immunol* 163: 4115-412

Dumitriu IE, Dunbar DR, Howie SE, Sethi T, Gregory CD (2009) Human dendritic cells produce TGF-beta 1 under the influence of lung carcinoma cells and prime the differentiation of CD4+CD25+Foxp3+ regulatory T cells. *J Immunol* 182: 2795-2807.

Durant L, (2010) Diverse targets of the transcription factor STAT3 contribute to T cell pathogenicity and homeostasis. *Immunity* 32: 605-615.

Eatough JP, Henshaw DL (1993) Radon and monocytic leukaemia in England. *J Epidemiol Com Health* 47: 506-507.

Engleman EG (1997) Dendritic cells: Potential role in cancer therapy. *Cytotech* 25: 1-8.

Ek-Vitorin JF, Burt JM (2013) Structural basis for the selective permeability of channels made of communicating junction proteins. *Biochim Biophys Acta* 1828: 51-68.

El Andaloussi A, Lesniak MS (2006) An increase in CD4+CD25+FOXP3+ regulatory T cells in tumors-infiltrating lymphocytes of human glioblastoma multiforme. *Neuro Oncol* 8:234-243.

Ernst PB, Garrison JC, Thompson LF (2010) Much ado about adenosine synthesis and function in regulatory T cell biology. *J Immunol* 185: 1993-1998.

Escobar A, Lopez M, Serrano A, Ramirez M, Perez C, Aguirre A, Gonzalez R, Alfaro J, Larrondo M, Fodor M, Ferrada C, Salazar-Onfray F (2005) Dendritic cell immunizations alone or combined with low doses of interleukin-2 induce specific immune responses in melanoma patients. *Clin Exp Immunol* 143: 555-568.

Eshhar Z, Waks T, Gross G, Shindler DG (1993) Specific activation and targeting of cytotoxic lymphocytes through chimeric single chains consisting of antibody-binding domains and the γ or ζ subunits of the immunoglobulin and T-cell receptors. *Proc Natl Acad Sci* 90: 720-724.

Ewen CL, Kane KP, Bleackley RC (2010) A quarter century of granzymes. *Cell Death and Diff* 19: 28-35.

Facciabene A, Motz GT, Coukos G (2012) T regulatory cells: Key players in immune escape and angiogenesis. *Cancer Res* 72: 2162-2171.

Fantini MC (2004) Cutting edge: TGF-B induces a regulatory phenotype in CD4+CD25+ T cells through FOXp3 induction and down-regulation of Smad7. *J Immunol* 172: 5149-5153.

Felcht M, Heck M, Weiss C, Becker JC, Dippel E, Muller CS, Nashan D, Sachse MM, Nicolay JP, Booken N, Goerdt S, Klemke CD (2012) Expression of the T-cell regulatory marker FOXP3 in primary cutaneous large B-cell tumor cells. *Br J Dermatol* 167: 348-358.

Fei F, Yu Y, Schmitt A, Rojewski MT, Chen B, Gotz M, Dohner H, Bunjes D, Schmitt M (2009) Dasatinib inhibits the proliferation and function of CD4+CD25+ regulatory T cells. *Br J Haematol* 144: 195-205.

Feinerman O (2010) Single-cell quantification of IL-2 response by effector and regulatory T cells reveals critical plasticity in immune response. *Mol Syst Bio* 6: 437-453.

Feng G, Nadig SN, Backdahl L, Beck S, Francis RS, Schiopu A, Whatcott A, Wood KJ, Bushell A (2011) Functional regulatory T cells produced by inhibiting cyclic nucleotide phosphodiesterase type 3 prevent allograft rejection. *Sci Trans Med* 3: 83ra40.

Finetti F, Baldari C (2013) Compartmentalization of signaling by vesicular trafficking: a shared building design for the immune synapse and the primary cilium. *Immunol Rev* 251: 97-112.

Fisson S (2003) Continuous activation of autoreactive CD4+ CD25+ regulatory T cells in the steady state. *J Exp Med* 198: 737-746.

Fontenot JD, Rasmussen JP, Gavin MA, and Rudensky AY (2005) A function for interleukin 2 in Foxp3-expressing regulatory T cells. *Nat. Immunol* 6: 1142–1151.

Foran E, Garrity-Park MM, Mureau C, Newell J, Smyrk TC, Limburg PJ, Egan LJ (2010) Upregulation of DNA methyltranferase-mediated gene silencing, anchorage-independent growth, and migration of colon cancer cells by interleukin-6. *Mol Cancer Res* 8: 471-481.

Forster R, Schubel A, Breitfeld D, Kremmer E, Renner-Muller I, Wolf E, Lipp M (1999) CCR7 coordinates the primary immune response by establishing functional microenvironments in secondary lymphoid organs. *Cell* 99: 23-33.

Frank NY, Margaryan A, Huang Y, Schatton T, Waaga-Gasser AM, Gasser M, Sayegh MH, Sadee W, Frank MH (2005) ABCB5-mediated Doxorubicin transport and chemoresistance in human melanoma. *Cancer Res* 65: 4320-4333.

Franks AL, Slansky JE (2012) Multiple associations between a broad spectrum of autoimmune diseases, chronic inflammatory diseases and cancer. *Anticancer Res* 32: 1119-1136.

Freiberg BA (2001) Staging and resetting T cell activation in SMAC's. *Nat Immunol* 3: 911-917.

Fredholm BB, IJzerman AP, Jacobson KA, Klotz KN, Linden J (2001) International union of pharmacology. XXV. Nomenclature and classification of adenosine receptors. *Pharmacol Rev* 53:527–552.

Fu C, Wang J, Xin X, Liu H, Xue S, Ma X, Jin Z, Sun A, Qiu H, Wu D (2013) Therapeutic effects of autologous hematopoietic stem cell transplantation in multiple myeloma patients. *Exp Ther Med* 6: 977-982.

Fu H (2014) Self-recognition of the endothelium enables regulatory T-cell trafficking and defines the kinetics of immune regulation. *Nat Comm* 5: 3436.

Fu W, Ergun A, Lu T, Hill JA, Haxhinasto S, Fassett MS, Gazit R, Adoro S, Glimcher L, Chan S, Kastner P, Rossi D, Collins JJ, Mathis D, Benoist C (2012) A multiply redundant genetic switch 'locks in' the transcriptional signature of regulatory T cells. *Nat Immunol* 13: 972-982.

Gaidot A, Landau DA, Martin GH, Bonduelle O, Grinberg-Bleyer Y, Matheoud D, Gregoire S, Baillou C, Combadiere B, Piaggio E, Cohen JL (2011) Immune reconstitution is preserved in hematopoietic stem cell transplantation coadministered with regulatory T cells for GVHD prevention. *Blood* 117: 2975-2983.

Gancedo JM (2013) Biological roles of camp: Variations on a theme in different kingdoms of life. *Biol Rev Camb Philos Soc* 88: 645-668.

Ganor Y, Teichberg VI, Levite M. (2007) TCR activation eliminates glutamate receptor GluR3 from the cell surface of normal human T cells, via an autocrine / paracrine granzyme B-mediated proteolytic cleavage. *J Immunol* 178:683–692.

Gao Z, et al. (2012) Synergy between IL-6 and TGF-B signaling promotes FOXP3 degradation. *Int J Clin Exp Pathol* 5: 626-633.

Garay J (2010) Crosstalk between PKA and Epac regulates the phenotypic maturation and function of human dendritic cells. *J Immunol* 185: 3227-3238.

Garbelli S, Mantovani S, Palermo B, Giachino C (2005) Melanocyte-specific, cytotoxic T cell responses in vitiligo: the effective variant of melanoma immunity. *Pigment Cell Res* 18: 234-242.

Gattinoni L, Powell DJ, Jr., Rosenberg SA, Restifo NP (2006) Adoptive therapy for cancer: building on success. *Natl Rev Immunol* 6: 383-393.

Gaur P, Qadir GA, Upadhyay S, Singh HK, Shukla NK, Das SN (2012) Skewed immunological balance between TH17 (CD4+IL17A+) and Treg (CD4+ CD25+ FOXP3+) cells in human oral squamous cell carcinoma. *Cell Oncol* 35: 355-343.

Gayed PM (2011) Toward a modern synthesis of immunity: Charles Janeway Jr. and the immunologist's dirty little secret. *Yale Jour of Bio and Med* 84: 131-138.

Gerhard M, Schmees C, Voland P, Endres N, Sander M, Reindl W, Rad R, Oelsner M, Decker T, Mempel M, Hengst L, Prinz C (2005) A secreted low-molecular protein form Helicobacter pylori induces cell-cycle arrest of T cells. *Gastroenterology* 128: 1327-1339.

Gerlo S, Verdood, P, Kooijman R (2013) Modulation of cytokine production by cyclic adenosine monophosphate analogs in human leukocytes. *J Interferon Cytokine Res* 30: 883-893.

Getnet D, Maris CH, Hipkiss EL, Grosso JF, Harris TJ, Yen HR, Bruno TC, Wada S, Adler A, Georgantas RW, Jie C, Goldberg MV, Pardoll DM, Drake CG (2009) Tumor recognition and self recognition induce distinct transcriptional profiles in antigen-specific CD4 T cells. *J Immunol* 182:4675-46-85.

Ghoreschi K, Laurence A, Yang XP, Tato CM, McGeachy MJ, Konkel JE, Ramos HL, Wei L, Davidson TS, Bouladoux N, Grainger JR, Chen Q, Kanno Y, Watford WT, Sun HW, Eberl G, Shevach EM, Belkaid Y, Cua DJ, Chen W, O'Shea JJ (2010) Generation of pathogenic T(H)17 cells in the absence of TGF-B signaling. *Nature* 467: 967-971.

Ghosh S, Hayden MS (2008) New regulators of NF-kappaB in inflammation. *Nat Rev Immunol* 8: 837–848.

Giao Q, Rosenberg SA (2013) Adoptive cell transfer for patients with metastatic melanoma: The potential and promise of cancer immunotherapy. *Can Con* 20: 289-297.

Goodman WA, Levine AD, Massari JV, Sugiyama H, McCormick TS, Cooper KD (2009) IL-6 signaling in psoriasis prevents immune suppression by regulatory T cells. *J Immunol* 183: 3170–3176.

Goodman WA, Young AB, McCormaick TS, Cooper KD, Levine AD (2011) Stat3 phosphorylation mediates resistance of primary human T cells to regulatory T cell suppression. *J Immunol* 186: 3336-3345.

Gold P (1970) The role of immunology in human cancer research. *Can Med Assoc J* 103: 1043-1051.

Goldstein LJ, Galski H, Fojo A, et al. (1989) Expression of a multidrug resistance gene in human cancers. *J Natl Cancer Inst* 81:116–24.

Gondek DC (2005) Cutting edge: Contact-mediated suppression by CD4+CD25+ regulatory cells involves a granzyme B-dependent, perforin-independent mechanism. *Immunol* 174: 1783-1786.

Gorelik L, Flavell RA (2002) Transforming growth factor-beta in T-cell biology. *Nat Rev Immunol* 2: 46–53.

Gorini S, Gatta L, Pontecovoro L, Vitello L, la Sala A (2013) Regulation of innate immunity by extracellular nucleotides. *Am J Blood Res* 3: 14-28.

Graf LH, Ferrone S (1989) Human melanoma-associated antigens. *Immunol Ser* 43: 643-679.

Graham DB, Akilesh HM, Gmyrek GB, Piccio L, Gilfillan S, Sim J, Belizaire R, Carrero JA, Wang Y, Blaufuss GS, Sandoval G, Fujikawa K, Cross AH, Russell JH, Cella M, Swat W (2010) ITAM signaling in dendritic cells controls T helper cell priming by regulating MHC class II recycling. *Blood* 116: 2308-3218.

Graham DY (2000) Helicobacter pylori infection is the primary cause of gastric cancer. *J Gastroenterol* 35: 90-97.

Grandoch M (2009) Epac inhibits apoptosis of human leukocytes. *J Leukoc Biol* 86: 847-849.

Grivennikov SI, Greten FR, Karin M (2010) Immunity, inflammation, and cancer. *Cell* 140: 883-899.

Gross A, McDollell JM, Korsmeyer SJ (1999) BCL-2 family members and the mitochondria in apoptosis. *Genes Dev* 13: 1899-1911.

Grossman WJ (2004) Human T regulatory cells can use the perforin pathway to cause autologous target cell death. *Immunity* 21:589-601.

Guerry, D., M.A. Alexander, M.F. Herlyn, L.M. Zeghngebot, K.F. Mitchell, C. M. Zmijewski, and E.J. Lusk. 1984. HLA-DR histocompatability leukocyte antigens permit cultured human melanoma cells from early but not advanced disease to stimulate autologous lymphocytes. *J. Clin. Invest.* 73: 267

Guerry D, Alexander MA, Elder DE, Herlyn MF (1987) Interferon-gamma regulates the T cell response to precursor nevi and biologically early melanoma. *J Immunol* 139: 305-312.

Guichelaar T, Mutis T (2013) Bone marrow provides and environment that prevents suppression of therapeutic graft-vs.-tumor immunity by regulatory T cells. *Oncoimmunol* 2: 7, e24659.

Hagness M, Henjum K, Landskron J, Brudvik KW, Bjornbeth BA, Foss A, Tasken K, Aandahl EM (2012) Kinetics and activation requirements of contact-dependent immune suppression by human regulatory T cells. *J Immunol* 188: 5459-5466.

Hahn S, Gehri R, Erb P (1995) Mechanism and biological significance of CD4 mediated cytotoxicity. *Immunol Rev* 146: 57-79.

Hall M (2010) The essence of communication in relationships. Back to the basics. *Trafford Publishing, Bloomington, IN.*

Han KL (2013) Adenosine A2A receptor agonist-mediated increase in donor-derived regulatory T cells suppresses development of graft-versus-host disease. *J Immunol* 190: 458-468.

Hanig J, Lutz MB (2008) Suppression of mature dendritic cell function by regulatory T cells in vivo is abrogated by CD40 licensing. *J Immunol* 180: 1405-1413.

Hao HY, Graham AL, Stengel RF (2012) Dynamics of a cytokine storm. *Plos One* 7: e45027.

Harding FA, McAurthur JG, Gross JA, Raulet DH, Allison, JP (1992) CD28-mediated signaling co-stimulates murine T cells and prevents induction of anergy in T-cell clones. *Nature* 356: 607-609.

Haribhai D, Edwards B, Williams ML, Williams CB (2004) Functional reprogramming of the primary immune response by T cell receptor antagonism. *J Exp Med* 200:1371-1382.

Hartwig A (2010) The role of DNA repair in benzene-induced carcinogenesis. *Chem Biol Interact* 184: 269-172.

Hasko G(1), Kuhel DG, Chen JF, Schwarzschild MA, Deitch EA, Mabley JG, Marton A, Szabo C (2000) Adenosine inhibits IL-12 and TNF- [alpha] production via adenosine A2a receptor-dependent and independent mechanisms. *FASEB J.* 14: 2065–2074.

Hasko G, Pacher P (2012) Regulation of macrophage function by adenosine. *Ather Throm and Vas Bio* 32: 865-869.

Hassin D (2011) Cytotoxic T lymphocyte perforin and Fas ligand working in concert even when Fas lytic action is still not detectable. *Immunol* 133: 190-196.

Hayden MS, Ghosh S (2008) Shared principles in NF-kappaB signaling. *Cell* 132: 344-362.

He JS, Gong D, Ostergaard HL (2010) Stored Fas ligand, a mediator of rapid CTL-Mediated killing, has a lower threshold for response than degranulation or newly synthesized Fas ligand. *J Immunol* 184: 555-563.

Heng D (1998) Bronchiolitis obliterans syndrome: incidence, natural history, prognosis, and risk factors. *J Heart Lung Trans* 17: 1255-1263.

Hemon P, Jean-Louis F, Ramgolam K, Brignone C, Viguier M, Bachelez H, Triebel F, Charron D, Aoudjit F, Al-Daccak R, Michel L (2011) MHC class II engagement by its ligand LAG-3 (CD233) contributes to melanoma resistance to apoptosis. *J Immunol* 186: 5173-5183.

Hendick SM (2012) FOXO transcription factors throughout T cell biology. *Nat Rev Immunol* 12: 649-661.

Herbeuval JP, Lelievre E, Lambert C, DY M, Genin C (2004) Recruitment of STAT3 for the production of IL-10 by colon carcinoma cells induced by macrophage-derived IL-6. *J Immunol* 173: 4630-4636.

Hernandez-Santos N, Gaffen SL (2012) Th17 cells in immunity to *Candida albicans. Cell Host Microbe* 11: 425-435.

Himer L, Csoka B, Selmeczy Z, Koscso B, Pocza T, Pacher P, Nemeth ZH, Deitch EA, Vizi ES, Cronstein BN, Hasko G (2010) Adenosine A2A receptor activation protects CD4+ T lymphocytes against activation-induced cell death. *FASEB J* 24: 2631-2640.

Hippen KL (2011) Generation and large-scale expansion of human regulatory T cells that suppress graft-versus-host disease. *Am J Transplant* 11: 1148-1157.

Hirahara K, et al. (2010) Signal transduction pathways and transcriptional regulation in Th17 cell differentiation. *Cytokine Growth Factor Rev* 21: 425-434.

Hirst CE, Buzza MS, Bird CH, Warren HS, Cameron PU, Zhang M, Ashton-Rickardt PG, Bird PI (2003) The intracellular granzyme B inhibitor, proteinase inhibitor 9, is up-regulated during accessory cell maturation and effector cell degranulation, and its overexpression enhances CTL potency. *J Immunol* 170: 805-815.

Hogan PG, Chen L, Nardone J, Rao A (2003) Transcriptional regulation by calcium, calcineurin, and NFAT. *Genes Dev* 17:2205–2232.

Hogg N, Patzak I, Willenbrock F (2011) Insiders guide to leukocyte integrin signaling and function. *Nat Rev Immunol* 11: 416-426.

Hong JJ, Rosenberg SA, Dudley ME, Yang JC, White DE, Butman JA, Sherry RM (2010) Successful treatment of melanoma brain metastases with adoptive cell therapy. *Clin Cancer Res* 16: 4892-4898.

Hori S (2010a) Developmental plasticity of Foxp3+ regulatory T cells. *Curr Opin Immunol* 22: 575-582.

Hori S (2010b) cRel: A pioneer in directing regulatory T-cell lineage commitment? *Eur J Immunol* 40: 664-667.

Horn J, Wang X, Reichardt P, Stradal TE, Warnecke N, Simeoni L, Gunzer M, Yablonski D, Schraven B, Kliche S (2009) Src homology 2-domain containing leukocyte-specific phosphoprotein of 76 kDa is mandatory for TCR-mediated inside-out signaling, but dispensable for CXCR4-mediated LFA-1 activation, adhesion, and migration of T cells. *J Immunol* 183: 5756-5767.

Hou WS, Van Parijs L (2004) A Bcl-2 molecular timer regulates the lifespan and immunogenicity of dendritic cells. *Nat Immunol* 5: 583-589.

Hsu TC (1983) Genetic instability in the human population: A working hypothesis. *Hereditas* 98: 1-9.

Huber S, Schrader J, Fritz G, Presser K, Schmitt S, Waisman A, Luth S, Blessing M, Herkel J, Schramm C (2008) P38 MAP kinase signaling is required for the conversion of CD4+CD25+ T cells into iTreg. *PLos ONE* 10: e3320.

Huber M, Heink S, Grothe H, Guralnik A, Reinhard K, Elflein K, Hunig T, Mittrucker HW, Brustle A, Kamradt T, Lohoff M (2009) A Th17-like developmental process leads to CD8(+) Tc17 cells with reduced cytotoxic activity. *Eur J Immunol* 39: 1716-1725.

Huehn J (2009) Epigenetic control of FOXP3 expression: the key to stable regulatory T-cell lineage. *Nat Rev Immunol* 9: 83-89.

Hurtado JC, Kim YJ, Kwon BS (1997) Signals through 4-1BB are costimulatory to previously activated splenic T cells and inhibit activation-induced cell death. *J Immunol* 158:26000-2608.

Ichiyama K, Yoshida H, Wakabayashi Y, Chinen T, Saeki K, Nakaya M, Takaesu G, Hori S, Yoshimura A, Kobayashi T (2008) Foxp3 inhibits RORgt-mediated IL-17A mRNA Transcription through direct interaction with RORgt. *Jour Bio Chem* 283: 17003-17008.

Ishigame H, Kakuta S, Nagai T, Kadoki M, Nambu A, Komiyama Y, Fujikado N, Tanahashi Y, Akitsu A, Kotaki H, Sudo K, Nakae S, Sasakawa C, Iwakura Y (2009) Differential roles of interleukin-17A and -17F in host defense against mucoepithelial bacterial infection and allergic responses. *Immunity* 30:108-119.

Ishikawa T, Kokura S, Sakamoto N, Matsumoto T, Funaki J, Adachi S, Okayama T, Uchiyama K, Handa O, Takagi T, Yagi N, Ando T, Uno K, Naito Y, Yoshikawa T (2011) Adoptive cellular therapy enhances the helper T cell response and reduces the number of regulatory T cells. *Exp Ther Med* 2: 737-743.

Itsekkson AM, Seidman DS, Zolti M, Lazarov A, Carp HJ (2007) Recurrent pregnancy loss and inappropriate local immune response to sex hormones. *Am J Reprod Immunol* 57: 160-165.

Ivanov II (2006) The orphan nuclear receptor RORgammat directs the differentiation program of proinflammatory IL-17+ T helper cells. *Cell* 126:1121-1123.

Iwata-Kajihara T (2011) Enhanced cancer immunotherapy using STAT3-depleted dendritic cells with high Th-1-inducing ability and resistance to cancer cell-derived inhibitory factors. *J Immunol* 187:27-36.

Jacob F, Perez Novo C, Bachert C, Van Crombuggen K (2013) Purinergic signaling in inflammatory cells: P2 receptor expression, functional effects, and modulation of inflammatory responses. *Purinergic Signal* 9: 285-306.

Jacobs JFM (2010) Dendritic cell vaccination in combination with anti-CD25 monoclonal antibody treatment: A Phase I/II study in melanoma patients. *Clin Cancer Res* 16: 5067-5078.

Jacobson KA, Hoffmann C, Cattabeni F, Abbracchio MP (1999) Adenosine-induced cell death: evidence for receptor-mediated signaling. *Apoptosis* 4: 197-211.

Janeway CA (1989) Approaching the Asymptote? Evolution and revolution in immunology. *Cold Spring Harbor Symposia on Quantitative Biology* 54: 1-3.

Janson PCJ (2008) FOXP3 promoter demethylation reveals the committed Treg population in humans. *PLoS ONE* 3: e1612.

Jatzek A, Tejera MM, Singh A, Sullivan JA, Plisch EH, Suresh M (2012) p27(kip1) negatively regulates the magnitude and persistence of CD4 T memory. *J Immunol* 189: 5119-5128.

Jena B, Dotti, G, Cooper LJN (2010) Redirecting T-cell specificity by introducing a tumor-specific chimeric receptor. *Blood* 116: 1035-1044.

Jenabian MA, Seddiki N, Yatim A, Carriere M, Hulin A, Younas M, Ghadimi E, Kuk A, Routy JP, Tremblay A, Sovigny J, Lelievre JD, Levy Y (2013) Regulatory T cells negatively affect IL-2 production of effector T cells through CD39/adenosine pathway in HIV infection. *PLOS* 9:e1003319.

Jenkins MK, Chen CA, Jung G, Muller DL, Schwartz RH (1990) Inhibition of antigen-specific proliferation of type 1 murine T cell clones after stimulation with immobilized anti-CD3 monoclonal antibody. *J Immunol* 144: 16-22.

Jeong MJ, Kim EJ, Cho EA, Ye SK, Kang GH, Juhnn YS (2013) cAMP signaling decreases p300 protein levels by promoting its ubiquitin/proteasome dependent degradation via Epac and p38 MAPK in lung cancer cells. *FEBS Lett* 587: 1373-1378.

Jijon UA (2013) Increased prevalence of circulating novel IL-17 secreting Foxp3 expressing CD4+ T cells and defective suppressive function of circulating Foxp3+ regulatory cells support plasticity between Th17 and regulatory T cells in inflammatory bowel disease patients. *Inflamm Bowel Dis* 12: 2522-2534.

Johnson LA (2009) Gene therapy with human and mouse T-cell receptors mediates cancer regression and targets normal tissues expressing cognate antigen. *Blood* 114: 535-546.

Johnston RJ Choi YS, Diamond JA, Yang JA, Crotty S (2012) STAT5 is a potent negative regulator of Tfh cell differentiation. *J Exp Med* 209: 243-250.

Jongstra J, Schall TJ, Dyer BJ, Clayberger C, Jorgensen J, Davis MM, Krensky AM (1987) The isolation and sequence of a novel gene from a human functional T cell line. *J Exp Med* 165: 601-614.

Jonuleit H, Schmitt E, Schuler G, Knop J, Enk AH (2000) Induction of interleukin 10-producing, nonproliferating CD4(+) T cells with regulatory properties by repetitive stimulation with allogeneic immature human dendritic cells. *J Exp Med* 192: 1213-1222.

Jonuleit H, Schmitt E, Schuler G, Knop J, Enk AH (2002) Infectious tolerance: Human CD25+ regulatory T cells convey suppressor activity to conventional CD4+ T helper cells. *J Exp Med* 196: 255-260.

Josefowicz SZ, Rudensky A (2009) Control of regulatory T cell lineage commitment and maintenance. *Immunity* 30: 616-625.

Joshi RP, Koretzky GA (2013) Diacylglycerol kinases: Regulated controllers of T cell activation, function, and development. *Int J Mol Sci* 14: 6649-6673.

June CH (2007) Principles of adoptive T cell cancer therapy. *J Clin Inves* 117: 1204-1212.

June CH (2011) Chimeric antigen receptor-modified T cells in chronic lymphoid leukemia. *N Engl J Med* 365: 725-733.

Kaizuka Y (2007) Mechanisms for segregating T cell receptor and adhesion molecules during immunological synapse formation in Jurkat T cells. *PNAS* 104: 20296-20301.

Kahn DA, Baltimore D (2010) Pregnancy induces a fetal antigen-specific maternal T regulatory cell response that contributes to tolerance. *PNAS* 107: 9299-9304.

Kanaporis G, Mese G, Valiuniene L, White TW, Brink PR, Valiunas V (2008) Gap junction channels exhibit connexin-specific permeability to cyclic nucleotides. *J Gen Physiol* 131: 293-305.

Kandalaft LE, Powell DJ Jr, Chiang CL, Tanyi J, Kim S, Bosch M, Montone K, Mick R, Levine BL, Torigian DA, June CH, Coukos G (2013) Autologous lysate-pulsed dendritic cell vaccination followed by adoptive transfer of vaccine-primed ex vivo co-stimulated T cells in recurrent ovarian cancer. *Oncoimmunol* 2: e22664.

Kao JY, Zhang M, Miller MJ, Mills JC, Wang B, Liu M, Eaton KA, Zou W, Berndt BE, Cole TS, Takeuchi T, Owyang SY, Luther J (2010) *Helicobacter pylori* immune escape is mediated by dendritic cell-induced Treg skewing and Th17 suppression in mice. *Gastroenterology* 138: 1046-1054.

Kastenmuller W (2011) Treg selectively control CD8+ T cell effector pool size via IL-2 restriction. *J Immunol* 187: 3186-3197.

Kennedy-Nasser AA, Ku S, Castillo-Caro P, Hazrat Y, Wu MF, Liu H, Melenhorst J, Barrett AJ, Ito S, Foster A, Savoldo B, Yvon E, Carrum G, Ramos CA, Krance RA, Leung K, Heslop HE, Brenner MK, Bollard CM (2014) Ultra low-dose IL-2 for GVHD prophylaxis after allogeneic hematopoietic stem cell transplantation mediates expansion of regulatory T ells without diminishing antiviral and antileukemic activity. *Clin Cancer Res* 20: 1-11.

Kershaw MH, Westwood JA, Parker LL, Wang G, Eshhar Z, Mavroukakis SA, White DE, Wunderlich JR, Canevari S, Rogers-Freezer L, Chen CC, Yang JC, Rosenberg SA, Hwu P (2000) A phase I study on adoptive immunotherapy using gene-modified T cells for ovarian cancer. *Clin Can Res* 12: 6106-6115.

Khandelwal S, Roche PA (2010) Distinct MHC class II molecules are associated on the Dendritic cell surface in cholesterol-dependent membrane microdomains. *J Bio Chem* 285: 35303-35310.

Kim H, Leonard J (2007) CREB/ATF-dependent T cell receptor-induced *FoxP3* gene expression: a role for DNA methylation. *JEM* 204: 1554-1551.

Kim HR, Na BR, Kwon MS, Ko YS, Han WC, Jun CD (2013) Dynamic motile T cells highly respond to the T cell stimulation via P13k-Akt and NF-κB pathways. *PLo S O*NE 8: e59793.

Kim, PS, Ahmed R (2010) Features of responding T cells in cancer and chronic infection. *Curr Opin Immunol* 22: 223-230.

Kim R, Emi M, Tanabe K (2007) Cancer immunoediting from immune surveillance to escape. *Immunol* 121: 1-14.

Kim EH, Suresh M (2013a) Role of P13K/Akt signaling in memory CD8 T cell differentiation. *Front Immunol* 4: 1-11.

Kim SY, Kang JW, Song X, Kim BK, Yoo YD, Kwon YT, Lee YJ (2013b) Role of IL-6-JAK1-STAT3-Oct-4 pathway in the conversion of non-stem cancer cells into cancer stem-like cells. *Cell Signal* 25: 961-969.

Kim WJ, Kim H, Suk K, Lee WH (2007) Macrophages express granzyme B in the lesion areas of atherosclerosis and rheumatoid arthritis. *Immunol Lett* 111: 57–65.

Klarquist J (2010) Reduced skin homing by functional Treg in vitiligo. *Pig Cell Mel Res* 23: 276-286.

Klein M, Vaeth M, Scheel T, Grabbe S, Baumgrass R, Berberich-Siebelt F, Bopp T, Schmitt E, Becker C (2012) Repression of cyclic adenosine monophosphate upregulation disarms and expands human regulatory T cells. *J Immunol* 188: 1091-1097.

Kochenderfer JN, Wilson WH, Janik JE, Dudley ME, Stetler-Stevenson M, Feldman SA, Maric I, Raffeld M, Nathan DA, Lanier BJ, Morgan RA, Rosenberg SA (2010) Eradication of B-lineage cells and regression of lymphoma in a patient treated with autologous T cells genetically engineered to recognize CD19. *Blood* 116: 4099-4102.

Koenen HJPM (2008) Human CD25highFOXP3 positive regulatory T cells differentiate into IL-17-poducing cells. *Blood* 112: 2340-2352.

Kolanowski ST, Dieker MC, Lissenberg-Thunnissen SN, van Schijndel GM, van Ham SM, Ten Brinke A (2010) TLR4-mediated pro-inflammatory dendritic cell differentiation in humans requires the combined action of MyD88 and TRIF. *Innate Immunol.* PMID: 23941760

Kolm I (2006) Dermoscopy patterns of halo nevi. *Arch Dermatol* 142: 1627-1632.

Komatsu N, Mariotti-Ferrandiz ME, Wang Y, Malissen B, Waldmann H, Hori S (2009) Heterogeneity of natural Foxp3+ T cells: A committed regulatory T cell lineage and an uncommitted minor population retaining plasticity. *PNAS* 106: 1903-1908.

Koreth J, Ritz J (2013) Tregs, HSCT, and GVHD: up close and personal. *Blood* 122: 1690-1691.

Korngold R, Sprent J (1978) lethal fraft-versus-host disease after bone marrow transplantation across minor histocompatability barriers in mice. Prevention by removing T cells from marrow. *J Exp Med* 148: 1687-1698.

Kornstein MJ, Brooks JSJ, Elder DE (1983) Immunperoxidase localization of lymphocyte subsets in the host response to melanoma and nevi. *Cancer Res* 43: 2749-2755.

Kouchkovsky D (2013) microRNA-17-92 regulates IL-10 production by regulatory T cells and control of experimental autoimmune encephalomyelitis. *J Immunol.* 191: 1594-1605.

Krensky AM, Clayberger C (2009) Biology and clinical relevance of granulysin. *Tissue Antigens* 73: 193-198.

Kriegel MA, Adam-Klages S, Gabler C, Blank N, Schiller M, Scheidig C, Kalden JR, Lorenz HM (2008) Anti-HLA-DR-triggered monocytes mediate in vitro T cell anergy. *Inter Immunol* 20: 601-613.

Krishnan A, Pasquini MC, Logan B, Stadtmauer EA, Vesole DH, Alyea E 3rd, Antin JH, Comenzo R, Goodman S, Hari P, Laport G, Qazilbash MH, Rowley S, Sahebi F, Somlo G, Vogl DT, Weisdorf D, Ewell M, Wu J, Geller NL, Horowitz MM, Giralt S, Maloney DG (2011) Autologous hematopoietic stem-cell transplantation followed by allogeneic or autologous haemopoietic stem-cell transplant in patients with multiple myeloma (BMT CTN 0102): a phase 3 biological assignment trial. *Lancet Oncol* 12: 1195-1203.

Kuhns DB, Priel DA, Gallin JI (2007) Induction of human monocyte interleukin (IL)-8 by fibrinogen through the toll-like receptor pathway. *Inflammation* 30:178–188.

Kushwah R, Hu J (2010) Dendritic cell apoptosis: Regulation of tolerance versus immunity. *J Immunol* 185: 795-802.

La Merrill M, Harper R, Birnbaum LS, Cardiff RD, Threadgill DW (2010) Maternal dioxin exposure combined with a diet high in fat increases mammary cancer incidence in mice. *Environ Health Perspect* 118: 596-601.

Langenhorst D, Gogishvili T, Ribechini E, Kneitz S, McPherson K, Lutz MB, Hunig T (2012) Sequential induction of effector function, tissue migration and cell death during polyclonal activation of mouse regulatory T-cells. *PLoS One* 11: e50080.

Lai W, Yu M, Huang MN, Okoye F, Keegan AD, Farber DL (2011) Transcriptional control of rapid recall by memory CD4 T cells. *J Immunol* 187: 133-140.

Lanteri MC, O'Brien KM, Purtha WE, Cameron MJ, Lund JM, Owen RE, Heitman JW, Custer B, Hirschkorn DF, Tobler LH, Kiely N, Prince HE, Ndhlovu LC, Nixon DF, Kamel HT, Kelvin DJ, Busch MP, Rudensky AY, Diamond MS, Norris PJ (2009) Tregs control the development of symptomatic West Nile virus infection in Humans and mice. *Jour of Clin Invest* 119: 3266-3277.

Laplante M, Sabatini DM (2012) nTOR signaling in growth control and disease. *Cell* 149: 274-293.

Latinis KM, Norian LA, Eliason SL, Koetzky GA (1997) Two NFAT transcription factor binding sites participate in the regulation of CD95 (fas) ligand expression in activated human T cells. *J Bio Chem* 272: 31427-31434.

Laurence A, Tato CM, Davidson TS, Kanno Y, Chen Z, Yao Z, Blank RB, Meylan F, Siegel R, Hennighausen L, Shevach EM, O'shea JJ (2007) Interleukin-2 signaling via STAT5 constrains T helper 17 cell generation. *Immunity* 26: 371-381.

Law RH, Lukoyanova N, Voskoboinik I, Caradoc-Davies TT, Baran K, Dunstone MA, D'Angelo ME, Orlova EV, Coulibaly F, Verschoor S, Browne KA, Ciccone A, Kuiper MJ, Bird PI, Trapani JA, Saibil HR, Whisstock JC (2010) The structural basis for membrane binding and pore formation by lymphocyte perforin. *Nature* 468: 447-451.

Lee JH, Ulrich B, Cho J, Park J, Kim CH (2011) Progesterone promotes differentiation of human cord blood fetal T cells into T regulatory cells but suppresses their differentiation into Th17 cells. *J Immunol* 187: 1778-1787.

Lee SK (2012) Th17 and regulatory T cells in women with recurrent pregnancy loss. *Am J of Reprod Immunol* 67: 311-318.

Le Floc'h A, Tanaka Y, Bantilan NS, Voisinne G, Altan-Bonnet G, Fukui Y, Huse M. (2013) Annular PIP3 accumulation controls actin architecture and modulates cytotoxicity at the immunological synapse. *J Exp Med* 210:2721-2737.

Lefranc M, Lefranc G (2001) The T cell Receptor Factsbook. *Academic Press, New York,* NY.

Leon B (2014) FoxP3+ regulatory T cells promote influenza-specific Tfh responses by controlling IL-2 availability. *Nat Commun* 5: 3495

Leverkus M (2003) MHC class II-mediated apoptosis in dendritic cells: a role for membrane-associated and mitochondrial signaling pathways. *Inter Immunol* 15: 993-1006.

Li L, Godfrey WR, Porter SB, Ge Y, June CH, Blazar BR, Boussiotis VA (2005) CD4+CD25+ regulatory T-cell lines from human cord blood have functional and molecular properties of T-cell anergy. *Blood* 106: 3068-3073.

Li L, Wang B, Frelinger JA, Tisch R (2008) T cell promiscuity in autoimmune diabetes. *Diabetes* 57: 2099-2106.

Li L, Kim J, Boussiotis VA (2010) IL-1B-mediated signals preferentially drive conversion of regulatory T cells but not conventional T cells into IL-17-Producing cells. *J Immunol* 185:4148-4153.

Liu, Z (2009) Potential role of TH17 cells in the pathogenesis of inflammatory bowel disease. *World J Gastroent* 15: 5784-5788.

Long SA(1), Cerosaletti K, Bollyky PL, Tatum M, Shilling H, Zhang S, Zhang ZY, Pihoker C, Sanda S, Greenbaum C, Buckner JH (2010) Defects in IL-2R signaling contribute to diminished maintenance of FOXP3 expression in CD4+CD25+ regulatory T-cells of type 1 diabetic subjects. *Diabetes* 59: 407-415.

Long SA (2011) An autoimmune-associated variant in PTPN2 reveals an impairment of IL-2 signaling in CD4+ T cells. *Genes Immun* 12: 116-125.

Longhi MP, Wright K, Lauder SN, Nowell MA, Jones GW, Godkin AJ, Jones SA, Gallimore AM (2008) Interleukin-6 is crucial for recall of influenza-specific memory CD4 T cells. *PLoS Pathog* 4: e1000006.

Lopez JA(1), Susanto O, Jenkins MR, Lukoyanova N, Sutton VR, Law RH, Johnston A, Bird CH, Bird PI, Whisstock JC, Trapani JA, Saibil HR, Voskoboinik I (2013) Perforin forms transient pores on the target cell plasma cell membrane to facilitate rapid access of granzymes during killer cell attack. *Blood* 121: 2659-2668.

Lopez-Bergami P, Kim H, Dewing A, Goydos J, Aaronson S, Ronai Z (2010) c-Jun regulates phosphoinositide-dependent kinase 1 transcription. Implications for Akt and protein kinase and melanoma tumorgenesis. *J Biol Chem* 285: 903-913.

Lotem M (2009) Autologous melanoma vaccine induces antitumor and self-reactiveimmune responses that affect patient survival and depend on MHC class II expression on vaccine cells. *Clin Cancer Res* 15: 4968-4977.

Lotze M, Custer MC, Sharrow SO, Rubin LA, Nelson DL, Rosenberg SA (1987) In vivo administration of purified human interleukin-2 to patients with cancer: Development of interleukin-2 receptor positive cells and circulating soluble interleukin-2 receptors following interleukin-2 administration. *Can Res* 47:2188-2195.

Leino O, Tainio M, Tuomistro JT (2008) Comparative risk analysis of dioxins in fish and fine particles from heavy-duty vehicles. *Risk Analysis* 28: 127-142.

Liang B, Workman C, Lee J, Chew C, Dale BM, Colonna L, Flores M, Li N, Schweighoffer E, Greenberg S, Tybulewicz V, Vignali D, Clynes R (2008) Regulatory T cells inhibit dendritic cells by lymphocyte activation gene-3 engagement of MHC class II. *J Immunol* 180: 5916-5926.

Lili Y, Yi W, Ji Y, Yue S, Weimin S, Ming L (2012) Global activation of CD8+ cytotoxic T lymphocytes correlates with an impairment in regulatory T cells in patients with generalized vitiligo. *PloS One* 7: e37513.

Lin Q (2005) Constitutive expression of JAK3/STAT3 in colon carcinoma tumors and cell lines. Inhibition of JAK3/STAT3 signaling induces apoptosis and cell cycle arrest of colon carcinoma cells. *Am Jour Pathol* 167: 969-980.

Lin XG, Zhou Q, Wang L, Gao Y, Zhang WN, Luo ZL, Chen BC, Chen ZH, Chang S (2011) Pregnancy estrogen drives the changes of T-lymphocyte subsets and cytokines and prolongs the survival of H-Y skin graft in murine model. *Chin Med Jour* 123: 2593-2599.

Liu J (2012) JNK-dependent Stat3 phosphorylation contributes to Akt activation in response to arsenic exposure. *Toxicol Sci* 129: 363-371.

Liu Z, Kim JH, Falo LD, You Z (2009) Tumor regulatory T cells potently abrogate antitumor immunity. *J Immunol* 182: 6160-6167.

Lo WL, Allen PM (2012) Self-awareness: How self-peptide/MHC complexes are essential in the development of T cells. *Mol Immunol* doi: 10.1016/j.molimm.2012.10.028. [Epub ahead of print]

Lombardi G, Luciano A, Riffo-Vasquez Y (2009) Dendritic cells. *Springer-Verlag,* Berlin Heidelberg, GBM.

Lu L, Ma J, Wang X, Wang J, Zhang F, Yu J, He G, Xu B, Brand DD, Horwitz DA, Shi W, Zheng SG (2010) Synergistic effect of TGF-B superfamily members on the induction of Foxp3+ regulatory T cells. *Eur J Immunol* 40: 142-152.

Luft T, Rodionova E, Maraskovsky E, Kirsch M, Hess M, Buchholtz C, Goerner M, Schnurr M, Skoda R, Ho AD (2006) Adaptive functional differentiation of dendritic cells: integrating the network of extra- and intracellular signals. *Blood* 107: 4763-4769.

Lund JM, Hsing L Pham TT, Rudensky AY (2008) Coordination of early protective immunity to viral infection by regulatory T cells. *Science* 320: 1220-1224.

Ma DY, Clark EA (2009) The role of CD40 and CD154/CD40L in dendritic cells. *Semin Immunol* 21: 265-272.

MacKenzie KF (2013) MSK1 and MSK2 inhibit lipopolysaccharide-induced prostaglandin production via an interleukin-10 feedback loop. *Mol Cell Biol* 33: 1456-1467.

Macon-Lemaitre L, Triebel F (2005) The negative regulatory function of the lymphocyte-activation gene-3 co-receptor (CD223) on human T cells. *Immunol* 115:170-178.

Maire C, Vercambre-Darras S, Devos P, D'Herbomez M, Dubucquoi S, Mortier L. (2013) Metastatic melanoma: spontaneous occurrence of auto antibodies is a good prognosis factoring a prospective cohort. *J Eur Acad Dermatol Venereol* 27:92-96.

Malek TR, Castro I (2010) Interleukin-2 receptor signaling: At the interface between tolerance and immunity. *Immunity* 33: 153-165.

Mandelcorn-Monson RL (2003) Cytotoxic T lymphocyte reactivity to gp100, MelanA/Mart-1, and tyrosinase, in HLA-A2-positive vitiligo patients. *J Invest Dermatol* 121: 550-556.

Marguti I, Yamamoto GL, da Costa TB, Rizzo LV, de Moraes LV (2009) Expansion of CD4+ CD25+ Foxp3+ T cells by bone marrow-derived dendritic cells. *Immunology* 127: 50-61.

Marijt EA (1993) Multiple minor histocompatability antigen disparities between a recipient and four HLA-identical potential sibling donors for bone marrow transplantation. *Hum Immunol* 37: 221-228.

Marks F, Klingmuller U, Muller-Decker K (2009) Cellular Signal Processing: An Introduction to the Molecular Mechanisms of Signal Transduction. *Garland Science,* New York, NY.

Maruyama T, Kono K, Mizukami Y, Kawaguchi Y, Mimura K, Watanabe M, Izawa S, Fujii H (2010) Distribution of Th17 cells and FoxP3(+) regulatory T cell in tumor-infiltrating lymphocytes, tumor lymph nodes, and peripheral blood lymphocytes in patients with gastric cancer. *Cancer Sci* 101: 1947-1954.

Matsuoka K (2010) Altered regulatory T cell homeostasis in patients with CD4+ lymphopenia following allogeneic hematopoietic stem cell transplantation. *J Clin Invest* 120: 1479-1493.

Matzinger P. (2002) The danger model: a renewed sense of self. *Science* 296:301–305.

Mayr B, Montminy M (2001) Transcriptional regulation by the phosphorylation-dependent factor CREB. *Nat. Rev. Mol. Cell Biol.* 2: 599–609.

McFarland HI (2012) Regulatory T cells in γ radiation-induced immune suppression. *PloS One* 7: e39092.

Meiraz A, Garber OG, Harari S, Hassin D, Berke G (2009) Switch from perfori-expressing to perforin-deficient CD8+ T cells accounts for two distinct types of effector cytotoxic T lymphocytes in vivo. *Immunol* 128: 69-82.

Mendoza-Naranjo A, Bouma G, Pereda C, Ramerez M, Webb KF, Tittarelli A, Lopez MN, Kalergis AM, Thrasher AJ, Becker DL, Salazar-Onfray F (2011) Functional gap junctions accumulate at the immunological synapse and contribute to T cell activation. *J Immunol* 187:3121-3132.

Merad M, Manz MG (2009) Dendritic cell homeostasis. *Blood* 113: 3418-27.

Michor F (2005) Chromosomal instability and human cancer. *Phil Trans R Soc* B 306: 631-635.

Middel P (2010) Chemokine-mediated distribution of dendritic cell subsets in renal cell carcinoma. *BMC Cancer* 10: 578-590.

Miech RP (2011) Immunophamacology of ulipristal as an emergency contraceptive. *International Journal of Woman's Health* 3: 391-397.

Mills KD (2003) The role of DNA breaks in genomic instability and tumorigenesis. *Immunol Rev* 194: 77-95.

Misra UK, Pizzo SV (2005) Coordinate regulation of forskolin-induced cellular proliferation in macrophages by protein kinase A/cAMP –response element-binding protein and Epac-Rap-1 signaling: effects of silencing CREB gene expression. *J Biol Chem* 280: 38276-38289.

Mirabet M (1999) Expression of A2B adenosine receptors in human lymphocytes: their role in T cell activation. *J Cell Sci* 112:491–502.

Mizukami Y (2008) CCL17 and CCL22 chemokines within tumor microenvironment are related to accumulation of Foxp3+ regulatory T cells in gastric cancer. *Int J Cancer* 122: 2286–2293.

Moldoveanu T, Grace CR, Llambi F, Nourse A, Fitzgerald P, Gehring K, Kriwacki RW, Green DR (2013) BID-induced structural changes in Bak promote apoptosis. *Nat Struct Mol Biol* 20: 589-597.

Molinero LL (2009) CARMA1 controls an early checkpoint in thymic development of FoxP3+ regulatory T cells. *J Immunol.* 182: 6736-6743.

Mondino A, Jenkins MK (1994) Surface proteins involved in T cell costimulation. *J Leukoc Biol* 55: 805-815.

Monks CR (1998) Three-dimensional segregation of supramolecular activation clusters in T cells. *Nature 395*: 82-86.

Monosalve M, Olmos Y (2011) The complex biology of FOXO. *Curr Drug Targets* 12: 1322-1350.

Moon EY, Pyo S (2007) Lipopolysaccharide stimulates Epac-1-mediated Rap1/NF-kappa pathway in Raw 264.7 murine macrophages. *Immunol Lett* 110: 121-125.

Morawski PA, Mehra P, Chen C, Bhatti T, Wells AD (2013) Foxp3 protein stability by cyclin-dependent kinase 2. *J Biol Chem* 288: 24494-24502.

Moreau-Aubry A, Fonteneau J, Labarriere N, Jotereau F, Houssaint E, Breathnach R (1997) Identification of a gp100 epitope recognized by HLA-A3 restricted melanoma infiltrating lymphocytes. *Int J Oncol* 10: 841-846.

Morgan RA, Dudley ME, Wunderlich JR, Hughes MS, Yang JC, Sherry RM, Royal RE, Topalian SL, Kammula US, Restifo NP, Zheng Z, Nahvi A, de Vries CR, Rogers-Freezer LJ, Mavroukakis SA, Rosenberg SA (2006) Cancer regression in patients after transfer of genetically engineered lymphocytes. *Science* 314: 126-129.

Morgan RA, Yang RA, Kitano M, Dudley ME, Laurencot CM, Rosenberg SA (2010) Case report of a serious adverse event following the administration of T cells transduced with a chimeric antigen receptor recognizing ERBB2. *Mol Ther* 18: 843-851.

Mori, Murakami-Mori K, Bonavida B (1999) Interleukin-6 induces G1 arrest through induction of p27(Kip1), a cyclin-dependent kinase inhibitor, and neuron-like morphology in LMCaP prostate tumor cells. *Biochem Biophys Res Commun* 257: 609-614.

Morlacchi S (2011) Regulatory T cells target chemokine secretion by dendritic cells independently of their capacity to regulate T cell proliferation. *J Immunol* 186: 6807-6814.

Morton DL (1974) BCG immunotherapy of malignant melanoma: Summary of a seven-year experience. *Ann. Surg* 180: 635-641.

Mrass P, Weninger W (2006) Immune cell migration as a means to control immune privilege: lessons from the CNS and tumors. *Immunol Rev* 213: 195-212.

Mukherji B, Nathanson L, Clark DA (1973) Studies of humoral and cell-mediated immunity in human melanoma. *Yale J Biol Med* 46: 681-692.

Munn DH, Sharma MD, Mellor AL (2004) Ligation of B7-1/B7-2 by human CD4+ T cells triggers indoleamine 2,3-dioxygenase activity in dendritic cells. *J Immunol* 172: 4100-4110.

Muranski P, Boni A, Wrzesinski C, Citrin DE, Rosenberg SA, Childs R, Restifo NP (2006) Increased intensity lymphodepletion and adoptive immunotherapy—how far can we go? *Nat Clin Pract Oncol* 3: 668-681.

Muranski P, Boni A, Antony PA, Cassard L, Irvine KR, Kaiser A, Paulos CM, Palmer DC, Touloukian CE, Ptak K, Gattinoni L, Wrzesinski C, Hinrichs CS, Kerstann KW, Feigenbaum L, Chan CC, Restifo NP (2008) Tumor-specific Th17-polarized cells eradicate large established melanoma. *Blood* 112: 362-373.

Nagata S, Goldstein P (1995) The fas death factor. *Science* 267: 1449-1456.

Nagata S (1996) A death factor-the other side of the coin. *Behring Inst Mitt* 97: 1-11.

Nagler A (1997) Immunotherapy with recombinant human interleukin-2 and recombinant interferon-alpha in lymphoma patients postautologous marrow or stem cell transplantation. *Blood* 89: 3951-3959.

Nembrini C, Abel B, Kopf M, Marsland BJ (2006) Strong TCR signaling, TLR ligands, and cytokine redundancies ensure robust development of type 1 effector T cells. *J Immunol* 176: 7180-7188.

Nguyen TL (2013) Autoimmune gastritis mediated by CD4+ T cells promotes the development of gastric cancer. *Cancer Res PMID:* 23378345.

Ning H, Shao QQ, Ding KJ, Gao DX, Lu QL, Cao QW, Niu ZH, Fu Q, Zhang CH, Qu X, Lu JJ (2012) Tumor-infiltrating regulatory T cells are positively correlated with angiogenic status in renal cell carcinoma. *Chin Med J* (Engl) 125: 2120-2125.

Njoo MD, Westerhof W (2001) Vitiligo. Pathogenesis and treatment. *Am J Clin De*rmatol 2: 167-181.

Neurath MF, Fintto S (2011) IL-6 signaling in autoimmunity, chronic inflammation and inflammation-associated cancer. *Cyto Growth Fac Rev* 22: 83-89.

Nopora A, Brocker T (2002) Bcl-2 controls dendritic cell longevity in vivo. *J Immunol* 169: 3006-3014.

Nurieva RI (2010) The E3 ubiquitin ligase GRAL regulates T cell tolerance and regulatory T cell function by mediating T cell receptor-CD3 degredation. *Immunity* 32: 670-680.

O'Gorman WE, Dooms H, Thorne SH, Kuswanto WF, Simonds EF, Krutzik PO, Nolan GP, Abbas AK (2009). The initial phase of an immune response functions to activate regulatory T cells. *J. Immunol.* 183, 332–339.

Ogino T, Shigyo H, Ishii H, et al. (2006) HLA class I antigen down-regulation in primary laryngeal squamous cell carcinoma lesions as a poor prognostic marker. *Cancer Res* 66: 9281–9289.

Ohta A, Kini R, Otha A, Subramanian M, Madasu M, Sitkovsky M (2012) The development and immunosuppressive functions of CD4+ CD25+ FOxP3+ regulatory T cells are under influence of adenosine-A2A adenosine receptor pathway. *Front Immunol* 3: 1-12.

Oldenhove G (2009) Decrease of Foxp3+ Treg cell number and acquisition of effector cell phenotype during lethal infection. *Immunity* 31: 722-752.

Oldham KA, Parsonage G, Bhatt RI, Wallace DM, Deshmukh N, Chaudhri S, Adams DH, Lee SP (2012) T lymphocyte recruitment into renal cell carcinoma tissue: a role for chemokine receptors CXCR3, CXCR6, CCR5, and CCR6. *Eur Urol* 61: 385-395.

Olkhanud PB (2011) Tumor-evoked regulatory B cells promote breast cáncer metastasis by converting resting CD4+ T cells to T regulatory cells. *Cancer Res* 71: 3505-3515.

Okamura Y, Watari M, Jerud ES, Young DW, Ishizaka ST, Rose J, Chow JC, Strauss JF 3rd (2001) The extra domain A of fibronectin activates Toll-like receptor 4. *J Biol Chem* 276:10229–10233.

Onishi Y, Fehervari Z, Yamaguchi T, Sakaguchi S (2008) Foxp3+ natural regulatory T cells preferentially form aggregates on dendritic cells in vitro and actively inhibit their maturation. *Proc Natl Acad Sci U S A* 105: 10113-10118.

Oosterhoff D, Lougheed S, van de Ven R, Lindenberg J, van Cruijsen H, Hiddingh L, Kroon J, van den Eertwegh AJ, Hangalapura B, Scheper RJ, de Gruijl TD (2012) Tumor-mediated inhibition of human dendritic cell differentiation and function is consistently counteracted by combined p38 MAPK and STAT3 inhibition. *Oncoimmunol* 1: 649-658.

Orlin JB, Ellis MH (1997) Transfusion-associated graft-versus-host disease. *Curr Opin Hematol* 4: 442-448.

Otten GR, Germain RN (1991) Split anergy in a CD8+ T cell receptor-dependent cytolysis in the absence of interleukin-2 production. *Science* 251: 1228-1231

Overwijk WW, Restifo NP (2000) Autoimmunity and the immunotherapy of cancer: targeting the "self" to destroy the "other." *Crit Rev Immunol* 20: 433-450.

Oviedo-Orta, E, Kwak BR, Evans WH, Eds. (2013) *Connexin Cell Communication Channels: Roles in the Immune System and Immunopathology.* CRC Press, Taylor & Frances Group, Boca Raton, FL. Oyarbide-Valencia K (2006) Therapeutic implications of autoimmune vitiligo T cells. *Autoimmun Rev* 5: 486-492.

Palmer DC (2008) Effective tumor treatment targeting a melanoma/melanocyte-associated antigen triggers severe ocular autoimmunity. *Proc Natl Acad Sci* 105: 8061-8066.

Pandiyan P (2007) CD4+CD25+Foxp3+ regulatory T cells induce cytokine depravation-mediated apoptosis of effector CD4+ T cells. *Nat Immunol* 8: 1353-1362.

Pandiyan P, Lenardo MJ (2008) The control of CD4+ CD25+ Foxp3+ regulatory T cell survival. *Biology Direct* 3: 1-12.

Pandiyan P, Conti HR, Zheng L, Peterson AC, Mathern DR, Hernandez-Santos N, Edgerton M, Gaffen SL, Lenardo MJ (2011) CD4+ CD25+ Foxp3+ regulatory T cells promote Th17 cells *in vitro* and enhance host resistance in mouse *Candida albicans* Th17 cell infection model. *Immunity* 34: 422-434.

Panther E, Dork T, Ferrari D, Di Virgilio F, Grimm M, Sorichter S, Cicko S, Herouy Y, Norgauer J, Idzko M, Muller T (2013) AMP affects intracellular Ca+ signaling, migration, cytokine secretion and T cell priming capacity of dendritic cells. *PLOS* 7: e37560.

Pardo J, Wallich R, Ebnet K, Iden S, Zentgraf H, Martin P, Ekiciler A, Prins A, Mullbacher A, Huber M, Simon MM (2007) Granzyme B is expressed in mouse mast cells in vivo and in vitro and causes delayed cell death independent of perforin. *Cell Death Differ* 14: 1768–1779.

Pardoll DM, Topalian SL (1998) The role of CD4+ T cell responses in anti-tumor immunity. *Curr Opin Immunol* 10: 588-594.

Park JH, Ryu JM, Han HJ (2011) Involvement of caveolin-1 in fibronectin-induced mouse embryonic stem cell proliferation: role of FAK, RhoA, PI3K/Akt, and ERK 1/2 pathways. *J Cell Physiol* 226: 267-275.

Parry GC, Mackman N (1997) Role of cyclic AMP response element binding protein in cyclic AMP inhibition of NF-kappaB-mediated transcription. *J Immunol* 159: 5450–5456.

Paustian C (2013) Extracellular ATP and toll-like receptor 2 agonists trigger in human monocytes an activation program that favors T helper 17. *PLOS* 8: e54804.

Pellegrini P, Berghella AM, Del Beato T Cicia S, Adorno D, Casciani CU, (1996) Disregulation of TH1 and TH2 subsets of CD4+ T cells in peripheral blood of colorectal cancer patients and involvement in cancer establishment and progression. *Cancer Immunol Immunother* 42: 1-8.

Pena SV, Krensky AM (1997) Granulysin, a new human cytolytic granule-associated protein with possible involvement in cell-mediated cytotoxicity. *Semin Immunol* 9: 117-125.

Pendergrast WJ, Drake WP, Mardiney MR (1976) A proper sequence for the treatment of B16 melanoma: chemotherapy, surgery, and immunotherapy. *J Natl Can Inst* 57: 539-544.

Pepper M, Jenkins M (2011) Origins of CD4+ effector and central memory T cells. *Nat Immunol* 12: 467-471.

Pinkoski MJ (2001) Granzyme B-mediated apoptosis proceeds predominantly through a Bcl-2-inhibitable mitochondrial pathway. *J Biochem* 276: 12060-12067.

Porter DL (2011) Chimeric antigen receptor-modified T cells in chronic lymphoid leukemia. *N Eng J Med* 365: 725-733.

Ramos CA, Dotti G (2011) Chimeric antigen receptor (CAR)-engineered lymphocytes for cancer therapy. *Expert Opin Biol Ther* 11: 855-873.

Rappaport SM, Kim S, Lan Q, Vermeulen R, Waidyanatha S, Zhang L, Li G, Yin S, Hayes RB, Rothman N, Smith MT (2009) Evidence that humans metabolize benzene via two pathways. *Environ Health Perspect* 117: 946-952.

Raskovalova T, Lokshin A, Huang X, Su Y, Mandic M, Zarour HM, Jackson EK, Gorelik E (2007) Inhibition of cytokine production and cytotoxic activity of human antimelanoma specific CD8+ and CD4+ T lymphocytes by adenosine-protein kinase A type I signaling. *Cancer Res* 67: 5949-5956.

Rass K, Reichrath J (2008) UV damage and DNA repair in malignant melanoma and nonmelanoma skin cancer. *Adv Exp Med Biol* 624: 162-178.

Rawlings DJ, Sommer K, Moreno-Garcia ME (2006) The CARMA1 signalosome links the signaling machinery of adaptive and innate immunity in lymphocytes. *Nat Rev Immunol* 6: 799-812.

Raynor J (2013) IL-15 fosters age-driven regulatory T cell accrual in the face of declining IL-2 levels. *Front Immunol* 4: 1-11.

Reya T (2001) Stem cells, cancer, and cancer stem cells. *Nature* 414: 105-111.

Rinsky R, Young RJ, Smith AB (1981) Leukemia in benzene workers. *Am J Ind Med* 2: 217-245.

Rivera SP, Saarikoski ST, Sun W, Hankinson (2006) Identification of novel dioxin-responsive genes by representational difference analysis. *Xenobiotica* 37: 271-279.

Rugegni P (2009) Melanoma with halo. *Clin and Exper Dermatol* 34: 747-750.

Rericha V (2006) Incidence of leukemia, lymphoma, and multiple myeloma in Czech uranium miners: A case-cohort study. *Environ Health Perspect* 114: 818-822.

Roncarolo MG, Gregori S (2008) Is FOXP3 a bona fide marker for human regulatory T cells? *Eur J Immunol* 38: 925-927.

Roselli M, Cereda V, di Bari MG, Formica V, Spila A, Jochems C, Farsaci B, Donahue R, Gulley JL, Schlom J, Guadagni F (2013) Effects of conventional therapeutic interventions on the number and function of regulatory T cells. *Oncoimmunol* 2:e27025.

Rosenberg SA (1975) Future prospects for immunotherapy. *Cancer* 36: 821-824.

Rosenberg SA, Packard BS, Aebersold PM, Solomon D, Topalian SL, Toy ST, Simon P, Lotze MT, Yang JC, Seipp CA (1988) Use of tumor-infiltrating lymphocytes and interleukin-2 in the immunotherapy of patients with metastatic melanoma. A preliminary report. *N Engl J Med* 319: 1676-1680.

Rosenberg SA, Yannelli JR, Yang JC, Topalian SL, Schwartzentruber DJ, Weber JS, Parkinson DR, Seipp CA, Einhorn JH, White DE (1994) Treatment of patients with metastatic melanoma with autologous tumor-infiltrating lymphocytes and interleukin-2. *J Natl Can Inst* 86: 1159-1166.

Rosenberg SA, Sherry RM, Morton KE, Yang JC, Topalian SL, Royal RE, Kammula US, Restifo NP, Hughes MS, Schwarz SL, Ngo LT, Mavroukakis SA, White DE (2006) Altered CD8+ T-cell responses when immunizing with multepitope peptide vaccines. *J Immunother* 29: 224-231.

Rubtsov YP, (2008) Regulatory T cell-derived interleukin-10 limits inflammation at environmental interfaces. *Immunity* 28: 546-558.

Rowe JH, Erteit JM, Aguilera MN, Farrar, MA (2011) Foxp3(+) regulatory T cell expansion required for sustaining pregnancy compromises host defense against prenatal bacterial pathogens. *Cell Host Microbe* 10: 54-64.

Rowshani AT, Strik MC, Molenaar R, Yong SL, Wolbink AM, Bemelman FJ, Hack CE, Ten Berge IJ (2005) The granzyme B inhibitor SERPINB9 (protease inhibitor 9) circulates in blood and increases on primary cytomegalovirus infection after renal transplantation. *J. Infect. Dis* 192: 1908–1911.

Ryba-Stanislawowaka M, Skrzypkowska M, Mysiliwiec M, Mysiliwska J (2013) Loss of balance between CD4(+)Foxp3(+) regulatory T cells and CD4(+)IL-17A(+) Th17 cells in patients with type 1 diabetes. *Hum Immunol* 74: 701-707.

Ryzhov S (2008) Adenosine A2B receptors in regulation of dendritic cell differentiation and function. *FASEB J* 22:1065.

Saeki H (1999) Cutting edge: secondary lymphoid-tissue chemokine (SLC) and chemokine receptor 7 (CCR7) participate in the emigration pathway of mature dendritic cells from the skin to regional lymph nodes. *J Immunol* 162: 2472-2475.

Salmi M, Jalkanan S (2012) Host CD73 impairs anti-tumor immunity. *Onc Immunol* 1:2: 247-248.

Safford M (2005) Egr-2 and Egr-3 are negative regulators of T cell activation. *Nature* Immunol. 6: 472-480.

Salek M, McGowan S, Trudgian DC, Dushek O, de Wet B, Efstathiou G, Acuto O. (2013) Quantitative phoshoproteome analysis unveils LAT as a modulator of CD3zeta and ZAP-70 tyrosine phosphorylation. *Plos One* 8): e77423.

Sallusto F, Geginat, J, Lanzavecchia A (2004) Central memory and effector memory T cell subsets: Function, generation, and maintenance. *Annu Rev Immunol* 22: 745-763.

Samstein RM (2012) Foxp3 exploits a preexisting enhancer landscape for regulatory T cell lineage specification. *Cell* 151: 153-166.

Sanborn KB, Mace EM, Rak GD, Difeo A, Martignetti JA, Pecci A, Bussel JB, Favier R, Orange JS (2011) Phosphorylation of myosin IIA tailpiece regulates single myosin IIA molecule association with lytic granules to promote NK-cell cytotoxicity. *Blood* 118: 5862-5871.

Sandoval S, Pigazzi M, Sakamoto KM (2009) CREB: A key regulator of normal and neoplastic hematopoiesis. *Adv Hematol* 2009: 634292.

Sands WA, Palmer TM (2008) Regulating gene transcription in response to cyclic AMP elevation. *Cell Signal* 20: 460-466.

Saraiva M, O'Garra A (2010) The regulation of IL-10 production by immune cells. *Nat Rev Immunol* 10: 170–181.

Sauer S, Bruno L, Hertweck A, Finlay D, Leleu M, Spivakov M, Knight ZA, Cobb BS, Cantrell D, O'Connor E, Shokat KM, Fisher AG, Merkenschlager M (2008) T cell receptor signaling controls Foxp3 expression via P13K, Akt, and mTOR. *PNAS* 105: 7797-7802.

Sawant DV, Vignali DA (2014) Once a Treg, always a Treg. *Immunol Rev* 259: 173-91.

Schatton T, Schotte U, Frank NY, Zhan Q, Hoerning A, Robles SC, Zhou J, Hodi FS, Spagnoli GC, Murphy GF, Frank MH (2010) Modulation of T cell activation by malignant melanoma initiating cells. *Cancer Res* 70: 697-708.

Schnurr M (2000) Extracellular ATP and TNF-alpha synergize in the activation and maturation of human dendritic cells. *J Immunol* 165: 4704-4709.

Schoorlemmer J, Jonk L, Sanbing S, van Puijenbroek A, Feijen A, Kruijer W (1995) Regulation of Oct-4 gene expression during differentiation of EC cells. *Mol Biol Rep* 21: 129-140.

Schumacher A, Zenclussen AC (2014) Regulatory T cells: Regulators of life. *Am J Reprod Immunol Mar* 24. doi: 10.1111/aji.12238.

Schutyser E, Struyf S, Van Damme J (2003) The CC chemokine CCL20 and its receptor CCR6. *Cytokine Growth Factor Rev* 14: 409-426.

Schwarz A, Schwarz T (2010) UVR-induced regulatory T cells switch antigen-presenting cells from a stimulatory to a regulatory phenotype. *J Invest Dermatol* 130: 1914-1921.

Schwartz RH, Jenkins MK (1987) Antigen presentation by chemically modified splenocytes induces antigen-specific T cell unresponsiveness in vitro and in vivo. *J Exp Med* 165: 302-319.

See AP, Han JE, Phallen J, Binder Z, Gallia G, Pan F, Jinasena D, Jackson C, Belcaid Z, Jeong SJ, Gottschalk C, Zeng J, Ruzevick J, Nicholas S, Kim Y, Albesiano E, Pardoll

DM, Lim M (2012) The role of STAT3 activation in modulating the immune microenvironment of GBM. *J Neurooncol* 110: 359-388.

Seigler HF (1979) Specific active immunotherapy for melanoma. *Ann Surg* 180: 366-371.

Serfling E (2012) NFATc1/aA: The other face of NFAT factors in lymphocytes. *Cell Com and Signal* 10: 1-10.

Sherr CJ, Roberts JM (1999) CDK inhibitors: positive and negative regulators of G1-phase progression. *Genes Dev* 13: 1501-1512.

Shirshev SV (2011) Role of epac proteins in mechanisms of cAMP-dependent immunoregulation. *Biochemistry* (Moscow) 76: 981-998.

Shuford WW (1997) 4-1BB costimulatory signals preferentially induce CD8 T cell proliferation and lead to the amplification in vivo of cytotoxic immune responses. *J Exp Med* 186:47-54.

Siegel AM, Heimall J, Freeman AF, Hsu AP, Brittain E, Brenchley JM, Douek DC, Fahle GH, Cohen JI, Holland SM, Milner JD (2011) A critical role for STAT3 transcription factor signaling in the development and maintenance of human T cell memory. *Immunity* 35: 806-818.

Sim GC, Martin-Orozco N, Jin L, Yang Y, Wu S, Washington E, Sanders D, Lacey C, Wang Y, Vence L, Hwu P, Radvanyi L (2014) IL-2 therapy promotes suppressive ICOS+ Treg expansion in melanoma patients. *J Clin Invest* 124: 99-110.

Simoncic PD, Lee-Loy A, Barber DL, Tremblay ML, McGlade CJ (2002) The T cell protein tyrosine phosphatase is a negative regulator of Janus family kinases 1 and 3. *Curr Biol* 12: 446-453.

Singh K, Kozyr N, Stempora L, Kirk AD, Larsen CP, Blazar BR, Kean LS (2012) Regulatory T cells exhibit decreased proliferation but enhanced suppression after pulsing with sirolimus. *Am J Transplant* 12: 1441-1457.

Singh SP (2008) Human T cells that are able to produce IL-17 express the chemokine receptor CCR6. *J Immunol* 180:214–21.

Slack EC, Robinson MJ, Hernanz-Falcon P, Brown GD, Williams DL, Schweighoffer E, Tybulewicz VL, Reis e Sousa C (2007) SYK-dependent ERK activation regulates IL-2 and IL-10 production by DC stimulated by zymosan. *Eur J Immunol* 37: 1600-1612.

Slamon DJ (1989) Studies of the HER-2/neu proto-oncogene in human breast and ovarian cancer. *Science* 244: 707-712.

Snyder LD, Palmer SM (2006) Immune mechanisms of lung allograft rejection. *Semin Respir Crit Care Med* 27: 534-543.

Soond DR, Slack EC, Garden OA, Patton DT, Okkenhaug K (2012) Does the P13K pathway promote or antagonize regulatory T cell development and function. *Front Immunol* 3: 1-8.

Soriano C, Mukaro V, Hodge G, Ahern J, Holmes M, Jersmann H, Moffat D, Meredith D, Jurisevic C, Reynolds PN, Hodge S (2012) Increased proteinase inhibitor-9 (PI-9) and reduced granzyme B in lung cancer: mechanism for immune evasion. *Lung Cancer* 77: 38-45.

Sprent J, Lo D, Gao EK, Ron Y (1988) T cell selection in the thymus. *Immunol Rev* 101: 173-190.

Strauss L, Bergmann C, Whiteside TL (2009) Human circulating CD4+ CD25high Foxp3+ regulatory T cells kill autologous CD8+ but not CD4+ responder cells by fas-mediated apoptosis. *J Immunol* 182: 1469-1480.

Steck DJ, Field RW, Lynch CF (1999) Exposure to atmospheric radon. *Environ Health Perspect* 107: 123-127.

Steinman RM, Banchereau J (2007) Taking dendritic cells into medicine. *Nature* 449:419–426.

Sumner WC, Foraker AG (1960) Spontaneous regression of human melanoma: clinical and experimental studies. *Cancer* 13: 79-81.

Su, MT, Lee IW, Chen YC, Kuo PL (2011) Association of progesterone receptor polymorphism with idiopathic recurrent pregnancy loss in Taiwanese Han population. J Assist Reprod Genet 28: 239-243.

Sun Z (2012) Intervention of PKC-theta as an immunosuppressive regimen. *Front Immunol* 3: 1-9.

Tadokoro C (2006) Regulatory T cell inhibit stable contacts between CD4 T cells and dendritic T cells in vivo. *J Exp Med* 203: 505-511.

Taflin C (2009) FoxP3+ regulatory T cells suppress early stages of granuloma formation but have little impact on sarcoidosis lesions. *Amer Jour Path* 174: 497-508.

Tak PP, Spaeny-Dekking L, Kraan MC, Breedveld FC, Froelich CJ, Hack CE. (1999) The levels of soluble granzyme A and B are elevated in plasma and synovial fluid of patients with rheumatoid arthritis (RA). *Clin. Exp. Immunol* 116:366–70.

Tao J (2008) Restoration of the expression of transports associated with antigen processing in human malignant melanoma increases tumor-specific immunity. *J Invest Dermatol* 128: 1991-1998.

Taylor SS, Kim C, Cheng CY, Brown SH, Wu J, Kannan N (2008) Signaling through cAMP and cAMP-dependent protein kinase: diverse strategies for drug design. *Biochim. Biophys. Acta* 1784: 16–26.

Teichman KY (1988) A little exposure to radon. *Stat Sci* 3: 374-376.

Thangavelu, G, et al. (2013) Control of in vivo collateral damage generated by T cell immunity. *J Immunol* 191: 1-6.

Thiery J (2011) Perforin pores in the endosomal membrane trigger the release of endocytosed granzymeB into the cytosol of target cells. *Nat Immunol* 12: 770-780.

Thompson LF, Tsukamoto H, Chernogorova P, Zeiser R (2013) A delicate balance. CD73-generated adenosine limits the severity of graft vs. host disease but also constrains the allogenic graft vs. tumor effect. *Oncoimmuno*l 2:1: e22107.

Thomas RM, Sai H, Wells AD, etal. (2012) Conserved intergenic elements and DNA methylation cooperate to regulate transcription at the IL-17 locus. *J Biol Chem* 278: 25049-25059.

Todi G, Rigo J Jr., Stenczer B, Vasarhelyi B, Molvarec A (2011) Increased prevalence of IL-17-producing blood lymphocytes in pre-eclampsia. *Am J Reprod Immunol* 66: 223-229.

Tokoyoda K, Tsujikawa K, Matsushita H, Ono Y, Hayashi T, Harada Y, Abe R, Kubo M, Yamamoto H (2004) Up-regulation of IL-4 production by the activated camp/camp – dependent protein kinase (protein kinase A) pathway in CD3/CD28-stimulated naïve T cells. *Inter Immunol* 16: 643-653.

Tone Y (2008) Smad3 and NFAT cooperate to induce Foxp3 expression through its enhancer. *Nat Immunol* 9: 194-202.

Toossi Z, Wu M, Rojas R, Kalsdorf B, Aung H, Hirsch CS, Walrath J, Wolbink A, van Ham M, Silver RF (2012) Induction of serine protease inhibitor 9 by Mycobacterium tuberculosis inhibits apoptosis and promotes survival of infected macrophages. *J Infec Dis* 205: 144-151.

Trapani JA, Thia KY, Andrews M, Davis ID, Gedye C, Parente P, Svobodova S, Chia J, Browne K, Campbell IG, Phillips WA, Voskoboinik I, Cebon JS (2013) Human perforin mutations and susceptibility to multiple primary cancers. *Oncoimmunol* 2: e24185-1-e24185-5.

Treilleux I (2004) Dendritic cell infiltration and prognosis of early stage breast cancer. *Clin Cancer Res* 10: 7466-7473.

Trenado A (2006) Ex vivo-expanded CD4+CD25+ immunoregulatory T cells prevent graft-versus-host-disease by inhibiting activation/differentiation of pathogenic T cells. *J Immunol* 176: 1266-1273.

Trinchieri G (2011) Innate inflammation and cancer: Is it time for cancer prevention? F1000 *Med Reports* 3: 1-6.

Tsukamoto H, Chernogorova P, Ayata K, Gerlach UV, Rughani A, Ritchey JW, Ganesan J, Follo M, Zeiser R, Thompson LF, Idzko M (2012) Deficiency of CD73/ecto- 5' – nucleotidase in mice enhances acute graft-versus-host disease. *Blood* 119: 4554-4564.

Tuomisto J, Pekkanen J, Kiviranta H, Tukiainen E, Vartiainen T, Viluksela M, Tuomisto JT (2005) Dioxin cancer risk- example of hormesis. *Dose-Respon* 3: 332-341.

Turesson C (2007) Systemic effects of rheumatoid arthritis. *US Muscloskel Rev:*64-66.

Turkington C, LiPera WL (2005) Encyclopedia of Cancer. *Facts On File,* Inc., New York, NY.

Uchi H, Stan R, Turk MJ, Engelhorn ME, Rizzuto GA, Goldberg SM, Wolchok JD, Houghton AN Uchi H, Stan R, Turk MJ, Engelhorn ME, Rizzuto GA, Goldberg SM, Wolchok JD, Houghton AN (2006) Unraveling the complex relationship between cancer immunity and autoimmunity: lessons from melanoma and vitiligo. *Adv Immunol* 90: 215-241.

Ueda K, Cornwell MM, Gottesman MM, et al. (1986) The mdr1 gene, responsible for multidrug-resistance, codes for P-glycoprotein. *Biochem Biophys Res Commun* 141: 956–62.

Ukena SN (2012) Human regulatory T cells of G-CSF mobilized allogeneic stem cell donors qualify for clinical application. *Plos One* 7: e51644.

Underhill DM, Goodridge HS (2007) The many faces of ITAM's. *Trends Immunol* 28: 66-73.

Vaeth M, Schliesser U, Muller G, Reissig S, Satoh K, Tuettenberg A, Jonuleit H, Waisman A, Muller MR, Serfling E, Sawitzki BS, Berberich-Siebelt F (2012) Dependence on nuclear factor of activated T-cells (NFAT) levels discriminates conventional T cells from Foxp3+ regulatory T cells. *PNAS* 109: 16258-16263.

van Helvoort A, Smith AJ, Sprong H, et al. (1996) MDR1 P-glycoprotein is a lipid translocase of broad specificity, while MDR3 P-glycoprotein specifically translocates phosphatidylcholine. *Cell* 87: 507–517.

Van Loosdregt J (2010) Regulation of Treg functionality by acetylation-mediated Foxp3 protein stabilization. *Blood* 115:965-974.

Vang AG (2013) Regulatory T-cells and cAMP suppress effector T-cells independently of PKA-CREM/ICER. *Biochem J* 456: 463-473.

Varma R, Campi G, Yokosuka T Saito T, Dustin ML (2006) T cell receptor proximal signals are sustained in peripheral microclusters and terminated in the central supramolecular activation cluster. *Immunity* 25: 117-127.

Veerapathran A, pidala J, Beato F, Yu XZ, Anasetti C (2011) Ex vivo expansion of human Tregs specific for alloantigens presented directly or indirectly. *Blood* 118: 5671-5680.

Vendetti S (2000) Anergic T cells inhibit the antigen-presenting function of dendritic cells. *J Immunol* 165: 1175-1181.

Vendramini-Costa DB, Carvalho JE (2012) Molecular link mechanisms between inflammation and cancer. *Curr Pharm Des* 18: 3831-3852.

Ventimiglia LN, Alonso MA (2013) The role of membrane rafts in Lck transport, regulation and signaling in T cells. *J Biochem* 454: 168-179.

Verbsky JW, Chatila TA (2011) T regulatory cells in primary immune deficiencies. *Curr Opin Allergy Clin Immunol* 11: 539-544.

Voo KS (2009) Identification of IL-17-producing FOXP3+ regulatory T cells in humans. *Proc. Nat'l Acad. Sci.* 106: 4793-4798.

Walch KT, Huber JC (2008) Progesterone for recurrent miscarriage: truth and deceptions. *Best Pract Res Clin Obstet Gynaecol* 22: 375-389.

Wan Q (2013) Probing the effector and suppressive functions of human T cell subsets using antigen-specific engineered T cell receptors. *Plos One* 8: e56302.

Wang HY, Peng G, Guo Z, Shevach EM, Wang RF (2005) Recognition of a new ARTC1 peptide ligand uniquely expressed in tumor cells by antigen-specific CD4+ regulatory T cells. *J Immunol* 174: 2661-2670.

Wang K (1998) BID. A proapoptotic BCL-2 family member, is localized to mouse chromosome 6 and human chromosome 22q11. *Genomics* 53:235-238.

Wang HT, Choi B, Tang MS (2010) Melanocytes are deficient in repair of oxidative DNA damage and UV-induced photoproducts. *Proc Nat'l Acad Sci* 107:12180-12185.

Waring P, Mullbacher A (1999) Cell death induced by the Fas/Fas ligand pathway and its role in pathology. *Immunol and Cell Bio* 77: 312-317.

Watanabe T, Wang S, Noritake J, Sato K, Fukata M, Takefuji M, Nakagawa M, Izumi N, Akiyama T, Kaibuchi K (2004) Interaction with IQGAP1 links APC to Rac1, Cdc42, and actin filaments during cell polarization and migration. *Dev Cell* 7: 871-883.

Weber M, Lupp C, Stein P, Kreft A, Bopp T, Wehler TC, Schmitt E, Schild H, Radsak MP (2013) Mechanisms of cyclic nucleotide phosphodiesterases in modulating T cell responses in murine graft-versus-host disease. *Plos One* 8: e58110.

Wekerle H (2001) Immune protection of the brain—efficient and delicate. *J Infect D*is 186 Suppl 2: 140-144.

Wen AY, Sakamoto KM, Miller LS (2010) Role of transcription factor CREB in immune function. *J Immunol* 185: 6413-6419.

Whibley N, Maccallum DM, Vickers MA, Zafreen S, Waldmann H, Hori S, Gaffen SL, Gow NA, Barker RN, Hall AM (2014) Expansion of Foxp3+ T-cell populations by Candida albicans enhances both Th17-cell responses and fungal dissemination after intravenous challenge. *Eur J Immunol* doi: 10.1002/eji.201343604.

Wieczorek G, Asemissen A, Model F, Turbachova I, Floess S, Liebenberg V, Baron U, Stauch D, Kotsch K, Pratschke J, Hamann A, Loddenkemper C, Stein H, Volk HD, Hoffmuller U, Gratzkau A, Mustea A, Huehn J, Scheibenbogen C, Olek S. (2009) Quantitative DNA methylation analysis of FOXP3 as a new method for counting regulatory T cells in peripheral blood and solid tissue. *Cancer Res* 69: 599-608.

Wierecky J, Muller MR, Wirths S, Halder-Oehler E, Dorfel D, Schmidt SM, Huntschel M, Brugger W, Schrader S, Horger MS, Kanz L, Brossart P. (2006) Immunologic and clinical responses after vaccinations with peptide-pulsed dendritic cells in metastatic renal cancer patients. *Cancer* 66: 5910-5918.

Wilkin F (2001) The P2Y11 receptor mediates the ATP-induced maturation of human monocyte-derived dendritic cells. *J Immunol* 166: 7172-7177.

Williams MA, Tyznik AJ, Bevan MJ (2006) Interleukin-2 signals during priming are required for secondary expansion of CD8+ memory T cells. *Nature* 441:890–893.

Wilson JM, Ross WG, Agbai ON, Frazier R, Figler RA, Rieger J, Linden J, Ernst PB (2009) The A2B adenosine receptor impairs the maturation and immunogenicity of dendritic cells. *J Immunol* 182: 4616-4623.

Wilson JM, Kurtz CC, Black SG, Ross WG, Alam MS, Linden J, Ernst PB (2011) The A2B adenosine receptor promotes Th17 differentiation via stimulation of dendritic cell IL-6. *J Immunol* 186: 6746-6752.

Winstead CJ, Reilly CS, Moon JJ, Jenkins MK, Hamilton SE, Jameson SC, Way SS, Khoruts A (2010) CD4+CD25+Foxp3+ regulatory T cells optimize diversity of the conventional T cell repertoire during reconstitution from lymphopenia. *J Immunol* 184: 4749-4760.

Wong S, Guerder S, Visintin I, Reich EP, Swenson KE, Flavell RA, Janeway CA (1995) Expression of the co-stimulator molecule B7-1 in pancreatic beta-cells accelerates diabetes in the NOD mouse. *Diabetes* 44: 326-329.

Workman CJ, Vignali DAA (2005) Negative regulation of T cell homeostasis by Lymphocyte activation gene-3 (CD223). *J Immunol* 174: 688-695.

Wu XZ (2008) Origin of cancer stem cells: the role of self-renewal and differentiation. *Ann Surg Oncol* 15: 407-414.

Yamazaki T, Yang XO, Chung Y, Fukunaga A, Nurieva R, Pappu B, Martin-Orozco N, Kang HS, Ma L, Panopoulos AD, Craig S, Watowich SS, Jetten AM, Tian Q, Dong C (2008) CCR6 regulates the migration of inflammatory and regulatory T cells. *J Immunol* 181:8391–401.

Yamashita Y, Honda S, Nishiharu T, Urata J, Takahashi M (1996) Detection of pseudocapsule of renal cell carcinoma with MR imaging and CT. *AJR Am Roentgenol* 166: 1151-1155.

Yao X, Ahmadzadeh M, Lu YC, Liewehr DJ, Dudley ME, Liu F, Schrump DS, Steinberg SM, Rosenberg SA, Robbins PF (2014) Levels of peripheral CD4 FOXP3 regulatory T cells are negatively associated with clinical response to adoptive immunotherapy of human cancer. *Blood* 119: 5688-5696.

Yee C, Thompson JA, Roche P, Byrd DR, Lee PP, Piepkorn M, Kenyon K, Davis MM, Riddell SR, Greenberg PD (2000) Melanocyte destruction after antigen-specific immunotherapy of melanoma: Direct evidence of T cell-mediated vitiligo. *J Exp Med* 192: 1637-1643.

Yolcu ES, Ash S, Kaminitz A, Sagiv Y, Askenasy N, Yarkoni S (2008) Apoptosis as a mechanism of T-regulatory cell homeostasis and suppression. *Immunol and Bio* 86: 650-658.

Zajchowski D, Band V, Pauzie N, Tager A, Stampfer M, Sager R (1988) Expression of growth factors and oncogenes in normal and tumor-derived epithelial cells. *Cancer Res* 48: 7041-7047.

Zanin-Zhorov A, Ding Y, Kumari S, Attur M, Hippen KL, Brown M, Blazar BR, Abramson SB, Lafaille JJ, Dustin ML (2010) Protein kinase C-Θ mediates negative feedback on regulatory T cell function. *Science* 328: 372-376.

Zarek PE (2008) A2A receptor signaling promotes tolerance by inducing T cell anergy and the generation of adaptive regulatory T cells. *Blood* 111: 251-259.

Zenewicz LA, Abraham C, Flavell RA, Cho JH (2010) Unraveling the genetics of autoimmunity. *Cell* 140: 791-797.

Zeytun A, Hassuneh M, Nagarkatti M, Nagarkatti PS (1997) Fas-Fas ligand-based interactions between tumor cells and tumor-specific cytotoxic T lymphocytes: A lethal two-way street. *Blood* 90: 1952-1959.

Zhang H, Conrad DM, Butler JJ, Zhao C, Blay J, Hoskin DW (2004) Adenosine acts through A2 receptors to inhibit IL-2 induced tyrosine phosphorylation of STAT5 in T lymphocytes: role of cyclic Adenosine 3',5' –monophosphate and phosphatases. *J Immunol* 173: 932-944.

Zhang M, Park SM, Wang Y, Shah R, Liu N, Murmann AE, Wang CR, Peter ME, Ashton-Rickardt PG (2006) Serine protease inhibitor 6 protects cytotoxic T cells from self-inflicted injury by ensuring the integrity of cytotoxic granules. *Immunity* 24: 451-461.

Zhang X, Chang Li X, Xiao X, Sun R, Wei H (2013) CD4(+) CD62L(+) central memory T cells can be converted to Foxp3(+) T cells. *PLoS One* 8(10):e77322.

Zhao JX, Zeng YY, Liu Y (2007) Fetal alloantigen is responsible for the expansion of the CD4(+)CD25(+) regulatory T cell pool during pregnancy. *J Reprod Immunol* 75: 71-81.

Zheng Y, Zha Y, Driessens G, Gajewski TF (2012) Transcriptional regulator early growth response gene-2 (Erg-2) is required for T cell anergy in vitro and in vivo. *J Exp Med* 209: 2157-2163.

Zhou L, Lopes JE, Chong MM, Ivanov II, Min R, Victora GD, Shen Y, Du J, Rubtsov YP, Rudensky AY, Ziegler SF, Littman DR (2008) TGF-B-induced Foxp3 inhibits Th17 cell differentiation by antagonizing RORgt function. *Nature* 453: 236-240.

Zhong XP, Guo R, Zhou H, Liu C, Wan CK (2008) Diacylglycerol kinases in immune cell function and self-tolerance. *Immunol Rev* 224: 249-264.

Zhu S, Qian Y (2012) IL-17/IL-17 receptor system in autoimmune disease: mechanisisms and therapeutic potential. *Clin Sci* (Lond) 122: 487-511.

Zorn E (2005) Reduced frequency of FOXP3+ CD4+ CD25+ regulatory T cells in patients with chronic graft-versus-host disease. *Blood* 106: 2903-2911.

Zou Q, Wu B, Xue J, Fan X, Feng C, Geng S, Wang M, Wang B (2013) CD8+ Treg cells suppress CD8+ T cell responses by IL-10-dependent mechanism during H5N1 influenza infection. *Eur J Immunol* doi: 10.1002/eji.201343583.

Zou T, Caton AJ, Koretzky GA, Kambayashi T (2010) Dendritic cells induce regulatory T cell proliferation through antigen-dependent and –independent interactions. *J Immunol* 185: 2790-2799.

Zou T, Satake A, Corbo-Rodgers E, Schmidt AM, Farrar MA, Maltzman JS, Kambayashi T (2012) Cutting edge: IL-2 signals determine the degree of TCR signaling necessary to support regulatory T cell proliferation in vitro. *J Immunol* 189: 28-32.

Author Contact Information

Dr. Michael A. Alexander
Widener University
One University Place, Chester, PA
Tel: 610-405-4795
E-mail: maalexander@mail.widener.edu

Index

B

C

D

E

F

G

H

I

N

O

P

Q

R

S

T

U

V

W

Y

Z